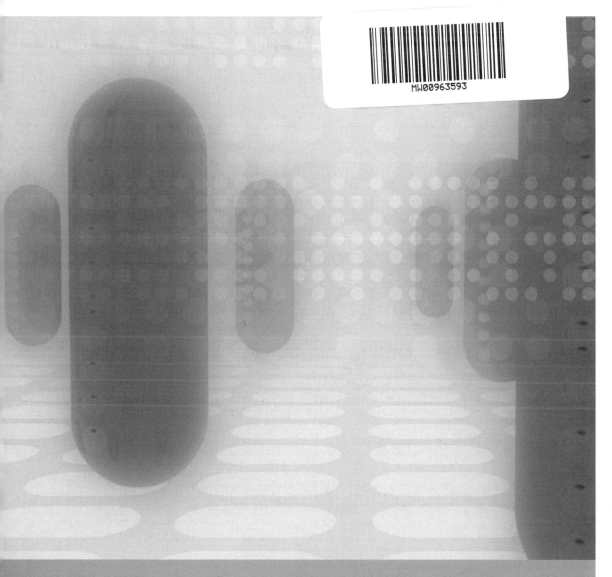

Health Informatics
Transforming Healthcare with Technology

Moya Conrick

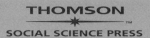

THOMSON
SOCIAL SCIENCE PRESS

Australia · Canada · Mexico · Singapore · Spain · United Kingdom · United States

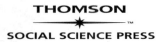

THOMSON

SOCIAL SCIENCE PRESS

Level 7, 80 Dorcas Street
South Melbourne, Victoria 3205

Email: highereducation@thomsonlearning.com.au
Website: www.thomsonlearning.com.au

First published in 2006
10 9 8 7 6 5 4 3 2 1
10 09 08 07 06

National Library of Australia
Cataloguing-in-Publication data

Conrick, Moya.
Health informatics: transforming healthcare with technology.

    Includes index.
    For tertiary students.
    ISBN 0 17 012731 1.

    1. Medical informatics. 2. Information storage and
    retrieval systems – Medical care. I. Title.

610.285

Editor: Bette Moore
Project editor: Chris Wyness
Publishing editor: Elizabeth Vella
Publishing manager: Michael Tully
Indexer: Julie King
Cover designer: Olga Lavecchia
Original cover concept: Patrick Jennings
Typeset in New Aster, Gill Sans, Franklin Gothic and Times Ten by Chris Ryan
Production controller: Jodie Van Teylingen
Printed in Australia by Ligare Book Printers

This title is published under the imprint of Thomson/Social Science Press.
Nelson Australia Pty Limited ACN 058 280 149 (incorporated in Victoria)
trading as Thomson Learning Australia.

The URLs contained in this publication were checked for currency during the production process.
Note, however, that the publisher cannot vouch for the ongoing currency of URLs.

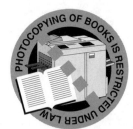

Contents

Part 6 – Health informatics supporting practitioners   345

Part 7 – Pushing the boundaries   405

Preface

Technology is one of the most pervasive and ubiquitous tools in healthcare today. It is not only transforming healthcare but also the professions within it. For those of us teaching health informatics over the years, being unable to steer students and other interested people to a comprehensive text on the subject has been trying. The idea for this text was conceived during a meeting with a broad range of stakeholders; it was born from frustration and nurtured by a number of people engaged in health informatics – some without even realising they were!

This book provides information, knowledge and skills necessary to understand the collection, storage, retrieval, communication and optimal use of health-related data, information and knowledge. It addresses a wide range of the most essential and current areas of health informatics and is divided into seven sections:

Chapter 1   introduces the basics of health informatics to the uninitiated.

Chapter 2   discusses the building blocks of data, information and knowledge and how these are modelled and manipulated for use in health information systems.

Chapter 3   considers the issues of leadership, planning, management and economics that are central to successful informatics implementations.

Chapter 4   builds on the fundamentals to introduce the ins and outs of information systems that might be employed in or used across health institutions or practices.

Chapter 5   considers the most pressing of the human factors in informatics, including workforce, consumer and philosophical issues.

Chapter 6   presents case studies from lived experiences of health informatics. These are wide-ranging and originate from the other side of Katherine (remote Australia) to the corridors of policy-making.

Chapter 7   concludes the text with a glimpse at informatics in genomics and a healthcare future increasingly dependent on technology for quality, cost effective outcomes.

It also recognises that health informatics is a tool that supports healthcare while demonstrating the interdependent and interconnected technologies that would be falsely isolated from each other.

I am still flabbergasted that I took on this task and can only look back on the merriment of the afternoon as the answer. However, the encouragement and help received during this project have made it worthwhile and very satisfying. Finding a name for the text was not difficult in some ways but challenging in another. Information technology is obviously transforming healthcare but the name health informatics often produces a 'glazing over' from the uninitiated or enthusiastic noises from the geeks!

My hope is that this text will have wide appeal to all healthcare workers as it is written in a reader-friendly style that makes it accessible and a resource that can be used at any time. It also exposes health informatics as the tool of practice that it is and not something for only the technically savvy.

Regards,
Moya

Online reading

INFOTRAC® COLLEGE EDITION
This book also contains InfoTrac search terms at the end of each chapter. To access this material please go to: **http://infotrac.thomsonlearning.com/**

To register:
1. Go to http://infotrac.thomsonlearning.com/
2. Click on Register New Accounts
3. Enter your access code found in the InfoTrac card that comes with this text.
   YOU WILL NEED TO CREATE A USERNAME
4. Fill out the registration form to activate your account.

Note: After registration is complete you will only need your username and password to log on.

Acknowledgements

A book like this does not just appear. It takes a lot of effort from many dedicated people and I would like to thank them all for their hard work.

I would particularly like to acknowledge the understanding, help and support of my sons Michael and Gerard because without it this book would still be a thought. I would also like to thank my late night companion, Blu, who kept me awake by grumping at possums.

Thanks also to Karen for her great artwork and Cath for being my sounding board and proof reader. However, this book owes its existence to the many authors who have helped me to put it together in the midst of their own busy lives and day jobs.

Dedication

I would like to dedicate this book to my Dad (who did so much for me), to my Mum for her support and patience and to my sons for being there.

Part I

The basics of health informatics

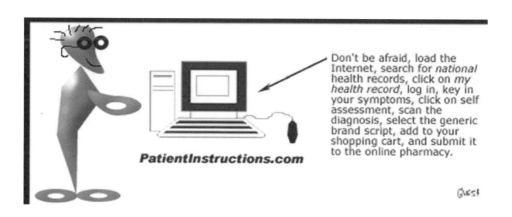

Don't be afraid, load the Internet, search for *national* health records, click on *my health record*, log in, key in your symptoms, click on self assessment, scan the diagnosis, select the generic brand script, add to your shopping cart, and submit it to the online pharmacy.

PatientInstructions.com

GUEST

1

Introduction to health informatics

Moya Conrick

> 'In attempting to arrive at the truth, I have applied everywhere for information, but in scarcely an instance have I been able to obtain hospital records fit for any purposes of comparison. If they could be obtained they would enable us to decide many other questions besides the ones alluded to. They would show subscribers how their money was being spent, what amount of good was really being done with it, or whether the money was not doing mischief rather than good.'
>
> (Florence Nightingale, 1859)
>
> What have we achieved since then?

Outline

This chapter introduces health informatics, an emerging discipline that is concerned about the management and processing of data, information and knowledge to support healthcare and healthcare delivery.

Introduction

The healthcare industry relies on data and information for every facet of its delivery. Huge amounts of data are generated and, because this occurs in a mostly unstructured paper environment, its use is restricted in supporting healthcare. Information technology (IT) has the capacity to transform the health industry and the way it manages its data, information and knowledge and to revolutionise the way in which clinicians work. The needs of clinicians should drive innovations that affect them and they must be vigilant overseers of any change to their practice bought about by technology.

Laboratory staff were the first users to access computer technology in healthcare, but it quickly spread to other areas when databases for the storage of client data such as laboratory results, demographics and human resource management data were introduced. These systems were service oriented and efficient in reducing administrative workloads. Most computers were stand-alone machines (unable to 'talk' to each other) and resulted in further fragmentation of information. The most a client could expect from this technology was a quick bill.

Based on experiences in other industries, the computer should offer the healthcare system greater flexibility, efficiency and effectiveness by reducing redundant data, duplicate testing and providing information at the point of care. The patient is now the focus of the computer and technological revolution in healthcare with electronic health records, individualised care plans and clinical pathways becoming a priority in recent implementations.

Large hospital information systems (HIS) are the norm and the fragmented stand-alone systems (legacy systems) are being phased out. The increased use of technology has implications for the whole of health, and includes administration, education, practice and research. Undoubtedly, technology is transforming the way in which all health professionals deliver patient care and health administrators manage their institutions.

Overview

Prior to the 1960s

As the computer industry grew in the early 1950s so did the use of computers in healthcare. Initially they had basic business office functions. Early computers were essentially large calculating machines, linked together and operated by paper tape and used teletype-writers to print their information (Proctor, 1992).

The 1960s

The introduction of cathode ray tube terminals, on-line data communication, and real-time processing added essential dimensions to the computer system making computers more accessible and 'user-friendly' (Proctor, 1992). Hospital information systems were developed primarily for financial transactions and as billing and accounting systems. Few machines were able to document and process health data. Progress was slow.

The 1970s

The healthcare system realised the great potential for technology to improve documentation and the quality of patient care. Computer applications for financial and management functions and patient care information systems were considered cost-saving technologies and rapid development began.

The 1980s

Informatics advanced greatly in healthcare. Nursing informatics was recognised as a speciality, resulting in the development of nursing information systems. Clinicians could document several aspects of patient records, including medical orders, vital signs, patient notes and discharge planning. The microcomputer was introduced and personal computers were made accessible, affordable and usable (Proctor, 1992).

The 1990s

Technology became an integral part of health and had a major impact on healthcare. Point-of-care devices were being developed and the potential of the Internet became evident. Clinical information systems were introduced and problems with data recognised. Efforts to standardise clinical language began. Technology greatly influenced the accessibility and availability of information for both patients and healthcare workers. Equity issues related to health literacy emerged as a major issue. Policy-making and legislation fell behind the introduction of the technology. The First World Congress on Medical Informatics took place.

21st Century

Some of the issues of the 90s remain. The potential for the use of technology in healthcare is now restricted by one's imagination – systems are smaller, faster and ubiquitous. Desktop computer systems have the capacity of the mainframe computers of a decade ago. Many governments are turning to technology in an attempt to reign in healthcare expenditure.

The birth of informatics

Informatics can be traced back to 1967 when Francois Gremy established a Technical Committee within the International Federation for Information Processing (IFIP). Then in 1983, Gorn coined the term 'informatics', which now underpins all definitions related to the use of computer science plus information science in healthcare. The International Medical Informatics Association (IMIA) was established under Swiss law in 1989 and in 1994, the First World Congress on Medical Informatics (MEDINFO) took place (IMIA, 2002). While medical informatics was at the forefront of this emerging discipline, it was soon realised that informatics was an issue for all of healthcare and that healthcare was far broader than medicine.

The overarching term became 'health informatics' and was defined as a combination of computer science, information science and health science designed to assist in the management and processing of data, information and knowledge to support healthcare and healthcare delivery (IMIA, 2002). It is a widely accepted convention that when informatics is used in conjunction with the name of a discipline, it denotes an application of computer science and information science to the management and processing of data, information and knowledge in the named discipline. Most healthcare professions have defined their own branches of Informatics, for example, Public Health Informatics is seen as the systematic application of information and computer sciences to public health practice, research, and learning (National Library of Medicine, 2001).

The development of Nursing Informatics as a discipline was slightly different and grew from Computers in Nursing groups in both the USA in 1968 and Australia in the '80s. The term Nursing Informatics was not in general use in nursing until the late 1980s. As with other disciplines, the definition of nursing informatics has evolved over time and reflects the developments in nursing practice and technologies. The most widely accepted definition comes from the International Nursing Informatics group IMIA-NI that redefined nursing informatics in 1998 as 'the integration of nursing, its information, and information management with information processing and communication technology, to support the health of people world-wide'.

Informatics organisations

IMIA is recognised as the major international organisation in health informatics and has ten working groups. Although IMIA retains its narrow title, it remains at the forefront of developments and has set up many working groups representing a cross-section of healthcare professionals. In 1992, the nursing working group recommended a change to its status and nursing became an informatics society within IMIA or IMIA-NI.

In Australia, informatics groups were formed along professional lines, for example, Computers in Nursing and the Australian Medical Informatics Association (AMIA), these had state based sub-groups that functioned independently. In 1993, with financial backing from nursing, the Health Informatics Society of Australia (HISA) was constituted in an attempt to draw these groups together. This body has affiliated most informatics groups and is now the most visible of the informatics organisations in Australia.

Relationship of health informatics to the healthcare system

Experience in areas of business and industry has shown that the appropriate deployment and use of information technology can result in improvements in efficiency and quality of service as well as greater customer satisfaction. There is no reason to assume that the health industry would be different.

The use of communications technologies, while essential to healthcare, also supports and empowers clients' decision-making and healthcare choices. The computer is an enabling tool and, for this reason, an understanding of its capabilities is necessary.

Informatics in clinical practice

Clinical practice has and will continue to benefit from the application of information technology in the workplace. Technology has opened up many avenues for connectivity and more expedient work practices for the practitioner. It has permeated all areas of practice and is changing the manner in which all clinicians work.

The widespread use of point-of-care devices for capturing source data should result in the collection of more accurate, reliable and legibility data, reduce transcription error (from scraps of paper etc), and trigger more numerous observations because of prompting or forced recall. The introduction of standards for technology and language will enable greater connectivity and understanding between clinicians while supporting data analysis and audit. The introduction of direct order-enter and complete pharmacy systems consisting of compliant carts and storage cupboards that use bar coders to ensure safe medication storage and administration, should have a major impact in healthcare.

Each year up to 140 000 Australians are admitted to hospital because of problems associated with the use of medicines.

(Commonwealth of Australia, 2003)

Electronic medications records will provide consumers with the opportunity to become active participants in their medication management and it will enable doctors and pharmacists – with patient consent – to make prescribing and dispensing decisions based on knowledge of previous prescriptions, the current medications regime, and previous medication reactions (Commonwealth of Australia, 2003). Great gains are envisioned at the hospital interface, where quick access to a patient's medication record could be life saving.

Information technology can deliver the tools that will profoundly effect clinical workflow and enhance and expand the clinician's ability to work with data and information. For example, Electronic Decision Support Systems maintain knowledge and augment the skills of the clinician by providing access to relevant, evidence-based information when and where it is needed. It also has the potential to greatly improve patient safety because the rapid changes in healthcare make it impossible for clinicians to carry around all information available to enable them to make informed decisions. Electronic decision support can assist by providing access to guidelines and pathways, built-in alerts, prompts for care, continuing patient monitoring and drug indexes. Links to current health information, journals and professional listservs can also be provided depending on the institution's policy.

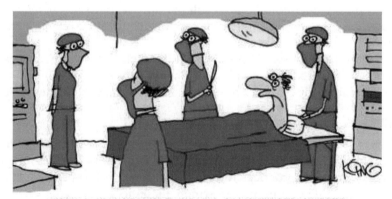

"Nurse, get on the internet, go to SURGERY.COM, scroll down and click on the 'Are you totally lost?' icon."

The introduction of an electronic record should enable healthcare workers much greater access to timely, reliable and accurate data. It is accepted that the patient record should contain all the evidence of the care, treatment and tests undertaken throughout a patient's episode of care. However, in the current paper system this is not always the case, because except for an ICD coded medical diagnosis and some medical tests, most of the data in the paper record lacks structure and is extremely difficult to retrieve (Walker, Frean, Scott & Conrick, 2003).

At the same time, the involvement of many specialty areas and health personnel with a single patient has always had inherent problems of disclosure as well as lost and misplaced files. In terms of security, an electronic health record should not create a situation any worse than the present paper system. In fact, access to the computer record is more restricted and has tight security planned for its introduction. Nonetheless, the community seems much less forgiving of computer error than human error.

Telehealth and eHealth

Worldwide, people living in rural and remote areas struggle to access timely, quality general health or specialist care. The urban sprawl, inadequate public transport and choked highways have all affected our ability to reach healthcare agencies in a timely fashion. An ongoing problem is also the practitioner shortage; telehealth or eHealth have enormous potential to provide some respite.

Innovations in computing and telecommunications technology have not only brought the world closer together, they have given clinicians the tools needed to provide patient care even when patients are geographically isolated. Telehealth will support nurses and other healthcare professionals working alone in remote communities and practitioners in other geographically dispersed areas. It has the potential to change the face of healthcare quite markedly over the next decade.

Informatics in research

Researchers will have unprecedented access to information and connectivity to de-identified, structured data and decision support systems. They will be able to interrogate the data, and query large well-constructed databases about the key indicators of care and maintain health information using database management tools. These databases will provide the healthcare system with the evidence that is needed to support claims about the outcomes of care, and for evidence-based practice.

Informatics in education

Technology supports autonomous learning while equipping students with the skills for self-directed, independent and life-long learning behaviours. Academics have many electronic tools to support their teaching. One of the most visible and flexible of these is technology-assisted learning that supports interactive learning and enables self-assessment. It also supports many different teaching strategies, with students engaging in self-paced self-learning, with greater control over the direction of their educational experiences.

Communication between computers has opened a new world of connectivity and access across the Internet and the World Wide Web. The volume of information available with a few keystrokes is staggering. It has also enabled educators to offer educational programs via the Internet to geographically dispersed students.

Informatics in management

Like any office automation, incorporating word processing, electronic mail, spreadsheets, presentation graphics and databases into daily work routines has made work easier for the healthcare manager. Information technology also assists in the management of personnel and departments, staffing, scheduling and resource allocation.

Undoubtedly, budgetary restraints are influencing the management of hospitals and other healthcare environments. Improvements from redesigned and automated systems will reduce costly errors and duplication. They will also provide better quality and timely information to managers so that they can better manage their institutions. Technology should support efficient, cost effective care and produce timely data for management, although it is now becoming evident that an oversupply or poor handling of data is just as limiting as an undersupply when making decisions.

Informatics, consumers and patients

Informatics has the capacity to empower patients and enable them to become autonomous participants in their healthcare. Access can be provided to their Electronic Health Record and the tools for patients to enter their own data into their record are available. Information technology can support patients being cared for at home and provide quality education to the community. It has enabled communication on a scale that has never been available before via for example, the Internet, email and computer conferencing.

Case study

Bill Johansen is 82 years old. He lives at Birdsville and has a remote-monitored pacemaker implanted. The pacemaker relays digital data about his cardiac rhythm through a portable transmitter over a telephone network to a receiving station in Germany that faxes the data about two minutes later to his cardiologist's clinic in Brisbane. Bill is alerted immediately if there is a problem or if his physician detects irregularities and he can be called into the hospital if necessary.

New roles in healthcare

The introduction of information technology systems in healthcare has created new roles for healthcare workers. One of these is the health informatician, who concentrates on improving efficiency using information technology and data management. Informaticians may have very little or no patient contact and no formal education background, but they often have to assume an educational role for clinicians, usually in information system concepts. They may also have an incidental role educating the technicians about healthcare.

Conclusion

Healthcare has been slow to embrace technology and is now beginning to realise the potential of computers and information technology to support the management of information. As healthcare grows more complex and people live more transient lifestyles, the ability to communicate effectively about patient care is crucial.

The tools of the health practitioner have undergone a revolution over the past few years and this is set to continue. The roles that healthcare workers have now will not be the same in fifteen years' time, and it may be that health professions as we know them may not exist. As a society, however, we run the risk of information overload and a greater divide between the information rich and the information poor.

Information and communications technology has the capability to address many of the business drivers in health. However, there are constraints and issues that limit the success of these solutions and all healthcare workers need to be aware of and work cooperatively to counter them. Information technology cannot replace good clinical decision-making or values, but it can offer the tools to support the delivery of quality, cost effective and timely care.

Review questions

1. What is your understanding of health informatics?
2. What should be the focus of informatics in healthcare?
3. What effects could information technology have on healthcare?
4. What is the clinician's role in health informatics?

Exercise

- Give examples of clinical, educational and administrative uses of health informatics.
- Discuss the use of technology by healthcare professionals.
- Is information technology able to replace the health worker? Why or why not?

Online reading

INFOTRAC® COLLEGE EDITION

For additional readings and review on health informatics, explore **InfoTrac® College Edition**, your online library. Go to: **www.infotrac-college.com** and search for any of the InfoTrac key terms listed below:

➤ Informatics
➤ Health information systems
➤ Health informatics
➤ Nursing informatics
➤ Medical informatics

References

Commonwealth of Australia (2003). *Facts Sheet*. Retrieved 22 March 2005 from http://www.health.gov.au/.

IMIA-NI (1998). Definition. Retrieved 4 February 2003 from http://www.imia.org/ni/.

International Medical Informatics Association (2002). Short Organizational History, 2004, from http://www.imia.org/history.html.

National Library of Medicine (2001). Public health informatics. Current Bibliographies in Medicine. Retrieved 5 February 2004 from http://www.nlm.nih.gov/pubs/cbm/phi2001.html.

Nightingale, F. (1859). *Notes on Nursing, What it is and What it is not*. Harrison 59 Pall Mall, Booksellers to the Queen, London.

Proctor, P. (1992). *Nurses, computers and information technology*, Chapman & Hall, Sheffield.

Walker, S., Frean, I., Scott, P. & Conrick, M. (2003). *Classifications and Terminologies in Residential Aged Care: An Information Paper*. The Ageing and Aged Care Division of the Commonwealth Department of Health and Ageing, Canberra.

2

IT and information management

Moya Conrick

> 'We've all heard that a million monkeys banging on a million typewriters will eventually reproduce the entire works of Shakespeare. Now, thanks to the Internet, we know this is not true.'
>
> (Robert Wilensky, 1996)

Outline

Information technology (IT) has the potential to transform healthcare delivery by providing information in a timely fashion, when and where it is needed. It also has the ability to reduce errors, costs, duplication and waste. This chapter discusses health IT and its use in the collection, storage, retrieval and transfer of clinical, administrative and financial health information electronically.

Introduction

Computer technology infrastructure is strikingly similar to other public infrastructures such as roads, hospitals, schools and so on, because they all require large investments in the hope of long-term benefits (Protti, 2005). It enables business activity that would otherwise not be economically feasible, but at the same time it is difficult to cost-justify in advance or to show value in hindsight.

However, we do know that without computer technology progress is difficult and that there is a delicate investment balance. Too little investment leads to project management problems, continued local inefficiencies, incompatibility, and wasted time and effort. Too much investment discourages end-user investment and involvement that may result in unused capacity and accusations of waste (Protti, 2005).

Information is the structure on which healthcare is built and attempting to manage it is as old as healthcare itself. A modern health system cannot function effectively with information locked in professional or organisational silos, nor can it be managed without computer systems because of the enormous amount of data that are generated. In fact, studies published by the Institute of Medicine and others have indicated that fragmented, disorganised, and inaccessible clinical information adversely affects the quality of healthcare and compromises patient safety (Heinrich et al., 2004).

Historically, finding effective ways of managing, accessing and standardising information has been problematic, with Nightingale bemoaning the lack of standardised and quality recorded information in 1859: '[we] apply everywhere for information, but in scarcely an instance ... have [we] been able to obtain hospital records fit for any purposes of comparison'. Little has changed since then.

Healthcare is an information-rich environment and all health workers have a responsibility to ensure the quality and reliability of health information, as it is fundamental to a quality health system. Governments, healthcare organisations, providers, consumers and communities increasingly require information for planning and managing healthcare delivery, policy development, the provision of advice (National Health Information Management Group, 2002) and for decision-making. Advances in technology have made the flow of information more available, comprehensive and useful, but it has also meant an explosion in the amount of data that can be collected, leading to an overload (infoglut) in some sectors.

IT can refocus healthcare into a truly consumer centric model which may mean that the manner in which the consumer interfaces with the health system might change dramatically. This is of course depends on the appropriate infrastructures and infostructures being in place.

Consumers already access vast amounts of online health information and some present to their provider with these as a basis on which to discuss their health issues. However, difficulties arise with the quality of these resources. Nonetheless, this does demonstrate increasing autonomy and a willingness by consumers to take more responsibility for their health choices. Slack (2004) regards the patient as one of the most under-utilised resources in medicine, but sees technology improving that nexus by enabling clinicians to better incorporate the patient into their practice.

The huge increase in the use of IT systems and the substantial investment in information management infrastructure is evidence of a strong belief that information management systems will improve patient care and deliver quality health outcomes (Conrick, Hovenga, Cook, Laracuente & Morgan, 2004). However, the changes that are accompanying the drive for IT solutions will also pose challenges to long-standing assumptions and practices.

Information as a dominant health resource

As healthcare grows more complex, and the boundaries between the professions and various health sectors become increasingly blurred, the ability to communicate effectively about patient care is paramount. Although healthcare relies on data and information for every facet of its delivery (Conrick et al., 2004), a significant proportion of clinicians and institutions are unable to communicate across locations and geographical settings.

The inherent characteristics of information make it a unique, crucial and invaluable resource. It increases with use, is not particularly resource hungry in comparison to other processes, and is sustainable, transportable, diffuse and shareable. Computer applications in the workplace assist managers and clinical decision-making by collecting and collating data and providing useable information as an output. Fundamental to this process is the method of collecting data, the type of data collected, and how it is described. It has been reported that the possible adverse effects on patient care may be highly significant if patient data is not consistently and accurately recorded (Currell, Wainwright & Urquhart, 2002).

There are limits to the growth of knowledge in healthcare because of the restrictions on the time that clinicians can devote to refining information. IT enables the development of large knowledge bases along with other resources for exchanging and storing information and knowledge. This is central to healthcare systems of the future.

IT in practice

The telephones has been an invaluable technology in healthcare for many years and is still the most dominant communication tools, being used for the majority of synchronous communications, triage and so forth.

The past few decades have seen major advances in the use of computers and communications technology, to the point where IT can determine the efficiency and effectiveness of communications, interaction and the management of data and information. There is evidence to support the use of IT to improve the safety and quality of care and support decision-making (Bates & Gawandee, 2003). IT can provide greater flexibility, greater access to quality information, reduced paperwork, a reduction in time spent by clinicians performing non-clinical tasks and improved decision-making. A computer system can store huge amounts of data and patients can be tracked, longitudinally or throughout their life, across all contact with the health system.

Despite growing evidence for the effectiveness of IT, clinicians remain sceptical. Much of this is based on the systems implemented over the past decade that have largely failed to offer any real benefits and, in some instances, have made clinical work more difficult. Some issues relate directly to the lack of terminals in the workspace and the competition for access to them. There has also been a lack of agreed protocols and mechanisms to support their use and, other than inputting data, clinicians have had little return from most systems.

The literature reports many instances of the unsuccessful introductions of health IT, with failures in both networks and computer systems reported (Kilbridge, 2003; Massro, 1993). There are many factors that can be linked to this, such as systems that were technology driven rather than user defined or meeting user requirements and stand-alone implementations that often required double handling of information (paper and electronic). In fact, with some of the implementations the use of paper and time spent on documentation escalated. Health also has many legacy systems that present challenges as most cannot interface with the newer systems being installed.

However, IT is pervasive. In the community nurses use handheld computers and mobile phone connections for emails, note-taking, caseload management, allocating resources, and tracking travel and visit times. Home carers use mobile devices to collect and upload information to client management systems. These systems reduce paperwork and save time. In remote locations, satellite phones are being used to provide roadside connections for specialist assistance. Many general practitioners and allied health and alternative therapists use IT for communications, files storage, and in electronic prescribing. Slack (2004) has also reported on the usefulness of patient-doctor e-mail in improving outcomes.

It is difficult to imagine what business and industry would be without computers and automation as they are so irrevocably entwined. These technologies are ubiquitous, expected and necessary; they have changed business forever. The same could be expected for health. Health institutions must accommodate the procedural and social change needed as the process for information management changes and evolves. The sensible application of IT in healthcare will ensure that information flows efficiently and effectively if it is appropriately managed at all stages of the life cycle.

Managing health information

Managing health information is a process that requires planning and decision-making, inside and outside of the technology. Key issues in the management of health information include:

- ensuring the privacy and security of data
- identification of consumers and practitioners
- standards and infrastructure
- systems and application interoperability and integration
- the provision of timely access to quality data for use in clinical decision-making, policy, planning and research.

As these issues are integral to health informatics they are dealt with in some depth later in this book. However, a short introduction will be offered here.

Security

The security of health data is critical to the success of any adoption of IT and covers three major areas; authentication, access, and containment. A person's identity must be authenticated and verified, access must be efficient and the user must have a unified view of information. The information itself must be controlled and contained appropriately, using pre-emptive and defensive techniques, to ensure its protection.

Access control

The unique identification of all clinicians is essential if data are to be valid and protected. Unique identification of providers will address most of the problems, but they have ramifications for privacy and liability when data are shared across boundaries. Appropriate security technologies must be in place to protect data from unauthorised access, along with appropriate user access, audit, policies and procedures (Conrick et al., 2004). There are a number of other issues for a unique identifier such as:

- standards for the characteristics of a unique ID
- how an ID is assigned (by clinician or organisation)

- development and maintenance of a registry
- the method to assign either a number or biometric data
- implementation costs
- continuity, such as processes and standards change
- historical records needing to be changed or mapped to the new ID
- privacy and confidentiality concerns (Conrick et al., 2004).

Standards

Widely accepted and implemented standards are needed to underpin the operation of key elements of information activities in the health sector, including electronic business transactions (e-commerce) and the development of a national system of electronic health records. However, for systems to interoperate and communication to seamlessly flow many different standards are required. These fall under the major groupings of systems, vocabulary, messaging and security.

Timely access to quality data

All health professionals engage in significant record-keeping activities that in the past have been paper-based and mostly handwritten. The problems of legibility, access and transportability of the paper records are well documented. One of the primary purposes of any information system is to acquire data, process it into useful information, and make the information available to whoever needs it, in a useful format and in a timely fashion.

Health workers have a responsibility to ensure the quality and reliability of data and information because governments, organisations, providers, consumers and communities have increasing requirements for it. Information forms the basis of the planning and management of health services, policy development, patient care and consumer advice.

Huge amounts of data are generated daily, not all of which needs to be shared but which needs to be available for safe care delivery and effective management. Information must be available 'just in time' and to a degree this rests with the interoperability between and within systems. It is a challenge to get the balance right.

Interoperability and integration

Arguably interoperability is the key to transforming healthcare. Seamless connectivity between clinicians allows information to follow the consumer from one point-of-care to another, across local and geographical boundaries. To enable this, systems must be able to 'talk to each other' – in other words, they must be interoperable and integrated. Three types of interoperability are required to achieve this, and all are underpinned by standards (Dibble, Walther, Jansen & Coiera, 2004).

Dibble et al. (2004) affirm that *basic interoperability* ensures that systems can physically communicate through a network. At this level of data exchange, a message can be sent from one computer and received by another without needing the receiver to interpret the data. Dibble et al. (2004) sees email as a prime example here. Technical interoperability is the second type and is often taken for granted, particularly since the advent of the Internet and the gradual demise of proprietary networks. Also called communication or functional interoperability, it ensures that information (or messages) can be exchanged over the network (Dibble et al., 2004).

The third type of interoperability is concerned with terminological or semantic interoperability, which is the ability of a receiving system to understand the information transmitted from the sending system. This is achieved through shared semantics where both systems have the same understanding of terminologies, their meanings and their context (Dibble et al., 2004).

Automation should produce legible, more accessible, and transportable records systems and information sharing, but robustness and integration have been a problem. Englebardt and Nelson (2002) point to the past practice of installing multiple systems without developing an integrated management strategy resulting in 'significant redundant data entry activities' and many complaints from healthcare professionals. A lack of integration also reinvigorated the 'silos' in healthcare, not so much by jurisdiction or purpose, but by computer system or personal computers.

Workforce issues

There are many related social and work factors involved in the implementation of IT into workplaces, such as a largely unprepared workforce and uncharted workflows. Few education and training programs are available at undergraduate or postgraduate level and there are very few informatics educators (Conrick et al., 2004). The area of general practice however, provides an example of where an investment in IT infrastructure and workforce capacity over a period of time has seen an increase in the use of IT and HI skills among general practitioners. This is both in absolute terms and relative to other areas of the medical workforce (Commonwealth Department of Health and Aged Care, 2003). However, it is essential that all practitioners have base informatics competencies for their professional areas of practice.

Workflow issues are critical in the implementation of IT, because without careful planning, the implementations meant to improve practice might have the opposite effect. Although it is recognised that implementations should be designed around best practice clinical workflow, little work on this has been undertaken. IT should not impede the workforce, it must instead assist rapid and intuitive data input and integrate seamlessly into work practices. The importance of interface and ergonomic design based on an understanding of clinician workflow cannot be understated because if designs are not compatible with work processes, workers will either not use the system or use it poorly. Workflow studies are required to determine 'best fit' information requirements for the health workforce.

Conclusion

The boundaries between disciplines have already begun to blur, new specialities have arisen, and responsibilities have changed. IT will continue to significantly redefine these boundaries as it supports healthcare workers by providing access to quality, timely data and information and to communication tools that are evolving on a daily basis. IT opens up new possibilities for the dissemination and use of information, and although it is not a panacea for all the problems in the healthcare system, it does have the potential to produce very positive outcomes.

Review questions

1. Why is information such a valuable resource in healthcare?
2. Discuss three types of interoperability.
3. What is a semantic network?

Exercise

'IT should not impede the workforce, rather it must facilitate rapid and intuitive data input and integrate seamlessly into work practices.' In light of this statement develop a flow chart with information flows for a healthcare group.

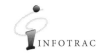

Online reading

INFOTRAC® COLLEGE EDITION
For additional readings and review on infrastructure and information management, explore **InfoTrac® College Edition**, your online library. Go to: **www.infotrac-college.com** and search for any of the InfoTrac key terms listed below:
➤ Health information technology
➤ Health informatics infrastructure
➤ Health Informatics Infrastructure

References

Bates, D, & Gawandee, A (2003). Improving safety with information technology, *New England Journal Medicine* (248), 2526–34.

Commonwealth Department of Health and Aged Care (2003). *Report on the health information workforce capacity think tank,* Canberra.

Conrick, M., Hovenga, E., Cook, R., Laracuente, T. & Morgan, T. (2004). *A framework for nursing informatics in Australia: a strategic paper,* Department of Health and Ageing, Canberra.

Currell, R., Wainwright, P. & Urquhart, C. (2002). *Nursing record systems: effects on nursing practice and health care outcomes,* The Cochrane Library Update Software, Oxford.

Dibble, C., Walther, M., Jansen, B. & Coiera, E. (2004). *How do I evaluate the interoperability of an EDSS?* Retrieved 24 February, 2005, from http://www.ahic.org.au.

Englebardt, S. & Nelson, R. (2002). *Health care informatics: an interdisciplinary approach,* Mosby Inc., Sydney.

Heinrich, J., Barsoum, G., Dievler, A., Khan, S., Price, R., Sanchez, Y. et al. (2004). *HHS's efforts to promote health information technology and legal barriers to its adoption,* Government Accountability Office report, United States Senate, Washington.

Kilbridge, P. (2003). Computer crash-lessons from a system failure, *New England Journal of Medicine* (348), 881–2.

Massro, T (1993). Intoducing physician order entry at a major academic medical center: impact on organisational culture and behaviour, *Academic Medicine* (68), 20–5.

National Health Information Management Group (2002). *Health information development priorities,* Department of Health and Ageing, Canberra.

Nightingale, F. (1859). *Notes on nursing, what it is and what it is not,* Booksellers to the Queen, Harrison 59 Pall Mall, London.

Protti, D. (2005). *Investing in computer technology is an investment in infrastructure – it's not unlike building motorways.* Retrieved 3 March, 2005, from www.informatics. nhs.uk.

RFDS. (n.d.). History of the Royal Flying Doctor Service. Retrieved 2 February 2005, from http://www.flyingdoctor.net/.

Slack, W. (2004). A 67-year-old man who emails his physician, *JAMA* (292), 2255–61.

Part 2

The building blocks of health informatics

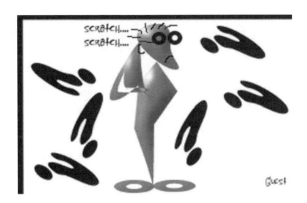

3

Health information interchange

Moya Conrick, Sue Walker, Peter Scott and Isobel Frean

Standards make an enormous contribution to most aspects of our lives –
although very often, that contribution is invisible. It is when there is an absence
of standards that their importance is brought home. The rail gauge problem
between New South Wales and Queensland requires no further comment.

Outline

Health is information intensive; it has many disparate groups with multiple perspectives and
subcultures. Each group sees things slightly differently, but they must all capture, communicate,
reliably retrieve and re-use information between each other and across multiple settings. This
chapter examines some of the methods used to represent data and to enable information
interchange across the health spectrum.

Introduction

The ad hoc collection of health data and the 'silos' in healthcare have little place in a
modern health system. There are now two powerful drivers shaping the face of health
and the manner in which data are collected: electronic health records and the need
to share data seamlessly across geographical settings. This should enable clinicians
to deliver efficient, effective and safer care to patients. However, one of the critical
issues arising from this vision is the requirement for standards across all platforms
and technologies.

What are standards?

Standards contribute to making the development, manufacturing and supply of
products and services more efficient and safer. When things go well, for example,
when systems and devices are safe and they work or if data are easily exchanged
between multiple systems, it is most often not by chance but because they conform
to standards.

The development of standards for health information management and information technology that are compatible with international standards activity is necessary for all nations contemplating the adoption of technology in healthcare. Without agreed standards, health information will remain locked away in small networks or 'silos' within jurisdictions, individual organisations or individual healthcare provider practices.

Standards are best applied where there is a genuine need and some gains can be realised. The approach taken in Australia is pragmatic and focuses on addressing the needs of the health sector rather than developing standards for standards' sake.

Australian standards developers

Australia has several standards committees, which in turn have various sub-committees and working groups. These organisations are necessary to set the direction and national priorities for standards development work.

Standards Australia (SA) is a major standards development organisation in Australia. It works in a similar way to the International Standards Organisation (ISO) with a mix of government and non-government organisations to deliver an integrated range of standards. It also reflects the committee structure of ISO having many specialised committees. IT-14 is the Health Informatics committee of SA and is comprised of membership from key stakeholder groups supported by SA. It has many working groups and technical committees.

The Australian Institute of Health and Welfare (AIHW) also develops health data standards, including meta-data standards. This organisation is responsible for the development and maintenance of the National Health Data Dictionary (NHDD) that identifies data elements from a number of national minimum data sets. It includes admitted patient care, admitted patient mental healthcare, admitted patient palliative care, alcohol and other drug treatment services, community mental healthcare, elective surgery waiting times, health labour force, and perinatal and injury surveillance. The AIHW's work in producing the NHDD is the result of an agreement between the cross-jurisdictional membership of the Health Data Standards Committee (HDSC), which has overseen health standards development for several years. The principal focus of the HDSC's work program is to highlight the need for healthcare consumers, providers and funders to have appropriate data available to facilitate planning, management and monitoring at the individual patient or client level and at an aggregated level (National Health Information Management Group, 2002).

Other standardising bodies in Australia include the National Electronic Health Transition Authority (NeHTA); a relative newcomer to the area. NeHTA is undertaking a governance role in standards development determining the direction and the development of national priority standards. It has also undertaken some data standards development within the Clinical Information Project.

Although data standards have been developed in Australia for years their adoption in health has not been widespread. However, there are a number of important standards that need to be confirmed, accepted and widely implemented if the eHealth agenda is to progress. Health information standards development must be adequately funded and systematically progressed in a co-operative, coordinated and innovative manner.

Australian standards are not developed in isolation. Members attend international meetings to keep abreast of developments in other countries and vice versa. Australia has taken a significant role in standards development internationally and representatives of Standards Australia chair committees in the International Standards Organisation (ISO) and lead projects being undertaken by that body and others.

International standards developers

ISO is the major international standards development organisation. It is a network of the national standards institutes of 148 countries, with one member from each country. It has a Central Secretariat that coordinates the standards development process. Like many of the national standards organisations it is non-governmental, and links the public and private sectors.

Many of its member institutes are part of the governmental structure of their countries, or are mandated by their government. Other members come from the private sector from partnerships of industry associations. ISO acts as a bridging organisation in which a consensus can be reached on solutions that meet the requirements of business and the broader needs of society, such as the needs of stakeholder groups including consumers and users (ISO, 2005). Standards Australia is a member of ISO.

Another international committee is the Digital Imaging and Communications in Medicine (DICOM) Standards Committee. This body creates and maintains international standards for communication of biomedical diagnostic and therapeutic information in disciplines that use digital images and associated data. The goals of DICOM are to achieve compatibility and to improve workflow efficiency between imaging systems and other information systems in healthcare environments worldwide.

The national standards bodies in the European Economic Community (EEC) and European Free Trade Association (EFTA) countries founded the European Committee for Standardisation (CEN). It contributes to the objectives of these bodies with voluntary technical standards that promote free trade, the safety of workers and consumers, interoperability of networks, environmental protection, exploitation of research and development programs, and public procurement (CEN, 2005). Australia also liaises and keeps abreast of CEN developments and vice versa.

Types of standards needed

Standards are required for interoperability and integration. Without these, the problems caused by the silos in healthcare will be exacerbated as no data exchange or communication can take place outside of a local computer network or system. In a complex area like healthcare this is unacceptable. Multiple standards are necessary and these can be categorised into four main areas: systems, vocabulary, messaging and security. Table 3.1 summarises these categories and they are further discussed at some length here.

Table 3.1: Categories of standards in healthcare

Systems standards Required for interoperability, integration performance and availability	• IT system and network operations • Devices interoperability • Systems interoperability • Telecommunications
Vocabulary standards Required for information management and meaningful collection, exchange, storage and re-use of clinical data.	• Data – description of data, structure • Classification • Vocabulary • Terminologies – Interface and Reference
Messaging standards Required to establish the format and sequence of data during transmission.	• Standards used for the interchange of data • IT system and network operations
Security standards Required to identify the practices necessary to maintain confidentiality, integrity and appropriate availability of health information.	• Data storage – structure and content for an electronic health record • Privacy, authentication, access control

System standards

The development of the national electronic summary health record (Health*Connect*) has highlighted the problems with the existing lack of interconnectivity in Australia and has become the impetus for a rush of important standards development work. It has also highlighted the need for interaction and common standards across systems to:

- inform other systems that information has been created, destroyed or modified
- receive information about new, deleted, or changed information
- request information from other systems
- respond to requests for information from other systems.

Significant cost savings can be realised across settings when systems share the same information. There are also less tangible savings and benefits that are difficult to quantify, but are nonetheless very real and clinically important. For example, it is very difficult to quantify quality of life issues or put a fiscal value on enabling patients to receive treatment in their own community.

However, sharing information can be problematic as the language of healthcare can be complex, unstructured, and diverse and can include regional and sub-domain variations. The only way to deal with this is by implementing data and vocabulary standards.

Vocabulary standards

The Health*Connect* agenda has also accelerated terminologies and vocabularies work in Australia and proposal for the adoption of standard terminologies across all health settings. These are essential for the electronic capture, exchange or transmission of health data. Presently this is partially achieved for patients who are admitted to hospitals as hospital data are currently coded using standard classifications, which aggregate health concepts *a posteori*. However, this limits the use of coded information for clinical decision-making and communications between clinicians at the point of care (Walker, Frean, Scott & Conrick, 2003).

Unlike humans, computers cannot communicate with each other using 'natural language'. They need to be told what things are and how they relate to each other; this requires the use of controlled terminologies. These terminologies sit behind the natural language that is visible to a user on the computer screen (Walker et al., 2003) and the user may be oblivious to their existence. They are an essential component of the computer system because they enable concepts to be stored and transferred electronically between different systems. Each concept has a unique identifier that has the same meaning to the sender and the receiver of the information. This means that the message is understood by the system and can be stored and retrieved as required.

Terminologies ensure that as data are entered, they are stored in such a way as to enable ready and reliable retrieval in a particular context, such as in care planning documentation (Scott, 2002) and for decision-making. Classifications have been used to describe grouped concepts such as symptoms, diagnoses and procedures in the acute care sector for many years, largely for non-clinical purposes. Considerable work is now underway to develop and implement terminologies across the disparate areas of healthcare to facilitate clinical use of the data. However, for this to occur data standardisation must be undertaken.

Data standards

Data are the building blocks of all data collections and these are the representation of real world facts, concepts or instructions in a formalised manner suitable for communication, interpretation or processing by human beings or by automatic means (ISO, 1999). Data or non-interpreted items may or may not be useful. Examples are '36' and 'blue', which without context or definition are meaningless.

> A long list of raw (un-coded) data is virtually useless in healthcare, however, data that are assigned a code can be manipulated and managed.

Coded data are used across healthcare in areas such as public health research, epidemiological studies at the population level and also for hospital management, funding and clinical purposes. They provide a means whereby the complexities of clinical practice can be described in a standard fashion, which lends itself to comparability, aggregation and analysis. They can also be used to pinpoint and access specific information and literature to inform clinical practice and support clinical decision-making.

Over the past century, collecting, retrieving and analysing data that is abstracted from individual patient medical records has been enabled by coding and classification systems. Classification systems in various forms are almost as old as healthcare itself.

Classifications

A classification is the categorisation of relevant natural language for the purposes of systematic analysis. It is a type of aggregating terminology, a logical system for the arrangement of knowledge. A fully developed classification scheme specifies categories of knowledge, provides the means to relate the categories to each other, and may specify in the code number all or the most important of the aspects and facets of a subject (US Library of Congress cited in Standards Australia (SA), 2003).

Classifications such the tenth revision of the International Statistical Classification of Diseases and Related Health Problems (ICD-10) and the Australian modifications of this classification (ICD-10-AM), incorporate generalist hierarchies of aggregation designed to make them useful for multiple purposes. These includes national statistical collections, management information, clinical research, epidemiology and reimbursement (SA, 2003).

Classifications enable the standardised collection of health information that:
- provides for the measurement of clinical care outcomes and supports an evidence-based approach to client assessment. Evaluating the outcomes of care requires the capacity to organise patient-based information from a variety of service delivery settings in both public and private sectors
- flows into case management and decision support software; facilitating coordinated care across sectors (acute care, emergency, other ambulatory and community health settings, non-acute settings)
- improves the monitoring of safety and quality in healthcare
- enables statistical analysis and reporting of health information for decision-making, policy development, service administration, financial management and health research (Walker et al., 2003).

Classifications, by their nature, often group diseases into single codes or categories with similar characteristics. While this is useful for specific purposes, such as statistical analysis and reporting, the coarse-grained nature of the resulting groups means that classifications are less useful at a clinical level. Innes and Bramley (1997) set down criteria for the development of classifications. These have been modified and are presented as Table 3.2.

Table 3.2: Criteria for classification development (based on Innes & Bramley, 1997)

Criteria	Attribute
Integrity	• Logical organisation • Each concept is unique • Each concept is relevant • Each concept has a clear meaning • Standardised terminology is used • Ability to compare data over time is not compromised
Retrievability	• Facilitates the retrieval of information
Flexibility	• Able to contract, or be modified to incorporate changes • There is a formalised mechanism for periodic updating • Changes to codes or concepts are compatible with the classification structure
Acceptability	• Easy access to the desired term • Adequate annotation or guidelines are available • Does not require more information than is available to the user
Comprehensive	• Comprehensive as possible • Appropriate 'catch all' categories are provided enabling all possible requirements to be classified somewhere
Standards	• Complies with relevant national and international standards

The form of the classificatory axes or ordering principles used in a classification are determined by the purposes for which the concepts are ordered (Scott, 2002) and because they are coarse grained, they are not meant to change much over time. The tabular disease list from ICD-10-AM (see Table 3.3) is a good example of an aggregate terminology and an excerpt of this is reproduced below.

Terminologies

In contrast to the 'lumpiness' or coarse-grained nature of classifications, a controlled clinical terminology is a more comprehensive vocabulary of health concepts and terms. Its purpose may be broader than that of a classification, being designed to provide a finer level of granularity in describing healthcare concepts (Scott, 2002). The level of granularity that is required depends on the purpose of the terminology. For instance, interface terminologies allow users to interact with computerised health records using the language or words that are the same as those that they normally employ. They are, however, a more structured form of natural language.

Table 3.3: Tabular disease list from ICD-10-AM

J20	Acute bronchitis

Includes: bronchitis:
- acute and subacute (with):
  - bronchospasm
  - fibrinous
  - membranous
  - purulent
  - septic
  - tracheitis
  - NOS, in those under 15 years of age
  tracheobronchitis, acute

Excludes: bronchitis:
- allergic NOS (J45.0)
- chronic:
  - mucopurulent (J41.1)
  - NOS (J42)
  - obstructive (J44.-)
  - simple (J41.0)
  - NOS, in those 15 years of age and above (J40)
  tracheobronchitis:
- chronic:
  - NOS (J42)
  - obstructive (J44.-)
  - NOS (J40)

J20.0	Acute bronchitis due to *Mycoplasma pneumoniae*
J20.1	Acute bronchitis due to *Haemophilus influenzae*
J20.2	Acute bronchitis due to streptococcus
J20.3	Acute bronchitis due to coxsackievirus
J20.4	Acute bronchitis due to parainfluenza virus
J20.5	Acute bronchitis due to respiratory syncytial virus
J20.6	Acute bronchitis due to rhinovirus
J20.7	Acute bronchitis due to echovirus
J20.8	Acute bronchitis due to other specified organisms
J20.9	Acute bronchitis, unspecified

Interface terminologies

A computer interface is the point at which the user and computer interact, so an interface terminology enables the user to enter and retrieve information through the computer system. The terms used in these terminologies are familiar to users and are formally linked by the computer to the underlying concepts in the reference terminology. Because there are usually a large number of terms, they are called 'finely grained'. Interface terminologies are meant to be dynamic and frequently updated. The developing Australian General Practice Vocabulary is a recent example of an interface terminology.

Interface terms and the concepts they identify can be related to each other in a reference terminology. This describes the relationships between concepts, as well as providing the unambiguous representation of health concepts (Walker et al, 2003).

Reference terminologies

A reference terminology is designed to uniquely represent concepts, by listing them and specifying their structure, relationships and, if present, their semantic and formal definitions. It normally has a meaningless unique identifier for terms and concepts with an alternate interface or synonymous terms linked to the preferred term. There may be external maps or pointers to classifications or aggregate terminologies (International Standards Organisation, 2002).

According to Walker et al. (2003), reference terminologies communicate information well, but they are not suited for counting information units for statistical purposes. Therefore, to communicate health information, and to count it accurately (for burden of disease studies, epidemiology, public health initiatives, resource planning and so forth), both classifications and terminologies are needed.

The Systematised Nomenclature of Medicine (SNOMED)-CT is a good example of a reference terminology. It aims to be a precise and comprehensive reference terminology for health and is a large, polyhierarchical mesh of uniquely identified concepts connected to each other by different types of relationships. The most common relationship type is a parent-child relationship (for example, influenza is a child of [or a type of] viral respiratory infection). One or more terms have concepts attached to them, and these may be described as preferred terms, abbreviations and synonyms.

SNOMED-CT aims to unambiguously represent around 350 000 concepts that are both pre- and post-coordinated. In other words, the combination of atomic concepts (for example, 'Family History' *and* 'Breast Cancer') is allowed along with multipart complex concepts being expressed as a *single* phrase (for example, 'Family history of breast cancer'). It also contains rich networks of semantic relationship links that taken together define a concept. Whether SNOMED-CT allows for the reliable retrieval of equivalent concepts expressed in differing ways is more contentious, and this needs to be examined further in the Australian context.

Figure 3.1 provides some real world examples and again shows the links between terminologies and classifications. Note the presence of rules that guide the mappings between concepts in the various levels.

Figure 3.1: Examples and links between the terminology types (MacIsaac, Scott & Saad, 2002)

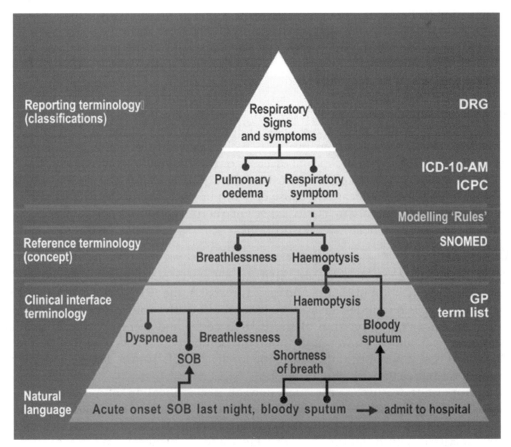

Recently another use has been found for reference and interface terminologies in the development of Archetypes or clinical constraint models for *open*EHR based Electronic Health Records (EHR). Heard (Chapter 16) discusses these further. The developers of standards relating to EHRs in Australia, Europe and the USA are involved in this project believing that Archetypes can be created for use in local EHRs. *Open*EHR is being trialled by the Health*Connect* Program Office.

An overview of the major classifications and terminologies used in Australia

The Australian Bureau of Statistics has been recording causes of death using the International Classification of Diseases (ICD) and its predecessors since 1907.

ICD-10

ICD-10 is a statistical classification released under the auspices of the World Health Organisation (WHO). It contains a limited number of mutually exclusive code categories that describe all disease concepts. ICD-10 has a hierarchical structure with subdivisions to identify broad groups and specific entities. The principal use of the ICD-10 is for international reporting of mortality data to the WHO, although many countries also use it for morbidity coding.

ICD-10 has been implemented in more than 120 countries for morbidity reporting purposes and slightly more for cause of death reporting. The ICD-10 is an alphanumeric coding scheme, which utilises one letter followed by two, three or four numeric characters. The classification has twenty-two chapters, most of which are associated with particular body systems, special diseases or external factors (WHO, 1992).

The Australian Bureau of Statistics introduced ICD-10 for the coding of data reported on medical certificates of cause of death in 1997. Use of the ICD-10 provides the opportunity to compare mortality experience across countries, across time, within Australia and between healthcare institutions.

ICD-10-AM

The *ICD-10 Australian modification* (ICD-10-AM) was developed by the National Centre for Classification in Health and has, as its basis, the ICD-10 (Volumes 1 and 3). To distinctively and uniquely classify diseases and health problems of local interest, Australian extensions to certain of the ICD-10 codes and some specific Australian codes have been added. However, the ability to compare data coded with ICD-10 and ICD-10-AM is still possible at the core code level. The ICD-10-AM disease codes have the same format as ICD-10 (NCCH, n.d.).

An important feature is the inclusion of a classification of procedures and interventions known as the Australian Classification of Health Interventions (ACHI). This is based on the Commonwealth Medicare Benefits Schedule (MBS) of fees for health services. A fifth volume has also been added, incorporating the Australian Coding Standards, which guide clinical codes in the use of the classification.

Australian uses

ICD-10-AM was introduced for hospital morbidity coding in 1998 in New South Wales, the Australian Capital Territory, Victoria and the Northern Territory and introduced in the remaining States in 1999. Therefore, all health information relating to the diagnoses treated and procedures provided in Australian hospitals is coded using this classification. Because of its compatibility with the ICD-10, it is possible for data coded using the ICD-10-AM to be compared with health information coded using the ICD-10.

ICPC-2 and ICPC-2-PLUS

ICPC-2, the second revision of the International Classification of Primary Care (ICPC), is a classification designed for use in primary care settings. It is a patient-oriented rather than disease or provider-oriented approach to classification.

ICPC-2-PLUS is an extended vocabulary of terms classified according to the ICPC-2. It includes terms used by Australian GPs to describe patient 'reasons for encounter' and problems managed. ICPC-2-PLUS has been designed for use in Australian computerised clinical systems, recall systems, disease registers and for secondary coding of clinical data.

Australian uses

ICPC-2-PLUS has been used in many general practice electronic health record and prescribing systems. It is also used for BEACH (Better the Evaluation and Care of Health), a general practice research project conducted by the Family Medicine Research Unit. In addition, it is used in various research and statistical collections, particularly those where there is self-reporting of patient problems.

Examples of domain-specific clinical classifications

In an electronic environment, it is essential that all clinicians can accurately communicate treatment plans, assessments, patient diagnoses and symptoms. They need to do this in an appropriately specific and accurate manner, using standard, accepted, and relevant terminology or terminologies.

Nursing

Nurses are recognised as key collectors, generators and users of patient/client information (Currell, Wainwright & Urquhart, 2002). However, without some type of organisation of data or use of a classification, the differences in nursing language can be quite marked and result in inappropriate interpretations of the patient record. This leads to the key process of nursing care being measured in different ways (Conrick, 1995). It was also known that if patient care is not consistently and accurately recorded, the possible adverse effects for the patient might be highly significant (Currell et al., 2002).

The development of a nursing language began in the early 1970s in the USA. Since then, American nurses have been joined by their European counterparts as the most active developers in the classification of nursing practice. Since 1998, various national nursing organisations (including the Royal College of Nursing Australia) and the International Council of Nurses (ICN) have supported these developments. However, Australia is yet to trial any of these data sets.

ICNP

The International Council of Nurses (ICN) and its member organisations have developed the International Classification for Nursing Practice (ICNP®).

The ICNP® provides a unifying framework into which local language and existing nursing vocabularies and classifications can be cross-mapped, enabling comparison of nursing data across organisations, across sectors within healthcare systems, and between countries (ICN, 2005). The newly released Version 1 is combinational, has non-semantic coding (the codes do not hold any meaning themselves) and numeric codes. It is a multi-axial single classification, with seven axes representing diagnoses, interventions and outcomes (ICN, 2005). To date, the ICNP® has been translated into twenty languages and therefore offers the opportunity to compare nursing data on an international level.

The ICNP® Program is developing 'ICNP® catalogues' that will consist of sets of nursing diagnoses, interventions, and/or outcomes that can be further tested and validated for specific use (ICN, 2005). For example, a catalogue may be a set of nursing diagnoses developed for Family Nursing and represented in ICNP®.

The ICN is planning mapping work between SNOMED-CT, NANDA, and the International Classification of Functioning Disability and Health (ICF) to ICNP®. Nursing experts have also been working with SNOMED to ensure nursing representation in this classification.

There are also a number of classifications used in America, for example, the North American Nursing Diagnosis Association (NANDA) International, the Nursing Interventions Classification (NIC) and Nursing Outcomes Classification (NOC) and SabaCare but, along with ICNP® these need to be trialled to gauge suitability for Australian use.

Allied health

Allied health professionals also need to order and manage their data in an electronic environment and individual professions have worked on this. Rhodes (Chapter 28) discusses this from a clinician's perspective. At a national level, the Health Professions Council of Australia (HPCA) group was a relatively early starter in data standardisation, with work on the National Allied Health Reference Standards Project undertaken in 1994.

This involved the collection of a variety of workload and output data by various HPCA groups. However, in common with other disciplines these were institution-specific, variously defined and infrequently standardised. Therefore, comparison between regions, states, or across like organisations was not possible. This was the impetus for the development of the Australian Allied Health Classification System (AAHCS), which offered:

- a common language to communicate key aspects of the business of allied health professionals to in-house senior management and government agencies
- a standardised system for allied health professionals to compare their clinical practices
- a rich database for research into allied health activities, interventions and outcomes
- the chance to benchmark services across organisations.

(National Allied Health Casemix Committee (NAHCC), 2001)

This project gave way to the Health Activity Hierarchy in 2001, but by then it had developed a common intervention/procedure classification system for allied health. It later contributed to the development of a generic framework and discipline-specific interventions and procedure codes in areas such as podiatry. The Australian Allied Health (Activity) Classification System (Version 1) was revised to reflect changes in the broader allied health interventions that have been integrated into the ICD-10-AM procedure codes to describe types of 'health services provided'.

'Indicators for Intervention' is a classification system that describes the condition or issue that leads to consumers using allied health services, and the reasons that AHPs are involved with healthcare of patients and the community. AHPs make extensive use of Diagnosis Related Groupings (DRGs), but there is wide acknowledgement that much of allied health activity is not well described or predicted by this procedure-based system as it is grounded in a medical/illness paradigm of care (NAHCC, 2001).

Community health terminology

The community health sector developed the first and only Australian Minimum Data Set for Nursing in 1991 and this is still in use today. The Australian Classification and Terminology of Community Health (CATCH) is also a recent development. CATCH is a terminology developed by clinicians for clinicians to facilitate clinical and service-related documentation for community health.

The National Centre for Classification in Health (NCCH) is developing CATCH in collaboration with the jurisdictions to populate software used in the Community Health Information Management Enterprise (CHIME). CATCH is composed of a hierarchical set of classification schemes and their component values that are specifically related to community health services. It has approximately 10 000 terms mapped to the community health concepts to allow clinicians to document, in terms familiar to them, clients' issues and subsequent treatments (NCCH, n.d.).

General Practice vocabulary

The General Practice (GP) Vocabulary is an interface terminology that has sourced about 180 000 clinical interface terms representing symptoms, problems, diagnoses and reasons for prescribing from a popular GP software program. The purpose of the project is to assist the development of software to enable GPs, even those with little training, to enter patient information in a structured way with minimal effort so that a computer is able to 'understand' the content of what has been entered. The GP has the benefit of access to decision support, relevant reports and analyses, clinical review (to facilitate quality of care assessment), and the ability to transfer and receive data electronically.

Minimum data sets

Minimum Data Set (MDS) development is undertaken in both administrative/management and clinical areas. MDSs are mostly used to support health service managers', policy-makers' or researchers' information needs because they contain insufficient elements to record the provision of care. An MDS is a list of data elements with uniform definitions and categories that contain the least number of data elements required in a data set to do a particular job (SA, 2003). Table 3.4 illustrates a simple MDS for an episode of care.

Table 3.4: A simple minimum data set

1: Age

2: Gender

3: Date of birth

4: Residential Address

5: Unique health record number of patient

6: Informal Carer Availability

7: Services provider

8: Unique number of principal provider

9: Diagnosis

10: Intervention

11: Outcome

12: Discharge or termination date

An MDS can be used to provide consistent, quality information within individual organisations and at state and national levels. It can enable comparisons at each level and assist in identifying problem areas, where improvements are needed, and subsequently allows the monitoring of progress following the introduction of quality improvement initiatives. Longitudinal data from an MDS will provide data for future planning by identifying successes, gaps or problems.

Data collected using an MDS can answer questions that previously might have been based on a 'guesstimate'.

Interest box

Based on data collected using an MDS, the Victorian Falls Prevention project was able to report a significant 64 per cent reduction in the number of falls and a 75 per cent reduction in falls causing injuries. They also reported 'small but significant improvements in most of the secondary outcome measures, including balance, gait and mobility, leg strength, fear of falling, and reduced number of medications taken' (National Ageing Research Institute, 2004).

Increasingly managers and health service executives are finding that more specific data are required to make informed decisions. The use of MDSs facilitates the capture of consistent, quality data and provides a mechanism for benchmarking within or across institutions. However, to use the data for external benchmarking requires the ability to exchange the data and, in this, messaging standards become vital.

Messaging standards

Information related to consumer healthcare is held in a variety of data formats and information structures using a range of computer applications and paper-based systems. The exchange of data or sending of electronic messages is challenging, particularly in health because of legacy systems, multiple computer formats, and multiple practitioners.

The exchange of data can take place on two levels:

1. The basic level where messages can be sent between computers and there is no need for data to be interpreted by the receiver. An example is the use of electronic mail (email).
2. The functional level where messages between computers are interpreted at the level of data fields. Here data passes from a structured field in one system to a comparably structured field in another. In this case neither system has any understanding of the meaning of the data. However, if both systems conform to a common messaging standard the data can be presented in a meaningful way to the user.

The use of common messaging standards is essential because it enables the communication and sharing of consumer healthcare information between disparate systems without customised interfaces. This process will enable the building of, and access to, electronic health records through the exchange of information in a consistent non-proprietary manner (Commonwealth of Australia, 2001). Australia has adopted the HL7 messaging standards as a way of assuring this.

HL7

Health Level 7 (HL7) is both the name of an international standards organisation and the name given to an international healthcare messaging standard. It takes its name from the seventh level of the ISO communications model for Open Systems. Level Seven, or the applications level, is where the clinical information in healthcare is handled. It is concerned with the definition of the data to be exchanged, the timing of the interchange, and the communication of certain errors, to the application. It supports functions such as security checks, participant identification, availability checks, exchange mechanism negotiations and, most importantly, data exchange structuring.

The HL7 domain is clinical and administrative data and it aims to:

> provide standards for the exchange, management and integration of data that support clinical patient care and the management, delivery and evaluation of healthcare services. Specifically, to create flexible, cost effective approaches, standards, guidelines, methodologies, and related services for interoperability between healthcare information systems.
>
> (HL7, 2003)

The Reference Information Model (RIM) is the cornerstone of the HL7 Version 3 development process. The RIM is a large object-oriented model of clinical data (domains). It identifies the life cycle of events that a message or groups of related messages will carry. It is a shared model across health domains and is the model from which all domains create their messages. The RIM is essential to increasing precision and reducing implementation costs in healthcare as it aims to explicitly represent the connections that exist between the information carried in the fields of HL7 messages (HL7, 2003).

To date Standards Australia has undertaken over 50 messaging projects including:
- referral-discharge messaging
- laboratory/radiology results and orders messaging
- pathology code set
- community health messaging
- drug prescription
- immunisation.

HL7 Version 2 has been widely adopted around the world as it enables the exchange of messages between proprietary and closed systems. Version 3 has been released but is not widely accepted at this time. In the UK, Netherlands and Canada for example, governments have mandated the use of HL7 Version 3 in the development of national electronic health information systems.

Security standards

Public Key Infrastructure (PKI) is being introduced into Australia to enable the exchange of health information in a secure way, particularly that contained in electronic health records. A number of projects have been initiated and some are yet to deliver outcomes and benefits. One drawback has been the lack of unique identifiers for patients and providers. NeHTA is now undertaking a project to correct this. Access to data has also been a vexed question particularly in the Health*Connect* trials where several different models have been trialled.

Conclusion

The recording of health data and the terms and concepts used are important, because these enable disparate health professional groups to communicate in a consistent, unambiguous, meaningful manner.

Because of the complex nature of health service provision in Australia and the multi-disciplinary nature of the care provided, it is important that any terminology used to describe healthcare in Australia reflects the work of all clinicians, administrators and managers. Developing the relationship between terminologies, pre-existing classifications and the underlying information models is crucial to furthering health informatics applications. The success of these endeavours will underpin a quality cost effective, health system.

Review questions

1. What types of standards enable electronic health information interchange? Give some examples.
2. What are the main differences between terminologies and classifications?
3. What are some pros and cons for adherence to global standards versus local point-to-point standards solutions?

Exercises

- Consider the statement 'terminologies are now software' (which comes from a paper by Alan Rector). Do you agree or disagree? Justify your answer.

- Go to www.openehr.org and read about archetypes. How could some nursing archetypes for example be useful? What would they look like? How would they incorporate nursing terminology standards?

- Go to www.hl7.org and click on 'What is HL7?'. Observe that the notions of a template and vocabulary standards are presented very early in the information. Read about these.

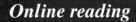

INFOTRAC® COLLEGE EDITION
For additional readings and review on information interchange, explore **InfoTrac® College Edition**, your online library. Go to: **www.infotrac-college.com** and search for any of the InfoTrac key terms listed below:

➢ Coding
➢ Classification
➢ Terminology
➢ Minimum Data Sets

References

Commonwealth of Australia (2001). *Setting the standards: a national health information standards plan for Australia,* Health Online, Canberra.

Conrick, M. (1995). *Issues in informatics: nursing within health* (Vol. 1), Centre for Research, Brisbane.

Currell, R., Wainwright, P. & Urquhart, C. (2002). *Nursing record systems: effects on nursing practice and healthcare outcomes,* The Cochrane Library Update Software, Oxford.

European Committee for Standarization (CEN) (2005). *What is CEN?* Retrieved 1 January, 2005, from http://www.cenorm.be/.

HL7 (2003). *What is HL7?* Retrieved 24 February 2005 from http://www.hl7.org/.

Innes, K. & Bramley, M. (1997). *Criteria for classification development,* National Codeset Project, Community Based Services, Sydney.

International Council of Nurses (ICN) (2005). ICNP® Version 1. Retrieved 3 June, 2005, from http://www.icn.ch.

International Standards Organisation (1999). ISO 2382–4. Information technology – Vocabulary – Part 4: Organization of data.

International Standards Organisation (ISO) (2002). ISO TS 17117. *Health informatics – controlled health terminology – Structure and high-level indicators.*

International Standards Organisation (ISO) (2005). *Introduction to ISO.* Retrieved 3 March, 2005, from http://www.iso.org/.

MacIsaac, P., Scott, P. & Saad, P. (2002). NCCH reproduced in *The Language of Health Concept Representation*, IT14–2.

National Ageing Research Institute (2004). *Evaluation of a minimum data set for Victorian Falls clinics,* Victorian Department of Human Services, Melbourne.

National Allied Health Casemix Committee (NAHCC) (2001). *The health activity hierarchy Version 1.1.* Retrieved 2 March, 2005, from http://www.dlsweb.rmit.edu.au/.

National Health Information Management Group (2002). *The Australian family of health and related classifications,* Commonwealth of Australia, Canberra.

NCCH (n.d.). *The Australian classification and terminology of community health.* Retrieved 28 May, 2005, from http://www3.fhs.usyd.edu.au/ncch/.

Scott, P. (2002). *An introduction to health terminologies,* National Centre for Classification in Health, Sydney.

Standards Australia (SA) (2003). *Health concept terminology data base,* Standard AS5021, Australia.

Walker, S., Frean, I., Scott, P. & Conrick, M. (2003). *Classifications and terminologies in residential aged care: an information paper,* The Ageing and Aged Care Division of the Commonwealth Department of Health and Ageing, Canberra.

World Health Organization (WHO) (1992). *International statistical classification of diseases and related health problems tenth revision* (ICD-10), Geneva.

4

Modelling healthcare information

Isobel Frean

'A reference information model is essential to ensure consistency and a shared understanding and to guide implementation decisions as to which health care concepts are integral to the terminology and which to the architecture.'

(Liaw, S-T et al., 2003)

Outline

Since the 1980s modelling in healthcare has assumed a pivotal role in defining the way we represent, store, retrieve and move healthcare data. Early approaches to modelling information in healthcare laid the foundations for the modelling methods of today. An understanding of these methods and one of the languages that underpin them, Unified Modelling Language (UML), is essential to understanding the way models are used to conceptualise healthcare data and information. This chapter discusses the issues of modelling and walks the reader through the UML language.

Introduction

National healthcare reforms at a time when fifth generation computer programs were offering potential solutions to the collection, storage and retrieval of healthcare information helped to confirm the role of information technology in the healthcare reform process (Abbott, 1992). These reforms gave rise to technical organisations whose role was to define how large organisations and nations would collect information that could better assist management in determining whether services at the local level were being delivered appropriately and effectively. For example, when faced with the need for a consistent approach to healthcare system development, the Information Management Centre (IMC) in the United Kingdom pioneered the development of the Common Basic Specification model (CBS) in 1990. This was a generic information model and process intended to become the de facto standard for system development across the National Health Service (NHS) (Jones, 1998).

While not providing the panacea required, the CBS served as a straw man upon which subsequent NHS and similar national and international efforts sought to build. Since the early 1990s there has been greater consistency between international efforts to model healthcare information through the use of common principles and methods. Today the nirvana of healthcare information interoperability, required for effective electronic health records delivery, will depend upon the continued convergence of these information models so that they may complement and perhaps one day map to each other.

What is modelling?

Modelling is exactly what it seems. It is the process of defining the real world using a conceptual construct – or model. Accordingly, models are developed to enable a better understanding of the business or activity for which a solution is required. Modelling therefore allows us to achieve four aims:

1. To visualise a system as it is or as we want it to be.
2. To specify the structure or behaviour of a system.
3. To provide a template to guide construction of a system.
4. To document decisions made in developing a system.

(Booch, et al., 1999).

A model may take the form of an architect's plans, a map of the Tokyo underground or an illustration of DNA genetic material or of a healthcare information system. In each case, the model allows the user to represent (to conceptualise) the complex details of a system or entity of concern, by breaking it down into simpler parts. Accordingly, there is rarely a simple model to represent any given real world 'thing'; typically several levels of model may be required and at the more granular level of detail several elements or views may be required. For example, a portion of DNA will be represented by the high level view of the helix. However, to understand the helix, models are required to describe each strand, each sequence of proteins in each strand and their relationship to other proteins, and eventually the molecular structure or the physical components of each protein.

Models can help us to capture the seemingly complex vocabulary or concepts required to define the healthcare information needs of an enterprise such as a state or national health system. At the other end of the spectrum, different types of models help to describe the unique data components required to define the responsibilities of entities (people, organisations or devices) in a system. As the four modelling principles below affirm, no one model is sufficient to describe the architecture of a real world event or process (Booch et al., 1999).

Four Principles of Modelling

1. The choice of what models to create has a profound influence on how a problem is attacked and how a solution is shaped.
2. Every model may be expressed at different levels of precision.

3. The best models are connected to reality.
4. No single model is sufficient. Every nontrivial system is best approached through a small set of nearly independent models.

The term *architecture* is also used when referring to information or data modelling. While the architecture of a healthcare information system will include models, the term is used more broadly to define the organisational structure of an information system (Rumbaugh et al., 1999). Accordingly the architecture of a state health department, for example, will outline the structure of the components to the system, how these are connected to each other (the organisational as well as the logistical connections) and reflect the policy or strategic decisions around which the system has been designed. Decisions related to the architecture of a system can be captured using models, subsystems, packages and components (Rumbaugh et al., 1999), as illustrated in Table 4.1.

Table 4.1: The architecture for a system is defined by models, subsystems, packages and components; and their relationships to each other

Architecture parts	Definition	Sample notation
Model	'A semantically complete abstraction of a system' (Rumbaugh, J. et al., 1999). To provide a complete abstraction of a real world system a model may comprise multiple different views, incorporate multiple use cases. The example illustrated is a Use Case Model.	

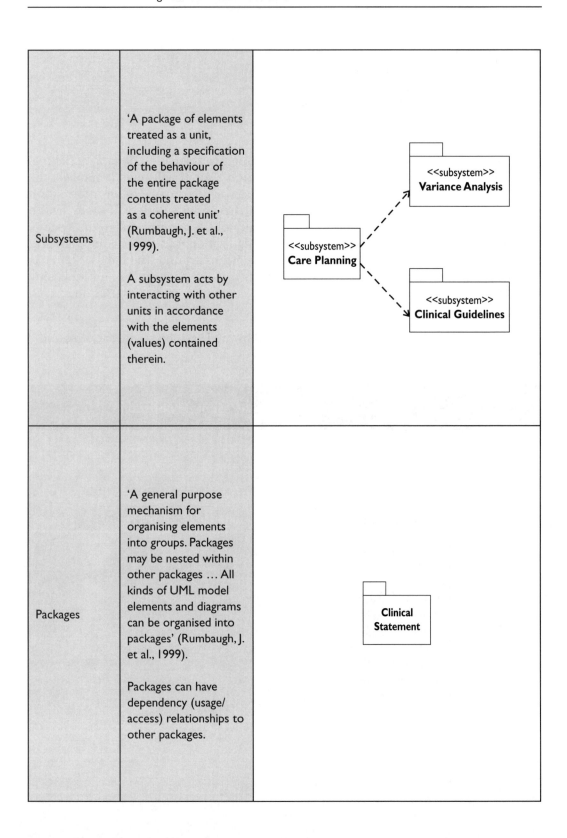

| Subsystems | 'A package of elements treated as a unit, including a specification of the behaviour of the entire package contents treated as a coherent unit' (Rumbaugh, J. et al., 1999).

A subsystem acts by interacting with other units in accordance with the elements (values) contained therein. | |
| Packages | 'A general purpose mechanism for organising elements into groups. Packages may be nested within other packages ... All kinds of UML model elements and diagrams can be organised into packages' (Rumbaugh, J. et al., 1999).

Packages can have dependency (usage/ access) relationships to other packages. | |

Components	'A physical piece of implementation of a system, including software code ... the physical units on computers that can be connected to other components, replaced by equivalent components, moved around, archived ...' (Rumbaugh, J. et al., 1999).	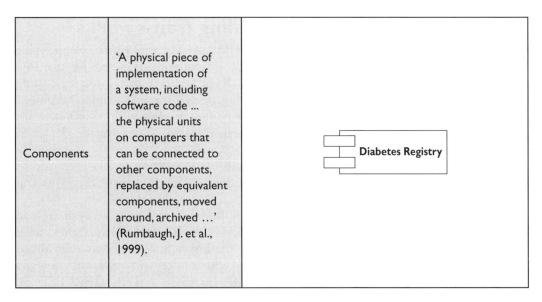

The terms information model and data model are often used synonymously as both are concerned with modelling data. However, an information model is really concerned with classifying information or semantic concepts, such as STATE OF HEALTH AND WELLBEING, ENABLING FACTORS, and ENVIRONMENT. Typically an information model is a conceptual or semantic model, while a data model (logical or physical) is concerned with classifying or grouping data items, such as PERSONS, PROCESSES, and OBSERVATIONS. Data models employ the principle of third normal form (TNF), by uniquely representing an item of data. Chu describes this in more detail in Chapter 5. A data model therefore unambiguously defines the data elements and their relationships within the structure being modelled. These different types of models are described in more detail below.

Enterprise architectures

Health information management and system design are concerned with a hierarchy of organisational structures, or architectures, for defining the why, what, when and where of information management across an enterprise – regardless of size. Organisational structures, their component parts and the relationship of these parts are represented using models and other elements such as packages and components. Together they form an *Enterprise Architecture*.

Enterprise architectures provide a global view of an enterprise. They comprise a package of interconnected models whose aim is to ensure that the mission of the enterprise, its business, organisational processes and systems flow through to the information technology (IT) strategy and investments of the enterprise. These models support the business development of an enterprise by describing the current and future drivers of the enterprise. Enterprise models are therefore important when large-scale redevelopment activities, such as the development of a national electronic health infrastructure, are being designed.

Healthcare information modelling frameworks

Healthcare information modelling today largely follows the enterprise architecture framework conceived by Zachman (1987) and subsequently adapted by the ISO Health Informatics Technical Committee (TC) 215 for health information modelling (AIWH, 2003). Zachman's matrix-like framework reflected the importance he placed on stakeholder involvement and contained inter-related models with different levels of abstraction to reflect six key stakeholder perspectives: planner, owner, designer, builder, subcontractor and the working system (SSC, 2003).

Zachman focused on maintaining a clear link between the models prepared at each level so that the resulting system delivered the original business objectives and principles.

Figure 4.1 provides a simplified view of the enterprise architecture approach to illustrate the more common contemporary models in healthcare. At the highest level of abstraction are context models, which define the big picture concepts relevant to the enterprise in question. In a healthcare system these models will represent concepts such as EVENTS, PEOPLE, ENVIRONMENT, GOVERANCE and RESOURCES.

Figure 4.1: Information modelling framework

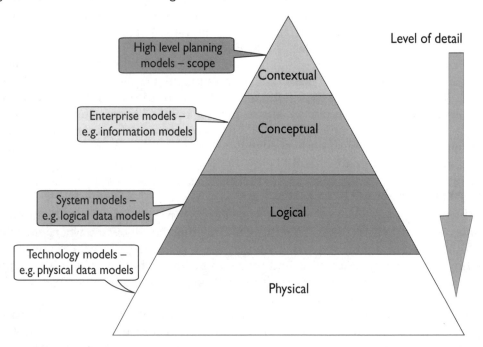

Context models do not provide any level of detail; rather they identify the concepts of interest; their relationship to each other; and the system vocabulary (the terms that are going to be used to describe things) so that these concepts are clearly and consistently defined and understood by others throughout the enterprise. Examples of context models in healthcare include the National Health Information Model (NHIM) Version 2, produced by the Australian Institute of Health and Welfare

(AIWH, 2003), illustrated in Figure 4.2, and the Contextual Health Data Model, produced by the Canadian Institute for Health Information (CIHI, 2001), illustrated in Figure 4.3.

Figure 4.2: Example of context model: Australian Institute for Health and Welfare (AIHW) National health information data model V2 *(Reproduced with permission of the AIHW)*

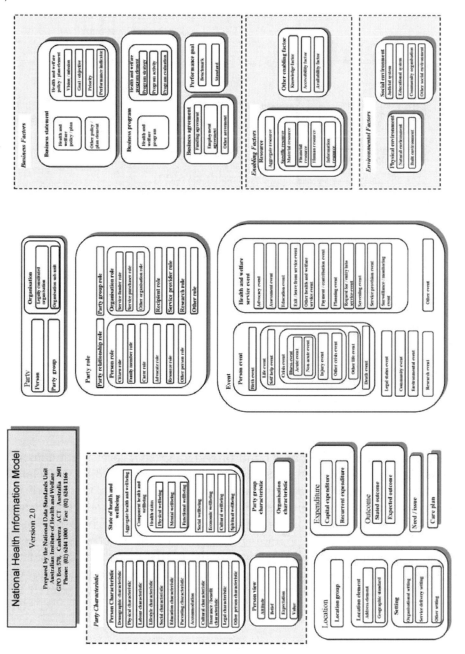

Figure 4.3: Example of context model: Canadian Institute for Health Information (CIHI) Contextual health data model *(Reproduced with permission of the CIHI)*

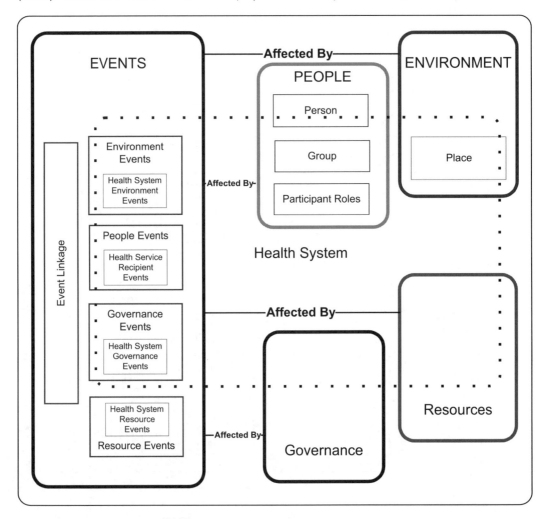

Conceptual models on the other hand provide a greater level of refinement of the enterprise concepts of interest than contextual models by detailing the relationships between the components that make up these concepts. Conceptual models are produced by and for system design stakeholders, who should include both the technical experts and the end users (clinicians). Conceptual models should derive from an existing contextual 'model' or strategic planning statement of the enterprise. An example of this is the CHII Conceptual Health Data Model (CHDM) Version 2.3, illustrated in Figure 4.4. This conceptual information model represents the higher order concepts derived from the CIHI context model as events or system activities, namely PEOPLE EVENTS, ENVIRONMENT EVENTS, GOVERNANCE EVENTS and RESOURCES EVENTS.

Figure 4.4: Example of conceptual model: Canadian Institute for Health Information (CIHI) Conceptual health data model *(Reproduced with permission of the CIHI)*

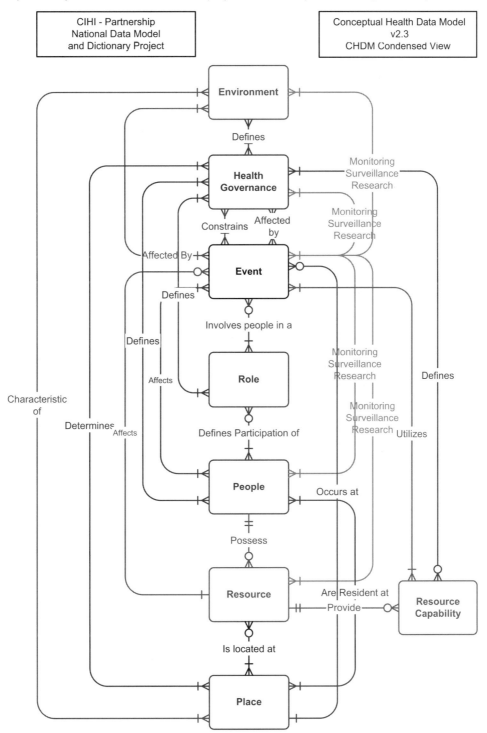

The next two levels of model abstraction, the *logical data model* and the *physical data model* (often referred to interchangeably) provide the details required by software developers to implement the objectives of the conceptual model. They provide the greatest level of detail about the data elements that make up the concepts of interest to the enterprise and their relationships to one another. Logical and data models are prepared by modelling experts (systems analysts), hopefully, working in close collaboration with end users.

In healthcare modelling, the systems modeller should be fully reliant on the input of clinicians to ensure that the data elements and the processes they are modelling reflect clinician consensus and workflow practices. Zachman's edict about the adoption of a holistic approach is particularly pertinent to healthcare information modelling because accuracy in representing clinical information in technical systems is paramount. Not surprisingly, many of those involved in data modelling in healthcare are clinicians who wish to ensure the accuracy and safety of the models to which they are contributing.

Logical models are software independent. They are critical for specifying and documenting the concepts or vocabulary of the healthcare domain and the structural (static) and behavioural (dynamic) ways in which those concepts exist and inter-relate. Physical data are also software independent; however they are concerned with modelling the physical and replaceable parts or components to an executable system.

Generic healthcare information models

In the 1980s, two drivers shaped the IT agenda in the United Kingdom and subsequently the evolution of healthcare information models. The first was the Korner Minimum Data Set (MDS) and related recommendations for improved information collection by the NHS. The second was the Griffith Report, which heralded a corporate approach to health service management by introducing non-clinician general managers who looked to information to inform their decision-making. The NHS Common Basic Specification (CBS) that set out a generic information model and process was an attempt to create a de facto standard for consistent NHS-wide systems development (Abbott, 1992) in part in response to these and other drivers.

However, Jones (1998) reveals that problems arose with the CBS, precisely because of its genericity, both in the process and the model itself. Jones, as part of the modelling team reviewing the CBS, developed a Formal Generic Model (FGM) for healthcare by defining a more scientific basis for the development of generic models. He found that there was no 'single all embracing methodology' that would meet the needs of all healthcare information modelling domains. His research demonstrated the need for generic models to use formal modelling notation and that these models should be used to define standards, which in turn must be subject to accreditation (Jones, 1998). He also concluded that system developers should build their *own* portfolio of tools and methods!

It is significant that at the time Jones was working, the Health Informatics Committee, TC251 of the European Standards Development Organisation (CEN), were developing generic healthcare information models and messaging standards to support emerging electronic health records. Today CEN and other open standards organisations (Health Level Seven, IEEE, DICOM, etc.) are succeeding in developing consistent methods, notations and tools for nationally and internationally compatible health information models by drawing upon the lessons learnt by those working in the 1990s.

Modelling notation and languages

Healthcare information/data models are portrayed using one of a handful of modelling notations. These notations or modelling languages enable the modeller to represent the many different business requirements of a healthcare system. The streamlining of modelling notations in the 1990s offered the opportunity for greater harmonisation between models within and across related healthcare enterprises. The experiences of the Australian Institute of Health and Welfare (AIHW) in this regard are illustrative. The modelling notations typically used for conceptual models are Entity-Relationship (E-R), Unified Modelling Language (UML) or Object-Role Modelling (ORM) notations. The E-R notation was seen as an effective, stable and relatively simple modelling convention in the mid 90s and the AIHW produced the National Health Information Model (NHIM) Version 1 using this notation (Chu, in Chapter 5, provides a brief description of the E-R diagramming notation and applies it to database development).

However, the AIHW abandoned the use of the E-R notation for Version 2 in favour of a contextual model because of the difficulties in representing relationships between entities at the national level (AIWH, 2003). The benefits from the NHIM Version 1, however, encouraged several state health departments to produce their own conceptual models. In 1996 the New South Wales Health Department released its Enterprise Information Model (EIM) using the E-R notation.

This model informed similar development in Queensland and West Australia. The latter EIM was released in August 2002 and is available on the West Australian Health Department's website along with useful examples of how it is being used to inform the development of more granular models and business processes (West Australian Government, 2002). Halpin's work on ORM is particularly illuminating, for those interested in learning more about this notation. However, knowledge of UML is also essential in reading and understanding modelling notations.

The emergence of Unified Modelling Language (UML)

At the time that generic information models for healthcare were being perused, software engineers were engaged in a significant battle over modelling notations. The outcome was the creation of the Unified Modelling Language (UML). While the E-R model remains the dominant notation for the conceptual design of databases, when modelling information in healthcare there is a need to understand the significance of UML and to read its simple notations/icons. An understanding of UML will also greatly assist in comprehending the Health Level 7 (HL7) Version 3 Reference Information Model (HL7, 2005) and the CEN prEN13606–1 EHR Reference Model (CEN/TC 251, 2005). These are arguably two of the most important health information models in the world. The following provides a brief history of UML.

Until object-oriented modelling languages emerged in the mid 1970s – late 1980s (Booch et al., 1999), concept models were difficult for all but the engineer responsible for developing them to understand. In the 'method war' of 1989 to 1994 multiple object–oriented modelling languages evolved as no one language satisfied the requirements of every modeller. These were followed several years later by the first object-oriented development methods (Rumbaugh et al., 1999). These methods included a holistic approach to modelling through a thorough analysis of a user's requirements and ensuring that these requirements (business processes) were reflected in the system design.

Three well-known examples of these development methods include Grady Booch's Booch method, Ivar Jacobson's Object-Oriented Software Engineering (OOSE) method and James Rumbaugh's Object Modelling Technique (OMT) (Booch et al., 1999). The method wars came to a head in the mid 1990s when Booch (working for Rational Software Corporation), Jacobson (Objectory) and Rumbaugh (General Electric) combined forces to achieve three goals.

1. To model systems, from concept to executable artifact, using object-oriented technique.
2. To address the issues of scale inherent in complex, mission-critical systems.
3. To create a modelling language usable by both humans and machines (Booch, G. et al., 1999).

Booch and Rumbaugh released the first public draft (V0.8) of UML in October 1995 and the following year Jacobson's OOSE method was rolled into the subsequent version. Following further development by a consortium UML Version 1.0 was released. The Object Management Group (OMG) standardised and adopted UML 1.1. They have since assumed a governance role for UML standards, including the management of the UML meta-model, used by organisations like HL7 to develop UML compliant stereotype models (like the HL7 RIM). The most current version of this now universally adopted modelling language is UML 2.

Understanding UML

UML is made up of objects, relationships and diagrams. In its entirety, the diagrams document the objects and their relationships to each other. In so doing UML can be used to document a system's architecture and model the activities of project planning or the workflow of a healthcare system. There are four key objects in UML: structural objects, used to represent the static features of the system or workflow being modelled; behavioural objects, used to represent the dynamic features of the system or model; groupings and annotational objects used respectively to organise components or packages of structural or behavioural objects and to describe or explain the elements in the model. While it is beyond the scope of this chapter to provide an in-depth examination of UML, the following sections highlight some of the main features of objects, relationships and diagrams.

The core concept of class is used to describe groups of objects. For example the concept of Entity describes groups of things (classes) that might be Living Subjects, Organisations or Devices. The class concept is represented in UML using a rectangle with a name, attributes and operations. Figure 4.5 illustrates a class entitled Living

Subject. The name is recorded in the top box. Names of more than one word are recorded without a space between the first and second word, but with the first letter of the second word capitalised as illustrated. The attributes, or the values of the properties of the class, are recorded in the middle box and the operations, or different behavioural states of the class, are recorded in the bottom box.

Figure 4.5: Illustration of UML class

LivingSubject
–Species
–Name
–ID
–Age
+Active()
+Inactive()

The life cycle of a class in response to events is the state machine and is an example of a behavioural object in UML. When modelling healthcare information flows as part of the process of documenting specifications for messaging standards, the state of a class will result in messages of different meanings. In the case, for example, of the act of care provision (CareProvision), a message or interaction in the created state indicates that the act of care provision has not yet commenced. Depending upon the events that impact the Care Provision Act, entitled Trigger Events by HL7, an interaction or message can specify whether a Care Provision Act has been created (but not yet activated), activated, completed, suspended or nullified. State can be illustrated using activity diagrams and state machine diagrams. Figure 4.6 illustrates the state machine for an act class in the HL7 Reference Information Model (RIM).

Figure 4.6: HL7 Version 3 act class state machine *(Reproduced with permission of HL7,)*

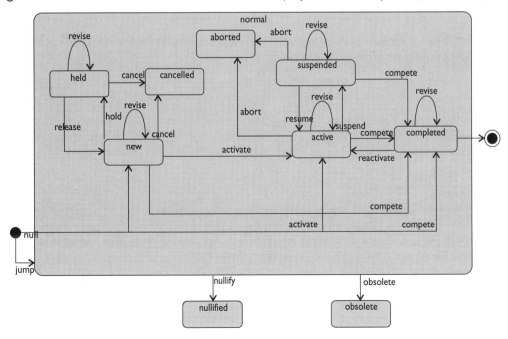

In UML, describing the relationships between things is a key function. There are four types of relationships: dependency, association, generalisation, and realisation.

A *dependency* is as it sounds, a relationship where a change to one object changes the meaning of something else. Dependencies are illustrated in models using a dashed line as shown in Figure 4.7. For example, a change in the assessed care requirements of a care recipient in residential aged care may mean a reduction in the subsidy rates paid by a government agency to the provider, in turn affecting the daily fees payable by the care recipient. This derived dependency is illustrated in Figure 4.7. The dependency relationship is pointed out using a UML 'note' box (a rectangle with a folded top right hand corner).

Figure 4.7: Illustration of UML dependency relationship

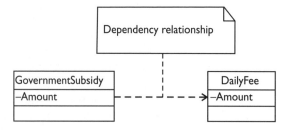

An *association* describes the link connecting two objects and is illustrated using a solid line, sometimes with a label and typically with a cardinality or numbering system to document the nature of the association. In the HL7 Version 3 RIM, there are six core classes, linked to one another through associations describing the types of structural relationships between each of these classes (Hinchley, 2003). These are illustrated in Figure 4.8.

Figure 4.8: Class diagram illustrating core HL7 Version 3 Reference Information Model (RIM) classes *(Adapted from Hinchley, 2003)*

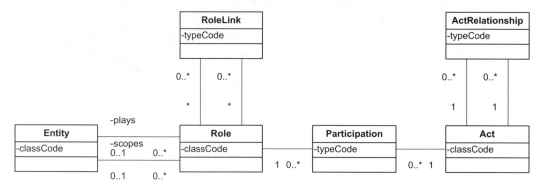

In the case of the link between the Entity class and the Role class in Figure 4.8, two associations are illustrated. One has the label 'plays' to indicate that an Entity plays a Role. The other label, 'scopes,' indicates that the Role class scopes or defines the various instances of the Entity class. Both have a set of numbers at either end of the association to explain further the scale or nature of these links. In the case of both the scoping and the play associations, there is a number set or cardinality of 0…* at the right hand end of the association to indicate that an entity may play zero or many different roles, or that an entity may scope (define) zero or many different roles. However, any one role can only be played or scoped by one entity, as indicated by the 0..1 cardinality at the left hand end of the association line.

Where the entity is a person, described as a LivingSubject in HL7, they may play multiple roles. While they might be a General Practitioner, they may also be a wife, a patient (when attending a breast screening clinic for example), and they may be the authorised legal representative for a parent. These are all instances of the role class played by the same entity. Where the entity is the Nursing Registration Board (NRB) for example, which in HL7 would be described as an Organisation, they would scope the roles of Registered Nurse, Enrolled Nurse etc. The cardinality of 0…1 at the other end of this association indicates that these roles of nurse are scoped by only one organisation, namely the NRB.

The third type of relationship in UML is *generalisation* and represents a most important concept in UML modelling. Here the objects in a child class can be substituted for the objects in a parent class. The child class shares the structure and behaviour of the parent class along with additional information. A generalisation is illustrated using a solid line with an open headed arrow pointing from the source class (the child) to the target (the parent) class, as shown in Figure 4.9.

Figure 4.9 Illustration of UML generalisation relationship

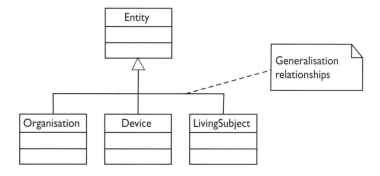

A *realisation* is used to describe the relationship between a classifier (such as a class, actor, interface, use case) where one classifier defines an action or function that the other will undertake. Realisations are most commonly illustrated using a dashed line with an open headed arrow. Figure 4.10 illustrates a situation where the CarePlan act class will implement the actions specified in the DiabetesGuideline act class.

Figure 4.10: Illustration of UML realisation relationship

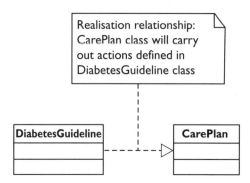

UML diagrams

At the beginning of this chapter models were described as comprising several components. When modelling complex systems like a healthcare system or a workflow carried out by healthcare providers, several diagrams make up the model. In UML there are nine important diagrams, which collectively help both the designer and users of the system to visualise the concepts being modelled from a range of perspectives. UML modelling tools have developed to the extent that the specifications described in these diagrams can be used to generate programming code, typically using eXtensible Markup Language (XML).

Accordingly, the UML diagrams provide a relatively simple way of breaking down elements of a system that can be verified by the eventual system user as reflective of 'the real world'. The relative simplicity of the UML notations and the use of diagrams to visualise structure, workflow, vocabulary and so on, should mean every nuance of every action or structure being modelled can be clearly defined and specified. A brief outline is provided below for each UML diagram. Readers are encouraged to consult any text or URL on UML to gain a more detailed understanding of each model.

A *class diagram* is the most common diagram used in object-oriented modelling and is used to describe the static structures of a system. Figure 4.8 above is a class diagram showing the static class structures of the HL7 RIM.

An *object diagram* models the instances (actual examples) of classes contained in class diagrams. Figures 4.7 and 4.10 are examples of object diagrams.

Use case diagrams also provide a static view of a system, but show the actors involved in a system. Use case diagrams are important for visualising the behaviours of a system. The model illustrated in line one of Table 4.1 is a use case diagram for a chronic disease management system focused around a diabetes program. It illustrates that the actors involved in this system include those involved in providing care to the patient (the doctor and the allied healthcare providers) as well as those involved in evaluating the effectiveness of the program, the Health Department, and those involved in receiving care, the patient.

The dynamic views of a system are illustrated using *interaction diagrams*, which visualise objects and their relationships to one another. These are used extensively when developing messaging standards to support interoperability. Interactions may be illustrated using *sequence diagrams* or *collaboration diagrams*. As the names imply, a sequence diagram illustrates the order in which a message flow or workflow takes place. A collaboration diagram emphasises the structural organisation of the objects that send and receive messages. Figure 4.11 illustrates a sequence diagram in which a sending system, the GP system, is requesting the receiving system, the allied healthcare provider's system, to accept responsibility for care for a patient.

Figure 4.11: Example of UML sequence diagram

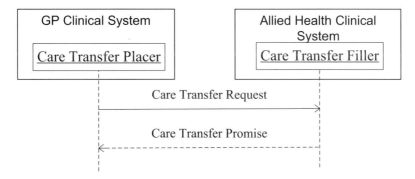

Also illustrated in this diagram are the *application roles* responsible within these collaborating systems for sending the particular interactions. In HL7 message specifications these application roles, together with the specifications defined in the message and the trigger event that initiates the sending of the message, make up the total instruction of a given message. Thus, a message specification in HL7 Version 3 involves a package comprising: an event (a state transition) in one computer system that creates the need for data to flow among systems (represented as a trigger event); a set of sending and receiving roles (application roles); and a data flow (represented as a message) (Harding & Russler, 2005). While not an example of a UML diagram, Figure 4.12 provides a schematic illustration of these components that go to make up a message in HL7. Some refer to the combination of these concepts as the 'dynamic model'.

A *state machine diagram*, illustrated in Figure 4.6, provides another view of the dynamic behaviour of a system. State machine diagrams illustrate the life cycle of a class (for example, a role or an entity) using transitions, events and activities. In HL7 messages the different state of an act, such as CareProvision, is defined using the term mood, a concept that derives from an understanding of the state or state transition of the class.

Figure 4.12: Schematic illustration of HL7 interaction components (dynamic model)

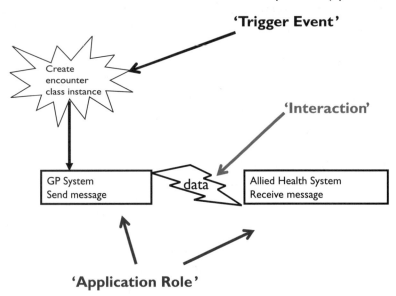

An *activity diagram* is a type of state diagram, in that it illustrates the flow of activity within a system. As they are relatively intuitive diagrams, an end user does not need to know UML to read an activity diagram and advise on its accuracy in portraying the function of a system or the flow of information. When documenting requirements for HL7 V3 message development, activity diagrams are used to provide a visual overview of the data flow within a *storyboard*. Figure 4.13 provides an example of an activity diagram in which a Registered Nurse working in a nursing home sends a request to a resident's General Practitioner seeking a review of a medication chart.

Component diagrams are used to model the static implementation view of a system. They are a type of class diagram except that they model components, interfaces and relationships (Booch et al., 1999).

Deployment diagrams are used to model the physical aspects of a system at the time of deployment. They are used to specify the construction of a system.

Modelling methodologies in healthcare

This chapter explains how the methods and models for conceptualising healthcare system development have been gradually converging. The main drivers for this have been the need to achieve semantic interoperability between computer systems in the interests of building safe and accurate electronic healthcare systems and records.

Now there is streamlining of approaches to the development of enterprise architectures for whole nations and a focus on the development of standardised approaches to healthcare modelling. One example of the latter is the HL7 Development Framework (HDF), a formal method for defining healthcare messaging requirements and for modelling these as message specifications that conform to international standards (HL7, 2004).

Figure 4.13: UML activity diagram illustrating the data flow associated with a request by a Nurse to a GP

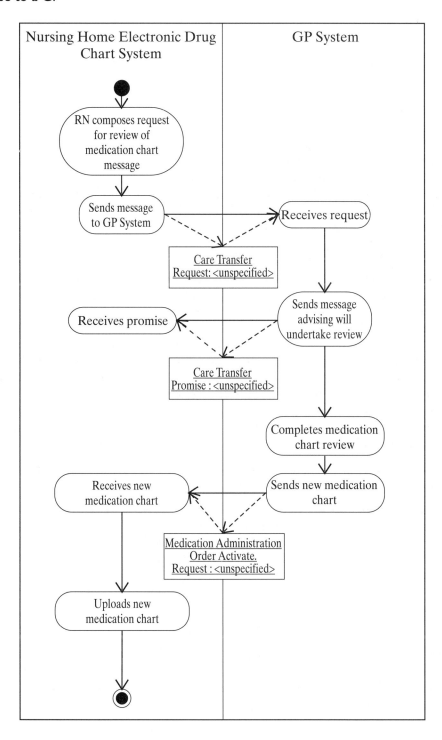

The HDF defines seven phases in the development of HL7 communications standards, these are:

1. Project Initiation
2. Requirements Documentation and Analysis
3. Specification Modelling
4. Specification Documentation
5. Specification Application
6. Specification Publishing
7. Implementation Profiling.

The HDF defines the methods, inputs and outputs of each phase, many of which involve the use of UML diagrams. To support the process, HL7 has developed a number of modelling tools, which are freely available to those developing specifications for HL7 communication standards. HL7 has been working on finalisation of the documentation of the HDF, including implementation guides for developers for the past two years and anticipates its formal release in early 2006.

Conclusion

Information models can be aligned with and inform other models to add coherence to the overall integration of healthcare information systems. They provide the basis for informing knowledge management. The emergence of common conceptual data models (HL7 RIM CEN EN13606–1, and openEHR) and common conceptual elements (CMETs and GPICs) will enable the collection, storage, analysis and sending of information and data across and between healthcare systems. UML has played a key part in this coalescing process, providing a method, for both the end user and the systems developer, to visualise the requirements of the system.

Once developers of healthcare systems architectures and standards have agreed on the methods for working with these emerging common conceptual models, it may be possible to contemplate the reality of semantic interoperability.

Review questions

1. What is an Enterprise Architecture and what purpose does it fulfil?
2. Describe the different types of models found in an information-modelling framework. Name one example in healthcare of each type of model.
3. Name examples of UML diagrams used to visualise the static and the dynamic features of a healthcare system.

Exercises

- Review the National Health Information Model Version 2 published by the Australian Institute of Health and Welfare (AIHW) accessible on the AHIW website: www.aihw.gov.au. List the main classes of interest and for each provide your own example of an instance of this class.

- Draw an UML activity diagram to describe the information flow associated with a request by a GP of a neurologist to see a patient with suspected head injury.
- Go to the HL7 website to review the HL7 Version 3 Reference Information Model (RIM): www.hl7.org. Identify the different colour schemes used to represent each of the six core RIM classes.

Online reading

INFOTRAC® COLLEGE EDITION

For additional readings and review on modelling, explore **InfoTrac® College Edition**, your online library. Go to: **www.infotrac-college.com** and search for any of the InfoTrac key terms listed below:

➤ **Information models**
➤ **Enterprise architecture**
➤ **Unified Modelling Language (UML)**

References

Abbott, W. (ed.) (1992). *Information Technology in Healthcare: A Handbook*, Longman Group, Harlow.

AIWH (2003). *National health information model Version 2*, Australian Institute of Health & Welfare, Canberra.

Booch, G. et al. (1999). *The Unified Modelling Language user guide*, Addison-Wesley, Boston.

CEN/TC251 (2005). Draft prEN13606–1 Health Informatics – Electonic health record communications Part 1: Reference Model, CEN, Brussels, March 2005.

CIHI (2001). *Conceptual Health Data Model v2.3*, Canadian Institute for Health Information, Ontario.

Harding, R. & Russler, D. (2005). In HL7 Working Group Meeting Orlando: HL7 Organisation.

Hinchley, A. (2003). *Understanding Version 3. A primer on the HL7 Version 3 Communication Standard*. Alexander Moench Publishing, Munich.

HL7 (2004). *Chapter 1: HL7 development framework v2.0.0*. Retrieved 5 July, 2005, from http://www.HL7.org.au

HL7 (2005). HL7 Version 3, September Ballot Site. Retrieved 5 September, 2005, from http://www.hl7.org/v3ballot/html/welcome/environment/index/htm.

Jones, M. (1998). *Formal generic modelling*, PhD thesis, Nottingham Trent University.

Rumbaugh, J. et al. (1999). *The Unified Modelling Language Reference Manual*, Addison-Wesley, Boston.

SSC (2003). *Architecture frameworks: Zachman*. Retrieved 5 July 2005 from http://www.software.org/.

West Australian Government (2002). *Enterprise information model v 2.1*. Retrieved 5 July, 2005, from http://www.health.wa.gov.au/.

5

Introducing databases

Stephen Chu

> 'One good reason why databases can do more work than people is that they never have to stop and answer the phone.'
>
> (Anonymous)

Outline

This chapter introduces the basic concepts of database management systems and their components in the healthcare environment. Data structure, modelling, and operations on health data are discussed along with some of the more commonly used database technologies. This chapter is not exhaustive and is written to trigger further research in the area. There are many database management texts and in-depth resources available to accommodate this.

Introduction

Until recent years, healthcare data have been captured in paper records with a rudimentary structure loosely organised into 'sections' such as clinical history, laboratory results, and clinical progress notes. Data items required for different sections of the records needed to be entered repeatedly due to the inherent constraints of paper, and an inability to dynamically cross-reference or link data stored. Data such as blood sugar level test results for example are redundantly recorded in the diabetic management chart, clinical progress notes, and dietician review charts. Redundant data entry is labour intensive and a major cause of data value and format inconsistency.

Many countries have begun implementing integrated care and chronic disease management programs because they generate significant cost benefits and quality improvements. The ability to share quality data is a key requirement if these programs are to succeed. Organising and storing healthcare data on database management systems (DBMS) is considered a cost-effective strategy that mitigates problems of paper data storage, greatly improving accessibility and sharing of healthcare data. As governments and the health industries of developed countries endorse electronic healthcare records (EHR) as key enabling technologies, databases and DBMS have emerged as two of the most important technologies in recent years.

Databases and DBMS are used by almost all industries to manage operational and executive or strategic planning data at all levels. Their uses vary from online transaction processing (OLTP) of operational data to online analytic processing (OLAP) of aggregated data in special databases (data warehouses).

Basic database concepts

Data are a representation of real world facts, concepts or instructions in a formalised manner suitable for communication, interpretation or processing by human beings or by automatic means (International Standards Organisation, 1999).

A database is an 'organised collection of logically related data' (Hoffer, Prescott & McFadden, 2002). The filing cabinet in a doctor's clinic can be seen as a 'database'. Patient medical records stored in the cabinet drawers are organised in alphabetical order and data in each medical record are organised in sections. In a computerised database, emphasis is on a structure that can adequately and dynamically link related data to support rapid retrieval and processing. Unlike the paper record, it is not important for patient data to be stored physically together.

A database management system (DBMS) is a computer program that facilitates the creation, maintenance and usage (storage, modification and extraction of data) of a computerised record (database). There are many different types of **DBMS** ranging from small systems that run on personal computers to complex systems on mainframe computers.

A knowledge-base presents knowledge about concepts that extends past the relationships that you need to define those concepts (Standards Australia, 2005)

A repository is a generic term used to denote any logically organised database capable of storing information and disseminating that information when requested to do so.

A database schema is a detailed specification of the overall structure of data to be captured by the database. A conceptual schema is a data structure specification independent of any database management technology. A physical schema contains the specifications for storing data defined in a conceptual schema in a database or a computer's secondary storage device.

Data independence is the immunity of (software) applications to change in physical representation (storage) of data and access techniques. In old/legacy systems, the application needs to be aware of the 'Patient Master' file that contains patient demographic and visit information that is indexed on the 'Unique-Patient-ID' field, the record sequence defined by this index and the application built around this knowledge. Any indexing structure changes require a corresponding modification of the application that uses the 'Patient Master' file. In modern systems, index implementation and data accessing become the responsibility of the database management systems. Any changes to the physical representation of data are of no concern to the application. Data independence is achieved.

File processing system

Before database technology was developed, computer applications used flat file structure or file processing system to store, manipulate and retrieve data. This file processing system was a very primitive database. To the computer, data stored in a file processing system is simply a long continuous string of characters/texts with no structured relationship. A comma can be used to separate each group of data stored within the file creating a comma-separated values file. The flat file model is the basis of spreadsheet design.

Systems or applications that use file processing systems are designed to meet the needs of specific groups of users or departments. Each system or application is likely to be developed independently and generally uses its own private file system, for example:

- patient master files store demographic, diagnosis and encounter data
- laboratory files store laboratory test orders and results data
- billing files store patient visit, charges and invoicing data.

As each of these systems or application has a data file, data sharing outside the system or application is almost impossible and the same data that are used by different applications need to be stored redundantly across different file systems. For example, the unique patient identifiers and patient demographic data are stored in all three of the file system examples above. Even in the same file system, data often are stored redundantly. Figure 5.1 demonstrates this in a fictitious patient master file table. As patients can have multiple encounters (or admissions) and because the data about each encounter have no structured relationship to each other, the patient identifier and some demographic data such as patient names and addresses need to be stored redundantly in the same file.

Figure 5.1: Data from a sample file processing system reorganised into table format

A file-based system

Patient Name	Address	Unique ID	Diagnosis	Admit Date	Disch Date
Alfred Thomas	34, South Road, Newmarket	AJT1302	Type 1 DM	01/03/00	10/03/00
Linda Cooper	12, Lakeside Road, Hamilton	KLM3216	Asthma	9/04/01	26/04/01
Judy Roberts	31, Long Drive, Epsom	BTK6219	Renal colic	30/05/01	10/06/01
Leanardo Key	21 Dorchester Road, Midbank	AAK1397	Gall stone	30/05/01	18/06/01
Michael Engelo	23, Meadowvale Road, Far Hill	TAA9628	Syncope	9/06/01	14/06/01
Rafael Romeo	6, Church Street, Onehunga	EZZ0821	Cholangitis	25/06/01	9/07/01
Donatelo Tabert	100, Beach Road, Long Bay	JWE3792	Chest pain	6/07/01	19/07/01
Wins Church	45, Redoubt Road Devonport	DDT2185	Stroke	20/07/01	28/09/01
Abe Lincoln	25, Allen Road, St. John's Park	GZL6270	AMI	5/08/01	19/08/01
Alfred Thomas	34, South Road, Newmarket	AJT1302	Leg ulcer	19/08/01	9/10/01
Linda Cooper	12, Lakeside Road, Hamilton	KLM3216	Pneumonia	25/01/02	6/02/02
Judy Roberts	31, Long Drive, Epsom	BTK6219	Renal stone	30/01/02	2/02/02

Duplicated data stored within or across file systems lead to high risk of inconsistency in data values. For example, when a patient changes his/her address, the changes may not be consistently applied across all files. Indeed, there is no guarantee that the change will be applied consistently to all patient address data recorded in the same file system.

The file description that defines the structure of the file processing system is stored within the application program that accesses the file. For example, the file description of the patient master file is stored within the 'Admission, Discharge and Transfer' (ADT) and any other application programs that use the file. Any changes to the file structure require changes to the file descriptions and data manipulation routines contained in all application programs that use the file. In addition, the file processing systems also lack the security features essential for multi-user and mission critical environments such as healthcare. A natural progression then is a move away from the file processing system to the technologically more advanced and robust DBMS.

Evolution of database systems

Data were first stored in file processing systems on computers in the 1960s. Not only were descriptions about the file structure stored within the applications that used the data, programmers had to write data manipulation routines to access and manage it. Data manipulation routines needed to be changed when views or use of the data changed. Large backlogs of user requests for new programs or changes to programs further compromised the productivity and usefulness of file processing systems. These problems led to the development of a DBMS in which the data and how they were stored were independent of the methods used for manipulating them.

The era of non-relational database (1968 to 1980)

While the file processing system persisted until the mid-1980s, this decade was dominated by the hierarchical and network database systems.

Hierarchical database

The architecture of the hierarchical database is based on the hierarchical data model with records (containing data) logically represented in a hierarchy of inverted (i.e. upside down) tree (Figure 5.2). The concept underpinning a hierarchical data model is that all data (contained in 'child' records) related to a 'parent' record (for example, 'PATIENT' in Figure 5.2) were part of that record and should be stored together with the parent record. Hierarchical databases are typically very fast and conceptually simple, but they were also quite inflexible and time consuming to query and complex to modify. They required very careful planning, excellent system coordination skills, and a high level of technical knowledge about the database and hierarchical data model.

Figure 5.2: The hierarchical model (A) and hierarchical database example (B)

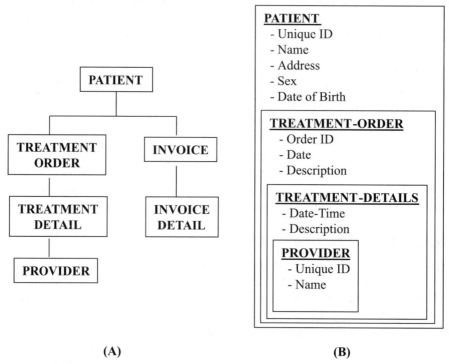

(A)   (B)

Network database

The Database Task Group of the COnference on DAta SYstems Languages (CODASYL) produced standard network specifications for a network schema, subschema and a data definition language (DDL). Although the network model attempted to address the limitations of the hierarchical model, its architecture closely resembles it but it had the added advantage of supporting multi-parent child nodes. The network model therefore appears as multiple inverted trees with shared branches (see Figure 5.3).

Figure 5.3: A network model representing staff-patient relationship in a department

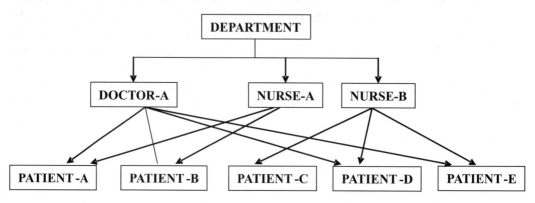

The network model was structurally complex and designers had to be very familiar with the database structure. The schema and subschema needed to be modified and revalidated if changes to the structure were required. Like the hierarchical model, the network database model failed to achieve data and structural independence. Although hierarchical and network databases still exist in legacy systems, they are now obsolete, at least from the technological perspective (Date, 2004).

The era of relational database (1970 onwards)

A relational database model was proposed in 1970 (Codd, 1970) and commercial relational database management systems (RDBMS) appeared in the 1980s. Their key feature is the complete separation of the logical and physical view of data. The logical data view in a relational model is set oriented. A relational set contains an unordered set of items, each set representing an Entity or Object of the real world. Each item then represents attributes that describe certain characteristics of that entity.

Relation is a mathematical term for table (Date, 2004) and a relational set is modelled as a table in the relational database. The table is the logical structure in a relational system, not the physical structure. At the physical level the system can store the data in any way, based on the best available technology, provided that it can map the stored data to tables at the logical level. At the logical level, the items of each relation are organised into tuples[1] (or rows). Each tuple is an aggregate of fields that contain atomic data values. A relation has a set of column names that correspond to the attribute names and forms the 'heading' of the relation. The rows are unordered and unnamed. A database consists of one or more relations that hold the data values and a system catalogue (also represented by tables) describing the database structure.

Figure 5.4A shows a simplified relational model created from the top level Health Level 7 Reference Information Model backbone classes (HL7, 2004). This simplified model is implemented as a set of relational database tables (Figure 5.3B). Each tuple in the individual relation represents an instance of the real world entity or object. The number of columns for each relation is determined by the number of attributes defined for the entity/object. The column header represents names of the attributes, for example Ord-ID (organisation ID), Org-Type (organisation type).

The different relations are logically linked to each other by the values of the 'primary-foreign' key pair (explored later in this chapter). There are no pointers connecting one relation to another. For simple illustration, consider the relations in Figure 5.5B, they are all logically linked by the key fields – 'Org-ID', 'Person-ID', and 'ID'.

The relational model defines a set of mathematical operations and constraints that can be applied to database tables. These are used to define business rules (user defined constraints). A DBMS can divide the requested operations (in the form of **S**tructured **Q**uery **L**anguage – SQL commands) into a number of independent tasks that can run on one or more Central Processor Units or even on distributed computers (parallel processing). RDBMS can support distributed data and distributed processing where relations or parts of relations may also be distributed, for example, the tuples of a relation can be partitioned and stored at distributed locations.

Figure 5.4: Relational model (A) and implementation as relational database tables (B)

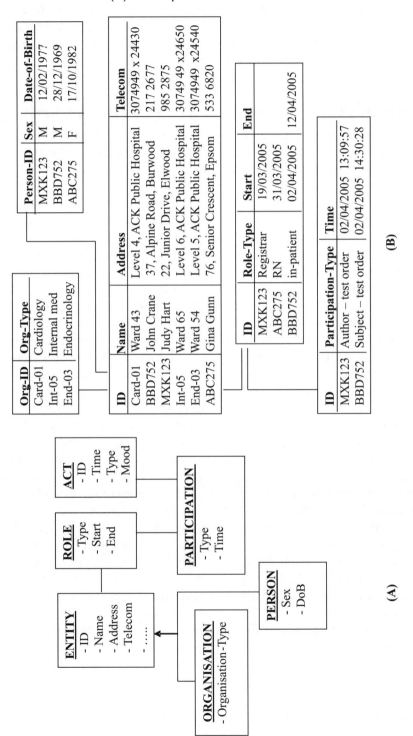

(A)

(B)

The healthcare industry generates increasingly large amounts of complex data including waveforms, digitised images of radiology images, ultrasound scans, audio and video files, etc. Even with structured textual data, complex components such as haemodynamic observations, respiratory and neurological assessments containing aggregates of individual assessment are often organised in complex hierarchies. Relational databases must break complex data sets into parts for storage within tables and simulate these complex objects by a number of 'join' operations. This approach can complicate modelling and often causes performance problems.

Increasingly, healthcare information system applications are developed in object-oriented languages to enhance the benefits of object-oriented features of reusable components and complex clinical objects. When attempting to persist (store) the objects in or retrieve them from relational databases, differences in object and relational models lead to the problem of impedance mismatch (Srinivasan & Chang 1997; Narang 2004; Pprabhu 2004). This means extra programming efforts are required when application logic is implemented using object-oriented language and data manipulations require the use of SQL.

When retrieving data from a relational database, there is the need to translate their representation to the in-memory representation using language (for example object-oriented language) specific to the application. Any updates to the database need to be explicitly translated from the in-memory representation back to the database representation. These activities lead to excessive and cumbersome processing. Therefore, there are strong pushes from the health informatics community, and indeed the information technology community, to move towards the object-oriented database technology.

The era of object-oriented database (1985 onwards)

This technology arises from the need to extend object-oriented programming language by adding persistence to the objects and to enhance the practical advantages of object-oriented applications. Before the era of object-oriented databases, object-oriented applications typically used RDBMS to store persistent data. Outside the computer assisted design (CAD) and computer assisted manufacturing (CAM) domains, object-oriented database technology has so far failed to capture the market interest and for this reason it is not persued in any detail here.

In the object-oriented DBMS (OODBMS), an 'object class'[2] is the equivalent of the 'relation' (or table) in the RDBMS. A tuple in a relation is similar to an object instance of a class with no operations. The operations of a class are computationally complete programming capabilities (that is a computationally complete structure and controls). RDMS provide some form of computational capabilities through stored procedures.

Users of object-oriented databases do not need to know the details of the attributes or to reference the primary key value when they insert a drug or test order into the database, rather, they use the 'make drug order' or 'make test order' operations of the Drug or Observation objects. The values of the orders persist in the object-oriented database following the successful invocation of the appropriate object operations. Therefore, details of the object (for example the internal structure and their methods/operations) are hidden from the users (principle of encapsulation).

Encapsulation is achieved by (a) the object having an internal/private memory that represents the internal structure and state of the object and (b) publishing a public interface. The advantage of encapsulation is that it allows the internal representation of the objects to be changed without rewriting the applications that use the objects. Any changes to an object's internal structure require corresponding changes to program codes that implement the objects operations. However, changes should be the responsibility of the object designer who initiates the changes to the internal structure. Therefore, encapsulation provides the benefit of data independence.

An object's public interface is published by the Class-Defining-Object (CDO) that defines the class to which a specific object instance belongs (Date, 2004). For example, a blood pressure observation object for Patient 'John Citizen' on 31 March 2005 at 0800 is an instance of the 'Blood Pressure' CDO. An interface specifies only the operations of a class visible to the external world without revealing its internal structure or implementation details (Lau, 2001; Narang, 2004). Figure 5.5 shows a sample public interface published by the ADT (admission, discharge, and transfer) object.

Figure 5.5: Public interface published by the ADT object

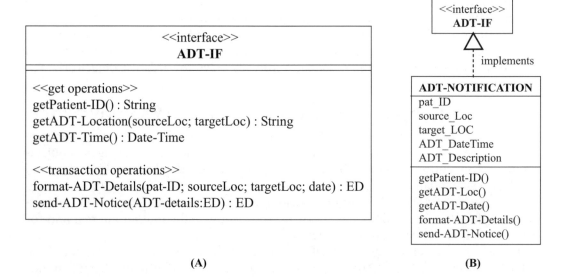

(A)   (B)

When data are persisted (stored) in relational databases, each row is identified by the value of the primary key. In the object-oriented systems, objects can be created, copied, accessed and deleted when a program is running as a process. The virtual memory addresses of the objects in the process are used for their identification and are known as Object ID (OID).

Figure 5.6: Data structure component of persistent objects (adapted from Date, 2004)

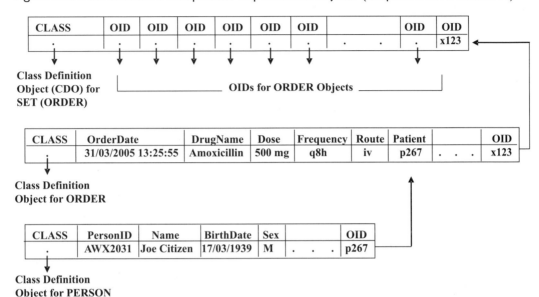

In object-oriented DBMS, OID will have to be persisted in addition to data. An OID refers to exactly one object in the database. When a program is running, an object is referenced by either the application or other objects using the object's OID. OIDs might also be needed for direct access to an object in a database. Figure 5.6 shows the use of OIDs in persisted objects and their data structure component.

The query and transaction processing of the object-oriented approach were unable to match the relational model (Dotsika, 2003). When populating or querying the database, these processes are preceded by object messaging and object method innovation. These processing overheads tend to make query and update transactions cumbersome. An OODBMS is typically tied to a specific object-oriented programming language via a specific application programming interface (API). This means that data in an OODBMS is typically only accessible from a specific language using a specific API (Obasanjo, 2001), which is usually not the case for relational databases.

Post-relational databases

The term 'post-relational' has been broadly applied to any data model or database that is developed after the advent of the relational model, but which is not object-oriented. It has been applied to 'multi-dimensional' databases, or nested relational, or object-relational databases (ORDBMS). In a multi-dimensional database, data are extracted from the database and loaded by multi-dimensional online analytical processing (multi-dimensional OLAP) into the cells of an intermediary structure, usually a multi-dimensional array (Date, 2004; Hoffer, Prescott & McFadden 2002, Pedersen & Jensen 2001). For example, to capture the measurements of the length of stay of patients with a different diagnosis treated by different physicians, the data can be 'conceptually stored' in a multi-dimensional array (see Figure 5.7). A multi-dimensional model is used in supporting online analytical processing (OLAP) to provide management decision support information. A nested relational database can store and retrieve multiple values, usually as a list, in a single field of a single record in the table (McClure, 1997), for example, the 'skills' field of a hospital employee, which contains a list of professional skills.

Figure 5.7: Sample data 'conceptually stored' in a multi-dimensional database

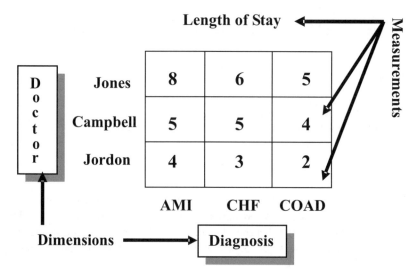

Extended relational and object relational are synonyms for database products that try to incorporate the good features of object systems into a relational database (Date, 2004; McClure, 1997). ORDBMS for instance extend the in-built basic data types (string, numeric, date, etc) to support more complex data types, such as time series data, biological data, engineering design data and spatial data. All persistent data are still stored in tables.

The physical database management system architecture

A database management system (DBMS) is a computer program that 'sits' between the user and the database (see Figure 5.8). It intercepts and executes requests from a user or a user program such as database maintenance (for example, which performs create, delete and modify data table structures, and maintains security and integrity functions) and data storage, retrieval and update requirements.

Figure 5.8: DBMS physical architecture

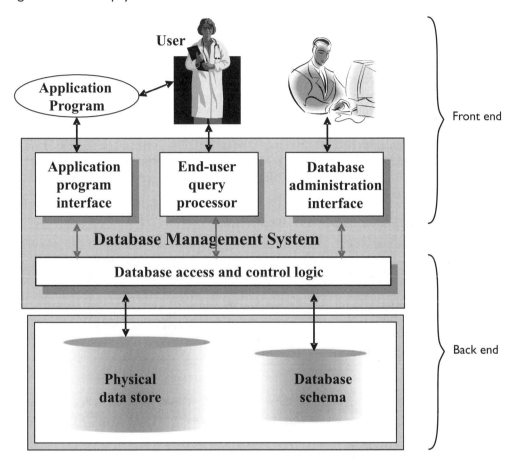

The DBMS physical architecture describes the software components used to interact with the database management system. These can be categorised into two basic groups: the front end and back end components. The front end manages the direct interaction with users and can be provided by DBMS vendors and/or third party software developers. The applications programs (for instance, electronic healthcare record system applications from third parties) are also general user interfaces that interact with the application programming interface (API). Power users will use the end-user query tools/forms provided by the DBMS vendors to interrogate the DBMS. The DBMS front end also has a set of tools for database administration and maintenance activities such as to create database tables, grant and revoke user access rights, perform database audits, etc.

The back end of the DBMS is the DBMS engine that contains the database access and control logic. The back end software components are responsible for managing the physical database including:

- providing support and mappings for database schema and the physical database structure

- maintaining concurrency control and data integrity
- providing security and access control
- analysing resources utilisation.

The ANIS/SPARC three-tier architecture

The development of databases involves a number of processes aimed at understanding the user requirements and views of the data, representing these views conceptually, and mapping these conceptual structures to a physical structure for storage in a database and the computer's secondary storage devices. In 1975, the American National Standards Institute/Standards Planning and Requirements Committee (ANSI/SPARC) developed an architecture that divided the DBMS into three levels of abstraction: the internal or physical level, the conceptual level, and the external (or view) level that is used today (see Figure 5.9).

Figure 5.9: The ANSI/SPARC three-tier DBMS architecture

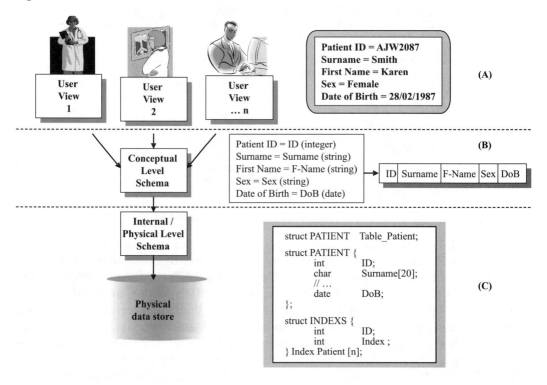

The external (or user view) level

The users' view of the organisation's database is considered in light of their roles and responsibilities within their domain of practice. Because organisations have multiple users (staff and health services consumers), there are multiple user views of the same set of data. Even in the same domain of practice there are many different user views. For example, a physician will view the clinical data slightly differently from a nurse or a physiotherapist. The top text box in Figure 5.9A depicts a simplified user view of a set of patient demographic data. The challenge for a database analyst and modeller is to translate/map the different user views to arrive at a robust conceptual schema.

The conceptual schema

A conceptual schema represents a logical view of the entire database as a unified whole (from all user views) and allows all data to be simultaneously viewed in a consistent manner. The conceptual schema is technology independent; it is not tied to any database management technology. The data definition language used to specify the conceptual schema only defines the information content (Figure 5.9), not the physical storage and data access details.

The internal or physical schema

The internal schema provides a low-level/detailed description of the physical database structure (Figure 5.9C). At this level, record type, methods of storage, integrity constraints, and optimisation such as indexing are defined, and information about stored files/ relations are represented. The specifications are bound to the underlying database management technology. The mapping process (from conceptual to physical schema) defines the correspondence between the records and fields of the conceptual view and the physical table, and data structures of the internal view. If the structure of the stored database is changed, then the conceptual ↔ physical mapping must also be changed accordingly to preserve the consistency between the two schemata. This mapping provides the physical independence for the database.

Data modelling for database development

The first step in database development is the modelling of user requirements and the development of a robust data model based on those requirements. The conceptual data model is often used to represent data from the user's viewpoint independent of the implementation technology. The entity-relationship diagramming notation is the de facto standard for conceptual data modelling (Hoffer, Prescott & McFadden 2002), while an enhanced entity-relationship model (E-R) is used to represent data and to capture more complex business rules that define or constrain the business processes and operations on the data. Frean discussed the importance of business rules in data modelling in Chapter 4 explaining that they govern how data are named, defined, handled/used and stored. The basic constructs of E-R model are 'entity' (and its attributes), and the 'relationship' between the entities.

An entity is a person, role (of a person or organisation), place, object, event, or concept about which the users and their organisations wish to maintain data. Common examples of entity in the healthcare environment include:
- Person: PERSON
- Role: EMPLOYEE, DOCTOR, NURSE, PHARMACIST, PATIENT
- Place: ORGANISATION, CLINICAL DEPARTMENT
- Object: EQUIPMENT, DRUG
- Event: ADMISSION, DISCHARGE, DIAGNOSTIC TEST
- Concept: DIAGNOSIS, TREATMENT, PROCEDURE, ROSTER.

An entity type is a collection of entities that share common properties or characteristics. For example, the entity type PERSON has a set of common properties such as name sex, date of birth, etc. An entity instance on the other hand is a single occurrence of an entity type. For example, John Citizen is an instance of the entity type PERSON. However, in modelling practice, the term entity is often used instead of entity type, and entity instance is often abbreviated as instance.

A strong entity type is one that exists independent of other entity types. A weak entity type is one whose existence depends on some other entity type called the identifying owner. It has no business meaning in an organisation (and the E-R diagram) without the entity type on which it depends (Hoffer, Prescott & McFadden 2002). For example, hospitals may offer fringe benefits such as a car and housing rental to their employees. The hospital's personnel database needs to record that EMPLOYEE is a strong entity type and BENEFIT is a weak entity type.

Each entity type has a set of attributes (properties) that have significant meaning to the organisation and users. For example, the TREATMENT entity type has a number of associated attributes: Treatment_ID, Description, Charge_Rate, Treatment_Date, etc. In the database, an entity instance has specific value associated with each attribute. The TREATMENT entity type has an entity instance with ID value = 'Rx-1234', Description value = 'bladder irrigation', Charge-Rate value = '$120'. A database can, therefore, be considered as a repository for all attribute values for all the entity instances.

Relationship is defined as an association that holds entity types together, while a 'relationship type' is a meaningful association between (or among) entity types that allows answers to questions not possible with entity types alone (Hoffer, Prescott & McFadden, 2002). The E-R diagramming notation for a relationship type is a diagram symbol containing the name of the relationship. A 'relationship instance' is an association between (or among) entity instances where each relationship instance includes exactly one entity instance from each participating entity type.

Figure 5.10 is a simplified E-R representation of the patient admission event capturing the entity types, the relationship between the entity types, and the business rules. The rectangles represent entity types and ellipses are notations used for attributes of the entity types.

In this example, the PATIENT_ADMISSION entity type has two subtypes – OUTPATIENT_ADMISSION and RESIDENT_ADMISSION. A subtype is an entity type that inherits all the attributes of its supertype (PATIENT_ADMISSION), and also possesses unique attribute(s) of its own that differentiates it from other subtypes from the same parent supertype. Figure 5.12 shows 'Checkback_Date' as an attribute unique to the OUTPATIENT_ADMISSION entity type. Business rules can also be represented through relationships between the entity types and certain constraints on their relationships (see Figure 5.11).

Figure 5.10: Simplified E-R model of patient admission event

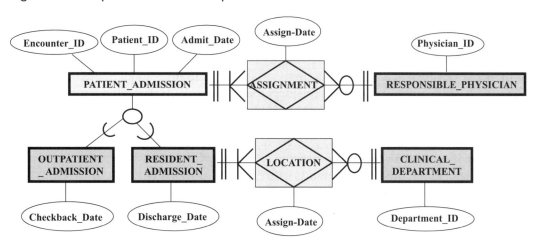

Figure 5.11: Sample business rules representation using E-R diagramming notations

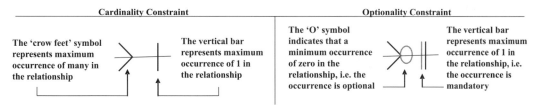

A logical data model is the intermediary step that is used to 'translate' the conceptual E-R model into a representation suited to DBMS implementation. The most common DBMS technology today is the relational data model and this is used as the logical data model. Figure 5.14 illustrates the conversion of entities from the Figure 5.12 E-R model fragment into a set of relations ready for implementation in a relational DBMS.

Figure 5.12: Conversion of a subset of entities from Figure 5.10 into logical data model

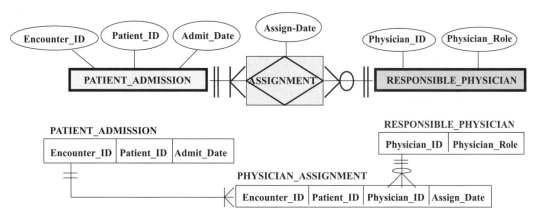

Users must be able to retrieve the data from the volumes of data stored in databases, based on certain data values stored in a tuple. To ensure the accurate execution of such activities, the relational database management system (RDBMS) uses a primary key. A primary key is an attribute (or combination of attributes) that uniquely identifies a tuple in a relation. In Figure 5.12, the RESPONSIBLE_PHYSICIAN entity has the primary key of Physician_ID. Sometimes, a single attribute is inadequate to uniquely identify a tuple in a relation. Consider the PATIENT_ADMISSION relation, the Patient_ID cannot uniquely identify a tuple as a patient can have multiple admissions. The Patient_ID + Admit_Date or Encounter_ID + Patient_ID combination would have to be considered as the primary key. When a primary key is formed by two or more attributes, it is known as a composite key.

This logical data model fragment is implemented physically in a RDBMS as tables (see Figure 5.15). Notice that in the RDBMS implementation, there is no physical connection between the tables. In the relational data model, associations between tables are defined through the use of the Primary-Foreign key pairs.

A foreign key is an attribute (or combination of attributes) in a relation (table) that serves as a primary key of another relation in the same database. The Physician_ID is a primary key in RESPONSIBLE_PHYSICIAN and also serves as foreign key in PHYSICIAN_ASSIGNMENT. The foreign key value is used to logically link data values from two relations together as in Figure 5.13.

Figure 5.13: Physical implementation of logical data model from Figure 5.14 in relational DBMS

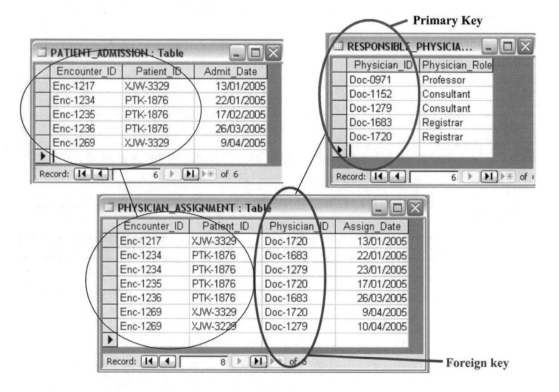

A key goal of data modelling is to create a database data structure free from redundancy – the problem that plagues the file processing system (see Figure 5.3). To ensure that this goal is achieved, the data structure can be validated through normalisation procedures. Normalisation involves examining the data structure for unnormalised or redundant patient data and removing any repeating data groups and functional dependent anomalies in the data structure. The repeating repeating data groups and functionally dependent data are separated from the other data group(s) by using a three-step process of Normalisation, in which redundancy free forms are generated.

A data structure free of repeating groups is in first normal form. The second step is to remove any partial functional dependency. This means removing any non-key attributes that are functionally dependent on part of a primary key. A data structure in first normal form and every non-key attribute is fully functionally dependent upon the primary key (not part of the key) is in the second normal form. Data structures in second normal form with no transitive dependency are in third normal form. Data structure in third normal form is generally considered sufficiently free of data structure anomalies and satisfactory for physical implementation in a database.

Data in third normal form are spread across a number of database relations (or tables) and a number of 'join' operations are required to retrieve inter-related data from the database. For example, to learn the diagnosis of a patient admitted on a certain date, the query procedure needs to 'join' the three relations – PATIENT, ADMISSION, DIAGNOSIS – to retrieve all required data (Figure 5.13).

Data manipulation

A highly flexible data manipulation mechanism is one of the key benefits of database technology. In relational DBMS, data manipulation is most commonly performed using the Structured Query Language (SQL). SQL is the de facto standard language for creating and querying RDBMS. It includes data definitions, control and manipulation operations and provides the key tools for 1) designing the physical database 2) maintaining and controlling the database and 3) implementing and manipulating the data stored there. Figure 5.14 illustrates these categories and the operations supported.

SQL data definition language is a powerful tool used to perform database creation and maintenance works. Once database tables are created, the data manipulation language (DML) can be used to populate (insert data into) the database tables and to manipulate data stored there. Common DML operations include: SELECT, INSERT, UPDATE and DELETE. Relational restrict (also known as 'SELECT') extracts specific rows from a table. It returns the results shown in Figure 5.15A. Project and join operations can also be performed on the data (Date, 2004).

The 'join' operation links two tables together based on common values in a common column. This operation allows inter-related data stored in different tables (as a result of normalisation) to be retrieved and presented in a single view (see Figure 5.15B). SQL statements can be executed through end-user query interface (by power users) and database administrative interface (by designers and administrators), or through applications as SQL commands embedded in application codes.

Figure 5.14: The three categories of SQL languages – DDL, DCL, DML (adapted from Hoffer, Prescott & McFadden, 2002)

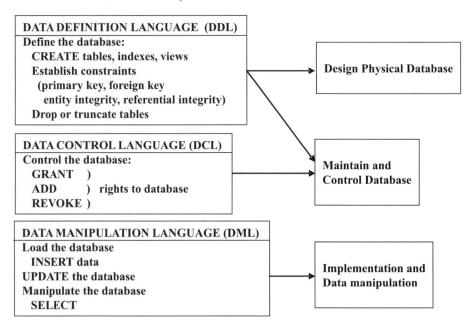

Figure 5.15: Result of sample SQL statements execution

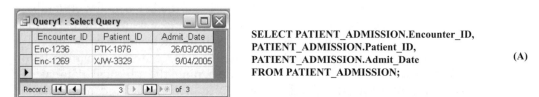

Data warehouse

A data warehouse is a subject-oriented, integrated, time variant, non-volatile collection used in support of management decision-making and business intelligence (Inmon & Hackathorn 1994). It is organised around the subjects of interest to the organisation (for instance, patient, clinician, clinical units, treatment, outcomes, time, etc). The source data are extracted from various operational databases and integrated into the warehouse database using consistent naming conventions, data format and encoding structures. Once data are loaded into the data warehouse, they cannot be updated, only periodically refreshed, hence data in a data warehouse are 'time variant' and 'non volatile'. Trends can be studied because the source data contains a time dimension. The process of creating a data warehouse from operational data stores is the subject of many texts and so is not discussed further here.

Data warehouses are underpinned by a four layer architecture consisting of (1) the operational data, (2) processing and transformation, (3) derived data, and (4) mining and visualisation layers. Figure 5.16 illustrates this architecture and the transformation processes. Well-designed healthcare data warehouses provide useful structures to represent and analyse relationships between outcomes, costs or resources consumptions (facts), and departments, clinicians, treatments or treatment categories (for example, surgical versus medical treatments), diagnosis or problems, and patient profiles or demographics.

Figure 5.16: A generic four-layer data warehouse architecture

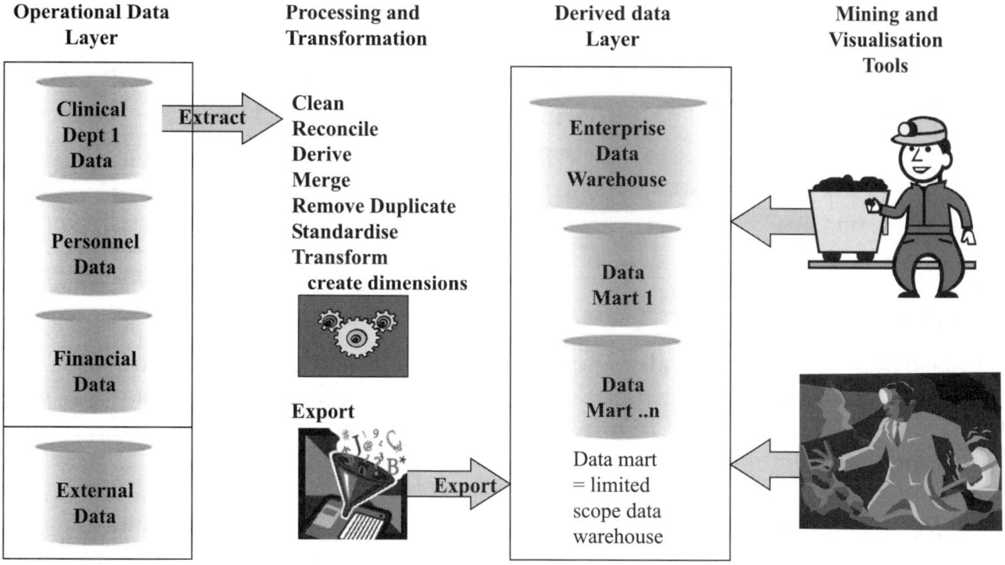

The star schema (also called dimensional schema) is a common and simple database design for data warehouses. It contains two types of tables – fact and dimension. The fact table contains quantitative measurements that represent specific aspects of business interest or activity, such as treatment outcomes, or treatment cost-effectiveness. Dimension tables contain qualifying characteristics that provide additional understanding or perspectives to given facts, for example, departments, clinician profiles, interventions and patient profiles. They are usually the source of attributes used to qualify, categorise, or summarise facts in queries or reports. Figure 5.17 contains a simplified star schema relating the Cost_Effect Fact Table to a number of dimension tables.

Each dimension table has a one-to-many relationship to the fact table. Relationships between the dimension and fact tables provide join paths that allow users to perform highly flexible queries on the data warehouse. For example, management can ask questions such as 'which surgeon from which department provides the most cost-effective surgical procedures for which diagnoses'?

Figure 5.17: Sample star schema containing surgical treatment cost-effectiveness as fact table and four dimensional tables.

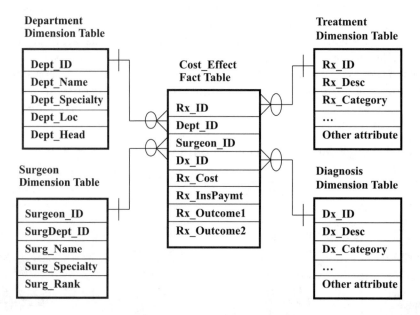

Database security

Database data security generally refers to the protection of data against unauthorised disclosure, alteration, or destruction. Data security is particularly important given the sensitive nature and legal requirements on healthcare data. Access to data can be easily controlled by:

- authentication technologies such as user ID, user determined and electronic token generated one-time-passwords, biometric identification, etc
- access privilege management, for instance role-based access control. Users can be granted access to data on 'need-to-know' basis determined by their role and responsibilities in the organisation. The data control language (DCL) provides commands for database administrators to grant and revoke user access rights to health data.

- database recovery facilities (Figure 5.18) are key mechanisms for ensuring data security. A number of security features are normally provided by DBMS:

Figure 5.18: Database recovery facilities

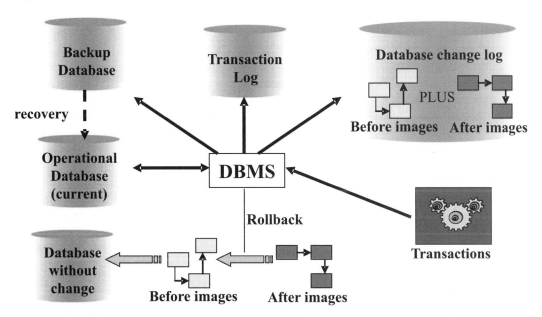

Backup facilities produce a backup copy of the entire database plus control and journal files and backups are scheduled to occur at the least busy time of the day. The most recent uncorrupted backup copy is used to restore the database in the event of hardware failure or natural disasters.

DBMS provide two journalling facilities – the transaction log and database change log. The transaction log contains a record of all transactions processed against the database. Details stored within this include types (for instance updates or inserts), time of transaction, network node number, user ID, and table and row ID. The database change log contains the before (old value) and after (new value) images of rows that have been modified by the transaction.

A checkpoint facility allows the DBMS to periodically freeze the DBMS transaction activities when all transactions in progress are completed and write a checkpoint record to a log file. The checkpoint record is a snapshot of the database and provides important information for restarting the system after a failure. As this is done regularly (several times per hour), at most only several minutes of data are lost in the event of system failure.

Transaction integrity is maintained by the 'COMMIT' or 'ROLLBACK' commands. Rollback (also known as backward recovery) is used to restore the database to the before-image state in case a transaction needs to be aborted, or is terminated abnormally.

Another important aspect of data security is auditing of users electronic footprints as they access data in the database. A security log is essentially a special file or 'database' in which the DBMS automatically keep track of all operations performed by users on the stored data. System and database administrators can inspect this audit log regularly.

Data integrity is often bundled as a data security issue. DBMS maintains data integrity through entity and referential integrity constraint, concurrency control, record locking and commit/rollback mechanisms.

Entity integrity specifies that no component of the primary key of any relation be allowed to accept null values. This constraint is intended to ensure that any tuple in any relation that contains data values must have a valid primary key value. Therefore, entity instances of the real world, represented in the database, can be identified by their unique primary key value.

Referential integrity specifies that the database must not contain any unmatched foreign key values. Enforcement of referential integrity constraint makes it impossible to delete a tuple in a relation whose primary key matches the value in the foreign key of another relation and therefore ensures data consistency in the database.

Concurrency control is a data integrity mechanism for ensuring that multiple transactions, triggered by different users who simultaneously access the same set of data in the database, do not interfere with each other. It is an important mechanism to ensure that data are not corrupted in multi-user environments such as healthcare. An example of concurrency control mechanism is record locking. When a tuple (or a set of tuples) in a database is accessed by one user, the tuple(s) is/are locked by the DBMS. Only this user has the privilege to update (i.e., change the values) of data in the tuple(s). Other users can only view data from the 'locked' tuple(s) but cannot change their data value. When the update transactions are completed, the lock on the tuple(s) is released.

Conclusion

Database management systems represent key infrastructure for clinical data repositories, electronic healthcare records, data warehouses and knowledge bases. The understanding of the strengths and constraints of different types of database technologies is critical to the selection, design, development and implementation of the information and knowledge management needs of different healthcare disciplines and sectors.

Review questions

1. Explain why an organisation would want to manage its data through a database environment?
2. What are some of the functions of a database?
3. What is the purpose of a data warehouse?

Exercises

*   Plan a database of your research articles.
*   Create a database of these articles.

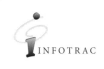

Online reading

INFOTRAC® COLLEGE EDITION

For additional readings and review on databases, explore **InfoTrac® College Edition**, your online library. Go to: **www.infotrac-college.com** and search for any of the InfoTrac key terms listed below:

➤ Data structure
➤ Relational model
➤ Object oriented model
➤ Database management systems
➤ Data warehouse
➤ Data mining

References

Codd, E. (1970). A relational model of data for large shared data banks, *Communications of the ACM*, Vol. 13, No. 6, June 1970, 377–87.

Date, C.J. (2004). *An introduction to database systems,* Addison-Wesley Publishing, Massachusetts.

Dotsika, F. (2003). 'From data to knowledge in e-health applications: an integrated system's for medical information modelling and retrieval', *Medical Informatics and the Internet in Medicine, 28*(4), 231–51.

Hoffer, J.A., Prescott, M.B. & McFadden, F.R. (2002). *Modern database management*, 6th edn, Prentice Hall, New Jersey.

HL7 (2004). *Reference Information Model.* Retrieved 21 August, 2003, from http://www.hl7.org/.

Inmon, W.H. & Hackathorn, R.D. (1994). *Using the Data Warehouse*, John Wiley & Sons, New York.

International Standards Organisation (1999). *ISO 2382–4. Information technology – Vocabulary – Part 4: Organisation of data*, Geneva.

Lau, Y.T. (2001). *The arts of objects: object oriented design and architecture*, Addison-Wesley, Boston.

McClure, S. (1997). 'Object database vs. object-relational databases', *IDC Bulletin*, No.14821E. Retrieved 23 February, 2005, from http://www.cts/jasmine/.

Narang, R. (2004). *Object Oriented Interfaces and database*, Prentice Hall of India.

Obasanjo, D. (2001). *An exploration of object-oriented database management systems.* Retrieved 22 February 2005 from http://www.25hoursaday.com/.

Pedersen, T.B. & Jensen, C.S. (2001). 'Multidimensional database technology', *Computer*, December, 40–46.

Pprabhu, C.S. (2004). *Object Oriented Database systems*, Prentice Hall of India.

Srinivasan, V. & Chang, D.T. (1997). 'Object persistence in object-oriented applications', *IBM Systems Journal, 36*(1). Retrieved 22 February, 2005, from http://www.research.ibm.com/.

Standards Australia (2005). *The language of health concept representation*, DR 04114, Sydney, Australia.

Endnotes

[1]   The term 'record' is often used synonymously with 'row' or 'tuple'. However, it (record) lacks the precision required by relational theory (Codd, 1970). When the term is used, it is often uncertain whether it is used to mean a 'record occurrence' or a 'record type'; a 'logical record'; or 'physical record'; a 'stored record' or a 'virtual record'. The relational model does not use the term 'record' (Date 2004). The preferred term is 'tuple'.

[2]   The term 'object class' is often used interchangeably with 'class' and 'object instance' is often used synonymously as 'object'. In this chapter, the terms 'class' and 'object' are used.

6

Knowledge management

Moya Conrick

> 'Knowledge is about people: Information is about systems'
> (Welch, 1997)

Outline

Harnessing the flow of essential health information is one of the most enduring challenges faced by all healthcare workers. The flood of information caused by an explosion of unstructured and sometimes unreliable information is overwhelming the workforce and requires careful management. The combination of machine-learning techniques and conventional knowledge acquisition from domain experts resolves many of the problems by enabling knowledge to be captured in knowledge bases. This chapter discusses the essence of knowledge and examines how technology is transforming knowledge management in healthcare.

Introduction

Healthcare workers satisfy the criteria proposed by Lee and Yang (2000) for knowledge workers; they are members of the workforce who possess competencies, knowledge and skills. They spend a great deal of time searching mountains of resources to ensure their work practices remain current, although the estimated fivefold increase in the size of the body of medical knowledge each year (Hanka & Fuka, 2000) makes this is a daunting task.

The availability of this volume of information has been a driver in the increase of clinical specialisation, as the depth of knowledge is exchanged for breadth, because keeping current across such an enormous body of literature is almost impossible. Added to this burden are the numerous governmental guidelines and reporting protocols, drug company information, alerts, warnings and so forth. Administration is not exempt from this glut that seems to continue unabated. Nevertheless, often the necessary information is not available to health workers in a useable fashion, when or where it is needed. The difficulties acquiring information have a direct impact on knowledge development because knowledge is increased through interaction with information (Standards Australia [SA], 2001) and relies on a complex blend of information analysis, synthesis and personal experiences.

Knowledge is crucial to healthcare because the ability to increase the knowledge base of health workers would significantly enhance the quality of care, care outcomes and the long-term sustainability of the system. Nonetheless, most employers are unaware of the richness and size of their acquired knowledge base and often lose it through attrition, high staff turnover, cost cutting and poor documentation (White, 2004).

Knowledge must be created, distributed, acquired, shared, reviewed, used and stored by the healthcare community; that is, it must be managed if it is to be useful. However, it seems implausible to talk of managing knowledge in terms of classical resource management because knowledge depends on an individual's cognitive process and it is stored in the mind. In fact Skryme (1997, p.24) argues that the 'management of tacit knowledge is an oxymoron'. Knowledge management (KM) is a contemporary philosophy comprising a number of elements derived from various disciplines, including human resources management, organisational learning, information management, and information technology (SA, 2001b).

However, the debate as to whether knowledge is managed or if technologies such as intranets and knowledge bases are simply 'supportive of knowledge exchange' continues. Snowden (2002, p.202) grounds this somewhat pointing out that:

- Knowledge can only be volunteered; it cannot be conscripted.
- People always know more than they can tell, and can tell more than they can write.
- People only know what they need to know when they need to know it.

McDermott (2002) argues that effective knowledge management depends more on cultural change and community building than information technology. Knowledge requires a human relationship to think about, understand, share and appropriately apply information to create solutions to problems. An automated environment that encourages creativity, learning, sharing and use of knowledge can be created. However, knowledge is not independent of other processes as it is derived from other sources. Hence, before discussing its management, it is worthwhile to examine the manner in which data and information are processed and knowledge is created.

The essence of data, information and knowledge

Terms like data, information and knowledge are often used interchangeably, but this should not be the case. Knowledge has a symbiotic relationship with data and information, but it is richer and more meaningful than both of these. These relationships are depicted in Figure 6.1.

As data have been discussed in Chapter 3 only a definition will be reiterated here. Data are formalised representation of real world facts, concepts or instructions suitable for communication, interpretation or processing by human beings or by automatic means (International Standards Organisation [ISO], 1999).

Information on the other hand, is an end product of data or sets of data that have been given form, filtered and/ or manipulated or interpreted making them useful for a particular task. Clinical information is unique and is:

about a subject of care, relevant to the health or direct treatment of that subject of care is recorded by or on behalf of a health care provider. Clinical information about a subject of care may also include information about the subject of care's environment or about related people where this is relevant.

(Standards Australia, 2005, p.18)

Knowledge is the body of understanding and skills that are mentally constructed by people (Standards Australia, 2001). It synthesised information with interrelationships identified and formalised. It combines rules, relationships, ideas (Johns, 2002) and experiences that guide actions and decisions. An example of knowledge would be that people over fifty are more likely to have particular diseases (Standards Australia, 2005).

Figure 6.1: Information processing cycle

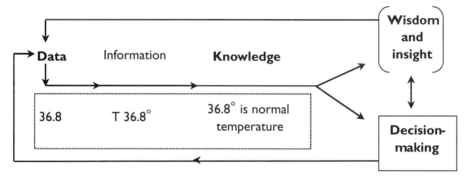

In organisational terms, knowledge is seen as 'know how', 'applied information', or 'information with judgment'. These definitions seem restrictive, because a modern healthcare organisation accumulates vast amounts of knowledge that provides a 'capacity for effective action' rather than an end point to the process (National Health Service [NHS], 2004). For instance, knowledge is used in the quality improvement cycle. While wisdom is not generally included in the information cycle, it is part of the cognitive cycle, using accumulated knowledge for further action. It is the final step in data conversion and occurs when a person understands which knowledge to use for what purpose (see Figure 6.1).

> 'Knowledge is experience. Everything else is just information.'
>
> (Albert Einstein)

Thinking processes comprise a theoretical component that has been well documented and will not be pursued here. However, the applied component derived from practice – the knowing how – is often a mixture of tacit, implicit or explicit knowledge that is more difficult to extract. In health professions, tacit knowledge is found in the 'folk' milieu of practice. It is expressed in the emotions felt when discussing a particularly satisfying, demanding or challenging case, is rarely recorded, and can only be accessed indirectly (Conrick, 2000). Tacit knowledge is not easily codified or shared because, according to Snowden's (2002, p.202) dictum, 'people always know more than they can tell'. Some authors divide tacit knowledge into 'technical' as in a skill or craft and 'cognitive', which includes beliefs, values, schemas, and mental models (Nonaka & Konno, 1998; Smith, 2001).

There is a clear distinction between tacit and explicit or codified knowledge (Nonaka & Nishiguchi, 2001; Sharma & Wickramasinghe, 2004; Smith, 2001) because explicit knowledge can be expressed in a document, a paper or computer in words, numbers, and formulae and is often technical, scientific or academic in nature (Wickramasinghe, Gupta, & Sharma, 2004). It is formalised, mostly well organised, readily available and can be documented into formal sources of knowledge. It is also easily transmitted or exchanged between individuals and groups (Nonaka & Takeuchi, 1995).

How knowledge is represented and managed

Knowledge representation is concerned with the interrelatedness of concepts within a domain. In information science and knowledge management, 'structural knowledge' is represented by a number of popular formalisms, e.g., semantic networks (Aronson & Rindflesch, 1998; Gangemi, Pisanelli & Steve, 2000), conceptual map/modelling, and ontologies (Gangemi, Catenacci & Battaglia, 2004) and these are discussed briefly here.

A semantic network is constructed by combining *semantic* links or formal representation of a relationship between two concepts, and applying this to define an individual concept. For example a:

- Fracture – has location – Scapula
  where 'has location' is the semantic link between fracture and scapula.

The combination of links, which apply to define an individual concept, provides a *semantic network* for example:

- Fracture – has location – scapula
  – is a disorder of – bone (Standards Australia, 2005)

Ontologies and *concept maps* are alike only in that they are about domain specific, explicit concepts and their relationships from a particular point of view. They represent concepts in a manner that is understandable and are conceptual schemas that organise thought.

Ontologies differ from concept maps in that they are an explicit specification of a conceptualisation (Gruber, 1993), concerned with the nature of the world, what things exist and the nature of reality. Applied ontologies include terminologies, classifications, knowledge bases, *metathesauri*, nomenclatures etc. (Kent, 2000). They are necessary for structured data entry into the electronic health record for health statistics, the aggregation of information, or can be integrated, for example, in a controlled vocabulary. In terms of knowledge engineering, ontologies are a consensus representation of the concepts used in a given domain (Kent, 2000). As a response to the plethora of knowledge and the way it is represented, knowledge management (KM) tools have evolved.

KM facilitates the processes by which both tacit and explicit knowledge is created, shared and used, and applies to the collective knowledge of the workforce. However, the transition from tacit to explicit knowledge may be unidirectional because deconstructing tacit knowledge and making the concepts explicit can have a very negative impact unless relationships are retained (Polanyi, 1966).

Nonetheless, KM treats intellectual capital as an asset that is an essential tool of modern healthcare (National Health Service, 2004; Wickramasinghe et al., 2004) and according to Arora (2002) it has three broad objectives:

1. leveraging the organisation's knowledge
2. creating new knowledge or promoting innovation, and
3. collaboration that enhances the skill level of employees.

KM can provide many benefits for organisations that plan carefully and those focusing on human factors, rather than technology alone, have a much greater chance of success (Arora, 2002). The most common KM programs involve the development of knowledge repositories, and the formation and nurturing of communities of practice. KM and the representation of knowledge are also central to technologies such as knowledge databases, decision support systems, protocol development, database design and all elements of electronic patient records.

Why manage knowledge?

The productivity of the knowledge worker is still abysmally low. It has probably not improved in the past 100 or even 200 years because all our work on productivity has been centered on the manual worker ... The way one maximizes the productivity of the knowledge worker is by capitalizing on their strengths and their knowledge rather than trying to force them into moulds.

(Drucker, 1998)

Knowledge management process

KM is based on the idea that an organisation's most valuable resource is the knowledge of its people (NHS, 2004). It also recognises all staff as 'knowledge workers', albeit to varying degrees, because nearly all jobs involve 'knowledge work', that is, they depend more on knowledge than manual skills. Therefore, the creation, sharing and use of knowledge are a significant activity for almost every person in health organisations (National Health Service, 2004).

The importance of knowledge in health is easily explained; health workers rely on knowledge to work effectively. Health provides an ongoing knowledge-rich environment in which each new situation is a potential learning opportunity. It has led to changing relationships with patients and new models of care that are forcing a rethink about health service delivery. According to the NHS (2004), knowledge must be constantly updated, renewed, shared, and used to improve practices or to change processes for the better, otherwise workers, organisations, patients and the general public ultimately suffer – 'We know this because it already happens'.

In health, managing knowledge has been implicit in education, internal communications, information technology, libraries and records management for a long time, but previously all facets have not been grouped under one overarching term. KM practices may range from a simple instruction pack to developing Communities of Practice that enable staff access to diverse information and knowledge. Bock (n.d.) and Wickramasinghe et al. (2004) differ slightly when describing KM. Figure 6.2 below is an adaptation of their work and presents the process of knowledge management as a four-part loop process that is discussed further below. It consists of:

- creation and elicitation
- capture (classify and modify) and storage
- dissemination
- application and exploitation.

Fig 6.2: Knowledge management loop (based on Bock, undated; Wickramasinghe et al., 2004)

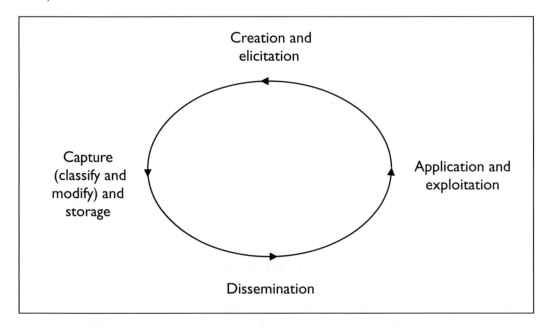

Creation and elicitation

The creation of knowledge is a cognitive process that has been the focus of books and debate for centuries. It is not addressed here for these reasons. Although elicitation is a fairly clear-cut term that refers to identifying and soliciting from the source, the process itself is often challenging.

Capture and storage

Capture is when knowledge is remembered or written and storage relates to its being entered into a computer system. Knowledge can be classified simply by the addition of keywords or by much more complex methods. The success of capture and storage is determined by how easily people can find and use the knowledge (Bock, n.d.; Wickramasinghe et al., 2004). Which media is used and how it is managed normally depends on what is being stored. Table 6.1 provides a brief commentary on this.

Table 6.1: Storing knowledge

Media	Comment
Human mind	Difficult to access
The organisation	Dispersed and distributed
Documents	From unstructured text to well structured tables and charts
Computer	Can be formalised, sorted, shared, well structured and well organised

Based on Drucker, P (1998). *Management's new paradigms*. Retrieved 2 February 2005 from http://wiredcotteges.com/managementthinkers/peterdrucker

The manner in which tacit and explicit knowledge can be elicited and captured is important because one of the greatest deterrents to sharing information and knowledge in healthcare is the 'siloing' of practice. This refers to the information and knowledge locked away by clinicians, disciplines or within organisational and jurisdictional boundaries. Socialisation and externalisation are seen as a vehicle for transferring tacit knowledge, because socialisation keeps the knowledge tacit during the transfer, and externalisation changes the tacit knowledge into more explicit knowledge (Nonaka & Takeuchi, 1995).

Tacit knowledge can be extracted by forming Communities of Practice. These are groups of experts who share an interest in a topic, an understanding of the issues, and who agree on common approaches to discussing them (Wenger & Snyder, 2001). These groups interact and build relationships while helping each other to solve problems and answer questions. They network across other teams and units to enrich their understanding of the issues and share information, insights, and best practices to develop knowledge. They also satisfy Arora (2002) and McDermott's (2002) concerns by addressing the social aspects of knowledge sharing.

Tools and knowledge bases for improving practice can be built and provide a basis for further exploration. This approach dismantles the silos, connects people, and enables the exchange of their current knowledge. Tacit knowledge becomes explicit and can be documented or codified and stored either on paper or electronically for further use (Arora, 2002). However, 'codifying and documenting this knowledge is not straightforward as it involves translating it from the context in which it was generated into the context for use' (Arora, 2002, p.242). However, once this is achieved it becomes a rich resource that can be managed and manipulated independent of the person who developed it. This is a fundamental task of KM (Lang, 2001).

A portion of data collected is in health statistical collections that are shared across organisational and geographical boundaries. These data become the basis of a wider knowledge that is used for the treatment of patients, both within and external to the organisation. When outside organisations share data there must be agreement on how they are described, and they must share a common language. Any codification strategy must be based on the premise that data must be stored, retrievable and reusable and it is crucial that the output is accurate, appropriate, and not corrupted in any way.

Scientific evidence stored in large data warehouses will be accessible to all clinical information systems and entering a patient diagnosis will produce the latest in scientific research, protocols, and clinical paths. Associated with warehousing data is data mining which transforms units of data into useable knowledge. These tools use mathematical operations to identify patterns in data (Young, 2000).

Archetypes provide a different method of storing knowledge and Heard discusses these in Chapter 16. These electronically generated documents provide a relatively simple way for clinicians to specify the structure, content and context of clinical information. They define how clinical information and knowledge is structured, stored and managed (Conrick, Hovenga, Cook, Laracuente, & Morgan, 2004).

Dissemination

Dissemination is the sharing and using of knowledge. Sharing explicit knowledge electronically is relatively easy, but the exchange of tacit knowledge requires a shared context, co-location, and again, a common language. In essence, it needs a face-to-face process before it can be shared (Nonaka & Takeuchi, 1995). Technologies such as video conferencing or desktop conferencing satisfy this requirement.

The most prevalent barriers to using knowledge are those between the knowledge provider and the knowledge seeker (Wickramasinghe et al., 2004). Therefore straightforward, user-friendly access and retrieval mechanisms must enable easy access to knowledge repositories to encourage their use.

In recent times, web-enabled knowledge repositories have become increasingly popular. They are relatively easy to access and provide the mechanism for a broad dissemination of information and knowledge using the Internet or Intranets. However, some of the largest repositories of knowledge and information are paper based and reside in libraries. These are not as accessible or as convenient as their electronic counterparts because of problems such as opening hours and competition for access and so forth. The Internet has a very large part to play in knowledge management, as it improves access to diverse resources immeasurably.

The Internet

Maintaining knowledge currency has always been difficult, particularly in the paper system. Many books are dated before they are published, staff shortages mean less time for research, and information overload has exacerbated the problem. Dynamic resource tools for 'knowledge and awareness discovery' enable the user to exploit the Internet to access, read and retrieve material from library catalogues, online databases and resources from millions of sites. The Internet has an expansive range of quality materials, but accessing these can be difficult and frustrating because of the huge amounts of information of unknown origin and provenance and a great deal of rubbish that also resides there (Conrick, 2002).

Providing an appropriate search algorithm is used, the Internet provides ready access to health information that enables clinicians to remain current, aware of the latest developments and to share knowledge about patient care and treatments. It consists of the surface web that is easily accessed by regular search engines and the deep web. This may require a specialised search engine because materials in the deep web are not written in hypertext mark-up language (html): the language of the surface web. The deep web is an estimated 500 times larger than the surface web, is highly specialised, 95 per cent fee free, and has a substantial proportion of government resources, databases and similarly structured materials (Conrick, 2002).

Knowledge awareness tools come in many forms and offer numerous approaches to remaining current. For example, timely alerting services apply a search algorithm defined by the user to monitor the Internet for the latest information, then sends email alerts to the user's computer, mobile phone or Personal Digital Assistant (PDA).

Specific subject based mailing lists; bulletin boards and forums enable people working in diverse geographical areas to share knowledge, as do Weblogs (Blogs) and News Aggregators. These also offer a great vehicle for establishing online knowledge communities.

Intranets

Organisational intranets are an integral part of hospitals as they automate. They enable the sharing of information and knowledge across different local area networks and computer platforms. They use web technology and are shielded from the general public. Access is usually restricted to specific customers and/or employees of the organisation that operate them. Intranets are powerful tools that provide staff with easy ways to access and build new knowledge (Blair, 2004). Organisations are able to identify expertise and experience among employees by locating the authors of documents on their Intranets. Published information is instantly available through a familiar browser interface in flexible formats (word-processed documents, HTML and PDF) because Intranets are not platform specific.

Most hospitals spend significant time and money developing, implementing and maintaining organisational policies that strengthen clinical governance along with improving patient safety and the outcomes of care. Healthcare is dynamic as is the knowledge that underpins it. However, constantly updating paper policies is a difficult, expensive and time-consuming task, but it is essential to health outcomes. Traditional paper-based dissemination of guidelines and policies are ineffective according to Williams et al. (2004), but are a rich source of evidence-based knowledge if they are standardised, based on the latest research evidence, and use document/ version control to reduce the risk of out-of-date information and knowledge being inadvertently used. Quick access to sources of evidence underpins the provision of quality care and this evidence can be locally sorted on Intranets (Conrick, Hovenga et al., 2004).

Exploitation and application

Knowledge becomes innovation when people learn to exploit and apply it (Bock, n.d.; Wickramasinghe et al., 2004) and a key measure of success is when employees use knowledge repositories to provide the highest quality decision-making and evidence-based care.

Knowledge creation, using the Communities of Practice discussed earlier, foster sharing, exploitation and application, and have much to offer healthcare. These communities should be encouraged because teamwork is essential in a modern health system and because the shortage of clinicians continues blurring the boundaries of practice. It is also acknowledged that the exploitation and application of knowledge occurs more readily in teams.

Interest box

- The more they (customers) use knowledge-based offerings, the smarter they get.
- The more you use knowledge-based offerings, the smarter you get.
- Knowledge-based products and services adjust to changing circumstances.
- Knowledge-based businesses' can customise their offerings.
- Knowledge-based products and services have a relatively short life cycle.
- Knowledge-based businesses' react to customers in real time.

(Davis & Botkin, 1994)

Conclusion

A modern healthcare system must provide access to high quality, current knowledge management and knowledge exchange systems to underpin decision-making and support best practice. These systems must be easily accessed, timely or perhaps 'just in time' and available wherever knowledge and information are needed. If knowledge is to be effective in improving health outcomes however, one cannot rely on technology alone but on the ability of the individual to act meaningfully on that knowledge.

Review questions

1. What are the types of knowledge?
2. How are they used?
3. Discuss the tools used for capturing, using and exploiting knowledge.
4. Discuss the integration of the different types of knowledge outlined in this chapter

Exercise

- Critically analyse the use of paper versus electronic knowledge management in healthcare.
- Log on to your local Intranet and find at least three knowledge resources. Discuss how these assist or could assist your practice.

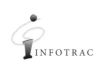

Online reading

INFOTRAC® COLLEGE EDITION
For additional readings and review on knowledge management, explore **InfoTrac®
College Edition**, your online library. Go to: **www.infotrac-college.com** and search for
any of the InfoTrac key terms listed below:
➤ Knowledge
➤ Knowledge management
➤ Information cycle
➤ Knowledge processing

References

Aronson, A. & Rindflesch, T. (1998). *Semantic knowledge representation project: a report to the Board of Scientific Counselors*. Retrieved 23 May 2005 from http://skr.nlm.nih.gov/papers/.

Arora, R. (2002). Implementing KM – a balanced score card approach, *Journal of Knowledge Management, 6*(3), 240–49.

Blair, J. (2004). Assessing the value of the internet in health improvement, *Nursing Times, 100*(35), 28–30.

Bock, W. (n.d.). *Knowledge management 101*. Retrieved 13 March 2005 from http://idm.internet.com/articles.

Conrick, M. (2000). *Students transitional experiences of problem based learning*. Unpublished Thesis, Griffith University, Brisbane.

Conrick, M. (2002). Looking for a needle in a haystack: searching the Internet for quality resources, *Contemporary Nurse, 12*(1).

Conrick, M., Hovenga, E., Cook, R., Laracuente, T., & Morgan, T. (2004). *A framework for nursing informatics in Australia: A Strategic Paper*, Department of Health and Ageing, Melbourne.

Davis, S., & Botkin, J. (1994). The coming of knowledge-based business, *Harvard Business Review*, 165–70.

Drucker, P. (1998). *Management's new paradigms*. Retrieved 2 February 2005 from http://wiredcotteges.com/managementthinkers/peterdrucker.

Gangemi, A., Catenacci, C. & Battaglia, M. (2004). Inflammation ontology design pattern: an exercise in building a core biomedical ontology with descriptions and situations. *Ontologies in Medicine*, 64–80.

Gangemi, A., Pisanelli, D. & Steve, G. (2000). Understanding Systematic Conceptual Structures in Polysemous Medical Terms. Paper presented at the Converging Information, Technology, and Health Care, AMIA Annual Symposium.

Gruber, T. (1993). A translation approach to portable ontologies, *Knowledge Acquisition, 5*(2), 199–220.

Hanka, R. & Fuka, K. (2000). Information overload and 'just-in-time' knowledge, *The Electronic Library, 18*(4), 279.

International Standards Organisation (ISO) (1999). ISO 2382–4. *Information technology – Vocabulary – Part 4: Organization of data*.

Johns, M. (2002). *Information management for health professionals*, 2nd edn, Delmar Publishers, Albany.

Kent, R. (2000). *The information flow foundation for conceptual knowledge organisation*. Paper presented at the 6th International Conference of the International Society for Knowledge Organisation (ISKO), Toronto, Canada.

Lang, J. (2001). Managerial concerns in knowledge management, *Journal of Knowledge Management*, 5(5), 7–15.

Lee, C. & Yang, J. (2000). Knowledge value chain, *Journal of Management Development*, 19(9), 783–93.

McDermott, R. (2002). *Knowing is a human act: how information technology inspired, but cannot deliver knowledge management*. Retrieved 22 May, 2005, from http://knowledgemanagement.ittoolbox.com/documents/.

National Health Service (NHS) (2004). *Knowledge management*. Retrieved 22 February, 2005, from http://www.nelh.nhs.uk/knowledge_management.

Nonaka, I. & Konno, N. (1998). The concept of Ba: building a foundation for knowledge creation, *California Management Review*, 40(3), 40–54.

Nonaka, I. & Nishiguchi, T. (2001). *Knowledge emergence*, Oxford University Press, Oxford.

Nonaka, I. & Takeuchi, H. (1995). *The knowledge-creating company: how Japanese companies create the dynamics of innovation*, Oxford University Press, New York.

Polanyi, M. (1966). *The tacit dimension*. Doubleday & Company, Inc., Garden City, NY.

Sharma, S. & Wickramasinghe, N. (2004). A framework for building a learning organisation in the 21st century, *International Journal of Innovation and Learning*.

Skryme, D. (1997). Knowledge management: oxymoron or dynamic duo? *Managing Information*, 4(7), 24–6.

Smith, A (2001). Knowledge management: classic and contemporary works, *Online Information Review*, 25(6), 407.

Snowden, D. (2002). Complex acts of knowing: paradox and descriptive self-awareness, *Journal of Knowledge Management*, 6(2), 100–11.

Standards Australia (SA) (2001). *Knowledge management: a framework for succeeding in the knowledge era*. HB275–2001, Sydney, Australia.

Standards Australia (SA) (2005). The language of health concept representation, *SDR 04114*. Sydney, Australia.

Wenger, E., & Snyder, W. (2001). *Cultivating communities of practice*, Social Capital Group.

White, M. (2004). Knowledge management involves neither knowledge nor management, *EContent*, 27(10), 39.

Wickramasinghe, N., Gupta, J., & Sharma, S. (2004). *Creating knowledge-based healthcare organizations*. Idea Group Publishing, Hershey.

Williams, J., Cheung, W., Price, D., Tansey, R., Russell, I., Duane, P., et al. (2004). Clinical guidelines on line: do they improve compliance? *Postgraduate Medical Journal*, 80, 415–19.

Young, M. (2000). Classifying the information, *Informatics for Healthcare Professionals*, F.A. Davis Company.

Part 3

Management considerations in health informatics implementations

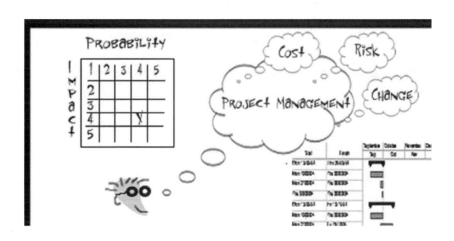

7

Introduction to the issues in leadership and management

Moya Conrick and Catherine Cameron

> 'While management calls for keeping an eye on the bottom line and short-term results, leadership means keeping an eye on the horizon and the long-term future.'
>
> (Daft, 1999 p.39)

Outline

Healthcare leaders and managers face unique challenges as they keep pace with the adoption of information and communications technologies (ICT) into their often complex, multidimensional healthcare organisations. This chapter discusses leaders and managers and examines some of these issues.

Introduction

The twenty-first century has an unprecedented opportunity and a responsibility to change the way the public and policy-makers think and act on issues of health and disease. The driving forces behind this transformation have been the availability of data and information that has led to the discovery and availability of knowledge, developments in technology and the interoperability of systems. The application of knowledge for the good of health provides the stimulus for motivating leaders, managers and policymakers to take action. While this is an era of ambiguity, uncertainty, and risk, it is also an era of spectacular advances in science and technology.

Healthcare and informatics require innovative leadership, management, and strategic, innovative partnerships. All of these are vital in an environment where cultural change affects healthcare and the general population and where there is fierce competition for shrinking resources. They are also vital in a system that is turning to technology as an answer to some of these challenges. These changes, and the drive for cost-effective healthcare, mean that modern health systems now emphasise the business of healthcare (Bekes et al., 2004). Managers in this system must make decisions about the future of healthcare in a data-rich technological age, but this cannot be done in isolation.

Basics of leadership and management

Often the terms leadership and management are used interchangeably, but this should not be the case. The attributes that distinguish leaders from managers are well described in the literature and while not mutually exclusive, do not necessarily occur in the same person. Managers can also have a variety of 'headship' titles such as the Director of Nursing or Medical Services, but again a title or designation does not make a leader. Only a person's behaviour determines whether a person occupies a leadership position.

Hagenow (2001) argues that managers are the stewards of an organisation's resources while leadership is about awakening and empowerment. Hersey and Blanchard (1993, p.5) distinguishes between the two by saying that leadership is 'any time one attempts to influence the behavior of an individual or group,' and management is 'working with and through individuals and groups and other resources to accomplish organisational goals'. These definitions emphasise that leadership and management are two very different concepts, and are not easily interchanged. Table 7.1 further illustrates these differences.

Figure 7.1: Differences between leaders and managers

Leaders	Managers
Are appointed or may emerge	Are appointed
Inspire the trust of others	Influence through formal authority
Look to the future	Concentrate on the present
Inspire change	Maintain stability
Mentor	Control others
Focus on process	Focus on people and relationships

The evolution of leadership and management

A brief outline of the evolution of management definitions demonstrates that the classic five functions – planning, organising, commanding, coordinating and controlling – of Henry Fayol in 1949 have been adapted and evolved over the years. In the 1960s, Mintzberg (1973) observed that the daily activities of managers did not always fit into the neat categories of the five managerial functions. He proposed ten interrelated roles. However, contemporary management sees the manager as planning, staffing, leading, organising and controlling organisational resources and the contemporary challenges bought by technology will see this evolve further.

Modern managers have to be multiskilled and eclectic. They must have the ability to set measurable goals and performance indicators, develop plans to meet these goals, supervise staff and measure their performance. They require project management expertise and must keep up to date with technology and its impact on their workforce.

Leadership

Many definitions of leadership have evolved over the years, but none seem to capture it in its entirety. Early discussions on leadership focused on the individual's characteristics and traits that were often thought to be hereditary (Kouzes & Posner, 1995). This 'Great Man Theory' approached leadership capacities as instinctive, fixed and cross-contextual. Skills and competencies were thought to be anchored in some internal personality or genetic set with which one was born. Hence the age-old question: 'Are leaders made or born?' (Avolio, 1999; Kouzes & Posner, 1995). Parts of this theory persist in some descriptors such as 'traits' of the leader and 'native trait' (Schwartz & Pogge, 2000).

From the 1940s through to the 1960s, behaviourism swept across the scene in academic and management circles. Here the emphasis was on what leaders did and their effect on others' behaviour (McGregor, 1960). The skills required here were efficiency, management and control in order to produce results. This led to Lewin (1951) and White & Lippitt (1960) isolating the leadership styles of authoritarian, democratic and laissez-faire. In contemporary leadership, however, these can be seen as more the ends and middle of a continuum. Marquis and Huston (2006) describe them in the following manner.

The *authoritarian* leader maintains strong control over the workforce and employs multiple rules. This leader motivates others by coercion and commands and makes decisions without involving them. Communication flows downward with an emphasis on differences in status ('I' and 'you') and criticism is punitive.

- results in well-defined group actions that are usually predictable. In turn people know what to do and when to do it, reducing the frustration group members feel
- productivity is usually high, but creativity, self-motivation, and autonomy are reduced
- useful in crisis situations or in very large bureaucracies such as the armed forces. It is alive and well in healthcare organisations.

The *democratic* leader is less controlling, involves others in decision-making, motivates by economic or ego awards and directs by suggestions and guidance. Communication flows up and down, there is an emphasis on 'we' rather than 'I' and 'you' and criticism is constructive.

- appropriate for groups who work together for extended periods of time
- promotes autonomy and growth in individual workers
- particularly effective when cooperation and coordination between groups is necessary
- usually more time-consuming because more people have to be consulted
- studies have shown it is quantitatively less efficient than authoritarian leadership.

The *laissez-faire* leader operates almost permissively, with little or no control exerted. They motivate by support when requested to do so and provide little or no direction. This person communicates between members of the group, as well as upward and downward, and disperses decision-making throughout the group while placing the emphasis on the group and does not criticise.

- can be frustrating because of non-directional leadership
- apathy and indifference can occur
- when all group members are highly motivated and self-directed, results in much creativity
- appropriate in situations when solutions to problems are needed through brainstorming for many alternatives.

According to Denis, Langley and Cazale (1996) complexity and chaos, advancements and disintegration, mark the organisational climate in almost every sector in today's environment and because of this there have been changes in leadership competencies and capacities. The idea of a leader working in a position of power has been diluted as the environment demands team- or community-centered views of leadership (Dentico, 1999). There has also been a move from hierarchical to collaborative models of leadership.

In 1978, Burns introduced the idea of transformational leadership in which leaders and followers have an almost symbiotic relationship. Here the leader identifies common values, is committed, inspiring, has a long-term vision, looks at effects and empowers others. Kouzes and Posner (1995, p 207) add to this with 'challenging the process, modelling the way and encouraging the heart'.

Leadership is now viewed as a process of developing and using a variety of skills and competencies rather than a position or role (Avolio, 1999). Yammarino and Bass (1990, p.159) provide four transformational leadership characteristics:

1. *Charisma*: 'I am ready to trust him/her to overcome any obstacle.'
2. *Individualised Consideration*: 'Gives personal attention to me when necessary.'
3. *Intellectual Stimulation*: 'Shows me how to think about problems in new ways.'
4. *Inspirational Leadership*: 'Provides vision of what lies ahead.'

Attributes of leaders and managers

Central to all the roles discussed above and to the process of leadership and management is the need for effective communication. This is particularly so in an environment where change and disequilibrium is commonplace, such as the health workplace. The introduction of technology into this mix excites some, but many are intimidated by technology and fearful of what it might mean for them.

Murdoch-Pera (2000) found that leaders' communication style determines their ability to relate to their success or failure. Communication needs to be congruent with the needs of the team, otherwise it creates dissatisfaction (Barter, 2002). These skills are also needed to surface, manage and negotiate conflict. Kerfoot (2001) believes that leaders who inspire their staff also motivate them and make them passionate about their work. Leaders also need to communicate respect to energise their staff and improve performance.

Murdoch-Pera (2000) believes that leaders must not only be trusting, they must also be trustworthy. She says that trust forms through honest communication, sharing information, giving and receiving feedback, and the internalising of trust in the work culture. Kerfoot (2001) agrees that the leader's ability to reproduce trust really matters because without it, people will not listen or hear. 'The process can be set back in a heartbeat by people at any level who see leadership as a process of intimidation, whose own lack of self esteem makes them unable to trust and let go' (Kerfoot 2001, p.42).

George et al. (2002) reveal that a leader's most important accomplishment is when staff assist in the change and planning processes. However, this must occur without coercion and staff should feel trusted and empowered to propose ideas and alternate solutions (George et al., 2002). When this happens, employees feel that they are doing something that matters; values and visions are shared, they learn more about the organisation (Swansburg & Swansburg, 2002), and are motivated to engage (Bittel 2003). They also feel a sense of empowerment when a leader demonstrates respect for them and their opinions.

Hanna (1999) feels that recognition is often a strong motivational factor, since all employees want to be recognised. Often they feel that they have something to offer and that they may possess skills that other staff members lack. Inclusive strategies and motivating staff often leads to greater satisfaction and improved performance. Staff feel valued and will stay in the organisation, they will also support rather that undermine the process. This is particularly important in the adoption of technology where disempowerment and disillusionment can lead to resistance and project failure.

As a precursor to discussion to leadership and management roles in HI implementation it is pertinent to provide some background to the Australian healthcare system as it will situate them in the environment in which they make decisions.

The Australian healthcare system

The Australian health care system is the product of a diverse range of economic, social, technological, legal, constitutional and political factors (Palmer & Short, 2000). It is a large and complex system consisting of several different types of service providers and organisations from both the public and private sectors. Historically most services have been planned in isolation from one another (Lewis, 2004) leading to a network of disparate organisations striving to provide quality healthcare services. Silos of information locked within professional and organisational boundaries have also served to fragment the system.

The health system also has a complex funding model and service responsibilities because of the involvement of all levels of government and the non-government sector in the provision of healthcare services. The power of the government sector varies; each has major functions of funding, providing, and regulating healthcare services and personnel (George & Davis, 1998). The Federal Government generally funds out-of-hospital services, while the state and territory governments support a broad range of other services. They jointly finance public hospitals and community care for the aged and disabled. Australia has a large private sector that provides healthcare services and is supported through government incentive schemes. Non-government religious and charitable organisations also provide healthcare services, particularly in relation to aged and community care.

State and territory government leaders have recently challenged the division of power between each level of government for a number of reasons including the confused governance arrangements for health that affect the planning, provision and coordination of healthcare services.

The acute care hospitals sector is by far the largest service provider and therefore receives the bulk of healthcare service funding. However, other service providers are challenging this. For example, the growth of long-term care institutions has paralleled the increase in the elderly population. People are living longer with poorer health and this is placing increasing demands on the long-term care sector and the health budget.

Moreover, there is an increasing trend toward home healthcare and initiatives to support seamless care. The National summary Electronic Health Record (Health*Connect*) project is being introduced in an attempt to integrate healthcare and support this agenda. It has the backing of all levels of government, has trialled many new technologies, and has spawned others catapulting Australia to the forefront of Electronic Health Record (EHR) developments worldwide.

Healthcare leaders and managers are acutely aware of the challenges of working in such a dynamic system and within budgets that often come from a variety of sources. Information and communication technologies are enabling technologies that support healthcare managers and these have the capacity to transform the face of healthcare.

The uses and benefits of information and communications technologies (ICT) in healthcare delivery are extensively cited in the literature (Hovenga & Lloyd, 2002; Tobin, 2003). This demonstrates the potential to reduce error and 'near misses' (that often result in extended lengths of stay), readmissions and duplication, all of which cost the system vast amounts each year.

The manager oversees all of the processes involved in the adoption of information technology and sometimes multi-million sums of money are involved. It is usually the manager who takes the risks and who is ultimately held accountable for decisions and outcomes.

Integration strategies

Strategies that focus on supporting the smooth transition of ICT into healthcare organisations are complex. They include strategic planning, effective project management, risk management strategies including cost benefit analysis, change management strategies, and identifying the professional roles and governance of ICT needs in organisations.

Gagnon et al. (2005) agree with Dixon-Hughes (Chapter 8) that it is vital to investigate the context prior to implementing ICT to ensure its success, and that understanding the organisation and stakeholders' readiness for the implementation of ICT is a vital consideration (Hebert & Korabek, 2004). Clearly, strategies for effective implementation need to include an analysis of the characteristics and the dynamics of the healthcare organisation and its socio-political background.

Integration of ICT in healthcare organisations is not exclusively the role of the healthcare manager. While strong leadership is required, appropriate staffing is also necessary, as managers work within teams to delegate specific tasks to those with expertise and the knowledge to carry out those activities.

The management considerations in health informatics implementations are critical for successful IT adoptions and for this reason they are discussed in dedicated chapters later in this book. However, a short introduction will be offered here.

Strategic planning

It is vital that the manager remain focused on the challenges that ICTs bring and respond to them by making strategic choices and redesigning healthcare organisations accordingly. An important component of strategic planning centres on information systems implementation and use (Hebda, Czar & Mascara, 2001). Strategic planning is a disciplined effort to produce fundamental decisions and actions that shape and guide what an organisation is, what it does, and why it does it, with a focus on the future (Bryson & Alston, 2004). Managers rely on teams of experts to assist with the execution of these plans but the manager takes overall responsibility.

Project management

Project management enables organisations to achieve their objectives. It provides managers with powerful tools that improve their ability to plan, implement and control activities and help them to use personnel and resources effectively. In terms of leadership skills, the project manager needs to be proactive and task focused to deliver specific outcomes; it is a directive role (Turner & Simister, 2000). The project plan can make or break an implementation.

Risk and information management

All businesses have inherent risk. Commonly healthcare organisations carry clinical, operational, financial, legal and external risks with the potential for huge impacts on the organisation. Risk management aims to protect organisations from loss and damage. It is part of the healthcare manager's role to ensure that strategies are in place to do this. A risk management plan enables managers to identify potential risks to the organisation and assists with strategic planning. It improves the use of resources while reducing the risk of litigation and ultimately can improve the quality of healthcare delivery.

Change management

Change is an inevitable part of life and the work environment but planned change is the exception rather than the rule. Change occurs whether one wants it to or not (Peters, 1991). Superimposed on the change to new models of healthcare and a mobile workforce is the accelerated adoption of information technology. Many health professionals are slow to embrace ICT tools into their practice and others are wary despite increasing evidence that supports its benefits (Audet et al., 2005). Healthcare managers need to be aware of these barriers and to plan for them.

However, in all areas of change, leadership is as important as the quality of the technology (Poon et al., 2004). Leaders must be firm believers in the benefits of technology and visibly demonstrate a commitment to the project; they can do this by becoming early adopters. They need to be effective and use simple strategies to manage the change that will inevitably come with ICT implementations. Leaders must also feel empowered to mandate use if significant benefits are determined.

During uncertainties and setbacks, leaders need to maintain and communicate a common vision, which should describe genuine reasons for the adoption of IT. These might include improvements in patient safety, quality and efficiency, and demonstrate gain for staff and the institution. Often staff will feel internal discord resulting from differences in ideas, values or feelings and conflict results (Marquis & Huston, 2006).

Conflict management

As complexity and ambiguity increases, conflict increases (Guy, 1986). It occurs naturally and it is expected by organisations. Conflict in itself is neither good nor bad. It should be neither avoided nor encouraged; it must be managed. The implementation of technology has the potential to cause situations that can derail the process.

Conflict produces distress when it occurs, but it can also lead to growth, energy and creativity by generating new ideas and solutions. If handled inappropriately, it can lead to demoralisation, decreased motivation and lowered productivity. Leaders have different roles from managers in managing conflict and the following roles adapted from Marquis and Huston (2006) describes the differences.

Leadership:

- is self-aware and conscientiously works to resolve intrapersonal conflict
- addresses conflict as soon as it is perceived and before it becomes felt or manifest
- seeks a win-win solution to conflict whenever feasible
- lessens the perceptual differences that exist between conflicting parties and broadens understanding about the problems
- assists subordinates in identifying alternative conflict resolutions
- recognises and accepts the individual differences of staff

- uses assertive communication skills to increase persuasiveness and foster open communication
- role models honest and collaborative negotiation efforts.

Management:

- creates a work environment that minimises the antecedent conditions for conflict
- appropriately uses legitimate authority in a competing approach when a quick or unpopular decision needs to be made
- when appropriate, formally facilitates conflict resolution involving subordinates
- accepts mutual responsibility for reaching predetermined supra-ordinate goals
- is prepared to negotiate for resources, including the advance determination of a bottom line and possible trade-offs
- addresses the need for closure and follow-up to negotiation
- pursues alternative dispute resolution when conflicts cannot be resolved using traditional conflict management strategies.

There is no doubt that conflict can or will arise with any implementation of technology. It is new, it has the capacity to change work practices, and many people will ask how management can justify expenditure on technology when beds are being shut and the workforce is struggling with high workloads. Leaders and managers need to use appropriate strategies to dissipate such conflict.

Professional roles and governance

Not only have healthcare managers had to adapt to new roles and responsibilities, new positions have emerged to cope with the increasing use of ICT in healthcare. Supporting the information-intensive healthcare organisation is a growing number of specialty staff. Governance is crucial in the success or otherwise of informatics implementations. It should perceive and consider all of the diverse requirements and views of stakeholders for projects to work. It provides the structure for accomplishing the aims, communicates a vision, and provides mechanisms for keeping goals visible and communicating progress and activities.

Financial management

Healthcare managers' decision-making incorporates clinical, management and financial factors. The benefits of ICT in healthcare management include the ability to provide high quality efficiency while attempting to maintain associated costs, ensuring adequate resource allocation and the monitoring of general financial management strategies.

Education and training

Leaders and managers must take responsibility for educating their workforce because nothing will destroy a project more quickly that disinformation or ignorance. Healthcare education is vital to change and to the adoption of new technologies. However, ICT can also play a vital role in recruiting and retaining healthcare workers

(Simpson, 2005) because of the perception of innovation and the ability of technology to support clinical practice.

All organisations must have an education, training and knowledge management plan in place. Duly qualified staff must oversee this as healthcare workers must understand and use health data, information and knowledge appropriately. Education sessions must be regular and positions must be backfilled to enable all employees to attend. Adequate resources are essential as is training on the technology used in the organisation.

Evidence-based decision-making

Managers must be flexible and their decisions must be based on evidence for decision-making to be effective. This includes ensuring that adequate decision support systems are in place or at least identified for deployment, and that tools to support financial management are available in each department within the organisation.

Conclusion

The common theme in each of the issues discussed above is that the manager's role in the adoption of information technology is multi-faceted, eclectic and demanding. They must oversee resource allocation, monitor and measure the effectiveness and the impact of the implementations, and ensure that adoptions run smoothly to deliver the desired health outcomes.

There is increasing recognition of the need for healthcare managers to be proactive with their integration of ICT into healthcare organisations. There are several significant drivers shaping current health services management: increasing use of information technologies, consumer expectations, decreasing resources and changing healthcare models. Knowledge of effective management strategies can assist managers in healthcare organisations to successfully integrate information technology to support a much-needed transformation of healthcare.

Review questions

1. What are the main challenges for health service managers in relation to information management?
2. Identify several roles ICT plays in healthcare organisations.
3. Why is ICT considered an important aspect of the strategic planning process?

Exercise

- Observe a leader and manager in your workplace or on clinical practice. Critically analyse at least three management functions and leadership roles that you observe. Particularly note communication used and interactions with the interdisciplinary team.

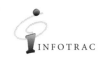

Online reading

References

Audet, A., Doty, M., Shamasdin, J. & Schoenbaum, S. (2005). Measure, learn, and improve: physicians' involvement in quality improvement, *Health Affairs*, 24(3), 843–52.

Avolio, B. (1999). *Full leadership development: building organizations*, Sage Publications, Thousand Oaks.

Barter, M. (2002). Follow the team leader, *Nursing Management*, 33(10), 54–8.

Bekes, C., Dellinger, R., Brooks D., Edmondson, R., Olivia, C. & Parrillo, J. (2004). Critical care medicine as a distinct product line with substantial financial profitability: The role of business planning, *Crit Care Med*, 32(5), 1207–14.

Bittel, L., Goodworth, C. & Veccio, R. 2003. *Leadership styles*. Retrieved 19 September, 2003, from http://www.see.ed.ac.uk/.

Bryson, J. & Alston, F. (2004). *Creating and implementing your strategic plan: a workbook for public and nonprofit organizations* (3rd edn), Jossey-Bass, New York.

Commonwealth of Australia (2005). Health*Connect*. Retrieved 15 July, 2005, from http://www.healthconnect.gov.au/.

Denis, J., Langley, A. & Cazale, L. (1996). Leadership and strategic change under ambiguity, *Organizational Studies*, 17, 673–699.

Dentico, J. (1999). Games leaders play: using process simulations to develop collaborative leadership practices for a knowledge-based society, *Career Development International*, 4(3), 17–18(12).

Fayol, H. (1949). *General and industrial management*, Pittman & Sons, London.

Gagnon, M., Lamothe, L., Fortin, J., Cloutier, A., Godin, G., Gagne, C. & Reinharz, D. (2005). Telehealth adoption in hospitals: an organisational perspective, *Health Organ Manag*, 19(1), 32–56.

George, V., Burke, L., Rodgers, B., Duthie, N., Hoffman, M., Koceja, V., Kramer, A., Maro, J., Minzlaff, P., Pelczynski, S., Schmidt, M., Wetsen, B., Kiekle, J., Brukwitzki, G. & Gehring, L. (2002). Developing staff nurse shared leadership behaviour in professional nursing practice, *Nursing Administration Quarterly*, 26(3), 44–60.

George, J. & Davis, A. (1998). *States of health: health and illness in Australia*, Addison Wesley Longman, Melbourne.

Guy, M. (1986) Interdisciplinary conflict and organizational complexity, *Hospital & Health Services Administration*, 31(1), 111–22.

Hagenow, N. (2001). Care Executives: Organizational intelligence for these times, *Nurs Admin Q*, 25(4), 30–36.

Hanna, L. (1999). Lead the way leader, *Nursing Management*, 30(11), 36–40.

Hebda, T., Czar, P., Mascara, C. (2001). *Handbook of informatics for nurses and health care professionals*, 2nd edn, New Jersey, Prentice Hall.

Hebert, M. & Korabek, B. (2004). Stakeholder readiness for telehomecare: implications for implementation, *Telemed J E Health*, 10(1), 85–92.

Hersey, P. & Blanchard, K. (1993). *Management of organizational behavior: utilizing human resources*, 6th edn, Prentice Hall, Englewood Cliffs.

Hovenga, E. & Lloyd, S. (2002). Working with information, in M. Harris (ed.), *Managing health services: concepts and practice* (pp.195–227), MacLennan and Petty, Sydney.

Kerfoot, K. (2001). From motivation to inspiration leadership, *Nursing Economics*, 19(5), 242–7.

Kouzes, J. & Posner, B. (1995). *The leadership challenge: How to keep getting extraordinary things done in organizations*. Jossey-Bass Publishers, San Francisco.

Lewin, K. (1951). *Field theory in social science*. Harper & Row, New York.

Lewis, J. (2004). Health service management: theory and practice, in Clinton, M (ed.), *Management in the Australian health care industry* (pp.97–119), Pearson Education Australia, Sydney.

Marquis, B. & Huston, C. (2006). *Leadership and management functions in nursing*, Lippencott Williams & Wilkins, Philadelphia.

McGregor, D. (1960). *The human side of enterprise*, McGraw-Hill, New York.

Mintzberg, H. (1973). *The nature of managerial work*, Harper and Row, New York.

Murdoch-Pera, B. (2000). Leadership: the key to quality outcomes, *Nursing Administration Quarterly*, 24(2), 56–61.

Palmer, G. & Short, S. (2000). *Health care and public policy: an Australian analysis*, 3rd edn, Macmillan Education Australia, South Melbourne.

Peters, T. (1991). *Thriving on chaos: handbook for a management revolution*, Harper Collins, New York.

Poon, E., Blumenthal, D., Jaggi, T. & Honour M. (2004). Overcoming barriers to adopting and implementing computerized physician order entry systems, in U.S. Hospitals. *Health Affairs*, 23(4), 184.

Schwartz, R. & Pogge, C. (2000). Physician leadership is essential to the survival of teaching hospitals, *The American Journal of Surgery*, 179, 462–8.

Simpson, R. (2005). Patient and nurse safety: how information technology makes a difference, *Nurs Admin Q*, 29(1), 97–101.

Swansburg, R. & Swansburg, R. (2002). *Introduction to management and leadership for nurse managers*, 3rd edn, Jones and Bartlett, Boston.

Tobin, G. (2003). Health care information technology: better care, better business, *Stud Health Technol Inform*, 92, 13–21.

Turner, J. & Simister, S. (2000). *Grower handbook of project management*. Grower, Vermont.

White, R. & Lippitt, R. (1960). *Autonomy and democracy: an experimental inquiry*. Harper-Row, New York.

Yammarino, E.J. & Bass, B.M. (1990). Long-term forecasting of transformational leadership and its effect among naval officers, in K. Clark & M. Clark (eds), *Measures of Leadership*, Library of America, West Orange, s.151–69.

8

Business planning and architectures

J. Richard Dixon-Hughes

'After you've done a thing the same way for two years, look it over carefully. After five years look at it with suspicion, and after ten years throw it away and start all over again.'

(Alfred E. Perlman, 1958)

Outline

Information and communications technology (ICT) now plays a vital role in most healthcare organisations, but still often fails to meet the needs of both organisations and end-users. Because of the intensely personal and highly specialised nature of their work, front-line clinical care providers often find it hardest to get full benefits from ICT initiatives. This chapter discusses how various ICT planning activities and ICT architectures are used to align ICT activities with organisational priorities and ensure that ICT investments meet business requirements and deliver successful outcomes.

Introduction

Previous chapters have discussed the acceleration of information exchange and the growing use of Internet applications in health. These are among the factors driving health service organisations to seek greater uniformity and control in their ICT activities, to ensure that they can deliver secure, reliable, accessible information systems that serve a wide diversity of users. Without a blueprint for integration and management of systems and information, even successful projects can become barriers to the wider interchange of information across the organisation and with key external stakeholders.

Formal ICT planning processes aim to deliver ICT outcomes that further an organisation's overall business objectives and better address its internal and external environment.

The planning and management of ICT activities can be undertaken at several different, but inter-related, levels. At the highest levels, ICT planning frameworks and ICT strategic plans align ICT activities with the organisation's strategic direction and operational needs. These high-level approaches are sometimes expressed as ICT policies, setting ground rules for coordination of ICT activities across the organisation and attempting to ensure that ICT initiatives are carried out in open and accountable ways that do, in fact, deliver benefits to the organisation.

Enterprise ICT architectures are another high-level expression of the relationship between an organisation's business goals and its ICT requirements. These involve the development of formal models to represent business processes and the information, applications and technology required to support them.

At an intermediate level, tactical ICT plans define how the portfolio of initiatives that flow from an organisation's ICT strategy are to be implemented, giving more detail on the initiatives and the resources, timetable and priorities for achieving them. Tactical plans often carry titles such as 'Annual IT Plan' and commonly schedule developments over a rolling two- or three-year period with updates every twelve months. In some organisations, a tactical ICT plan may represent the highest form of ICT planning that is regularly undertaken.

Each major ICT initiative must usually be further justified by a business case that confirms the benefits, resources, timetable and responsibilities associated with the initiative and also the controls that will be applied to ensure that it achieves its goals. A business case is aimed at securing approval for an initiative and in many smaller organisations may be the only type of ICT planning that is used.

At a lower level planning and project management activities are used to manage individual ICT initiatives. The project management techniques described in other chapters of this book are aimed at ensuring that initiatives are achieved on time, within budget, and deliver benefits over their operational life.

Health informatics promises significant improvements in the delivery of healthcare and the management of healthcare facilities. Health informaticians and health workers to varying degrees therefore need a sound appreciation of ICT planning processes in order to:

- anticipate activities that may be required to get health informatics onto an organisation's ICT agenda
- progress initiatives through planning and approval processes
- be informed when working on ICT planning activities.

We will now consider in more depth some of the ICT planning activities introduced above.

ICT planning frameworks

In governing their information resources, enterprises such as major corporations and government agencies often establish ICT planning frameworks. Such frameworks typically prescribe processes that units within the enterprise are to follow when planning their ICT activities. Features often found in ICT planning frameworks include:

- statements identifying the strategies, goals and objectives to be progressed through information management and ICT initiatives
- a requirement for the framework to be applied throughout the enterprise, sometimes supported by legislation or corporate governance requirements
- a scope that encompasses management of information resources and the organisation of information services, as well as ICT issues
- processes and principles for systematic planning, management and review of ICT resources and programs, including requirements for organisational units to engage in regular ICT planning and measure ICT performance and outcomes
- identification of the internal and external relationships and activities to be supported by ICT
- processes to facilitate integration of information management and information processing activity across the organisation and to avoid duplication.

An ICT planning framework may be encapsulated within broader information management policies designed to ensure that information resources are effectively exploited and that information collection, retention, use and maintenance are well managed in accordance with legal requirements (such as laws governing records management and archiving, privacy of personal information, or audit of budget allocations).

Examples of ICT planning frameworks include the Information Management Strategic Plan (Department of Defense, 1999) and the New South Wales Government's IM&T Blueprint (2000).

ICT strategic planning

The main objective of ICT strategic planning is to align an organisation's ICT activities with its strategic direction and ensure that ICT investments make genuine contributions to improved operational effectiveness. More specifically, ICT strategic planning aims to define how computer systems and communications technology can best support the organisation, what initiatives need to be undertaken to deliver these outcomes, and the priorities, resources and timescales for these initiatives. A further objective of ICT strategic planning is to define technology standards and management structures needed to support ICT within the organisation.

ICT strategic planning is only one facet of an organisation's overall strategic planning process. Strategic planning may be defined as 'the process of developing a plan which will guide the implementation of an organisation's long-term objectives and goals' (NSW Premier's Department, 1992). An organisation's overall strategic plan is often referred to as its 'Corporate Strategic Plan'.

Within this context, ICT Strategic Planning may be defined as 'the component of the strategic planning process which defines the information and communications technology needs and priorities of an organisation in order to maximise the benefits it receives from current and future investments in ICT'.

In a health service organisation, corporate strategy is normally focused on clinical services and their relationship to the evolving needs of the organisation's consumer populations, clinical providers and funding bodies. Other important facets may include personnel, clinical training, support services, research, business development, the competitive environment and the financial situation. Changing needs arising from the corporate strategic plan become drivers to be addressed in developing the ICT strategic plan.

Corporate strategic planning is typically characterised as a layered process similar to that depicted in Figure 8.1 in which the ICT and other sectoral strategic plans are driven by (and contribute to) a corporate strategic plan, which is derived from the corporate goals, which flow from an organisation's mission statement.

Figure 8.1: Corporate strategic planning hierarchy

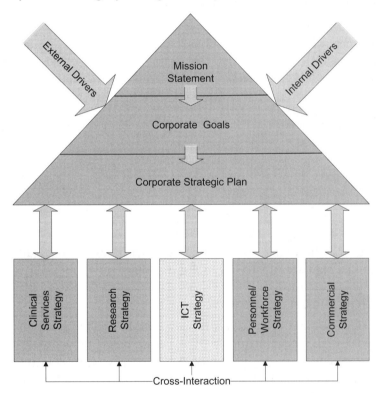

Strategic planning horizon and update of plans

Strategic planning should serve the organisation, rather than the organisation serving the plan. Accordingly, organisations facing different circumstances have quite different ideas about what constitutes appropriate strategic planning horizons, even within a single industry. Because it would be expected to drive changes requiring major long-term investments, a corporate strategic plan would be expected to have a planning horizon of five to ten years, and be reviewed every two to three years.

Because of rapid changes in ICT and the difficulty of realising benefits from longer-term ICT initiatives, an ICT strategic plan should focus on investments over a two- to five-year period and be updated every one or two years. The time taken to develop an

ICT strategic plan will vary according to the complexity of the organisation and its needs, with most requiring three to six months from commencement to approval.

In practice, the mission of most health service organisations can be encapsulated in a relatively simple statement and usually remains fairly constant over time. So, why do ICT strategic plans need to be updated so often? The answer lies in the other sources of change – the internal and external factors affecting the ability of the organisation to realise its stated goals, the implications of these factors, and the need to revise priorities in line with new goals and objectives.

The ICT strategic planning process

There are many different approaches to ICT strategic planning but most generally follow similar lines, with changing emphasis depending on the specific needs of each organisation. We shall consider an ICT planning process carried out as five major stages, each of which concludes with feedback from the organisation.

- Stage 1 – Initiate project
- Stage 2 – Analyse strategic ICT situation
- Stage 3 – Develop ICT strategic requirements
- Stage 4 – Develop ICT strategic plan
- Stage 5 – Activate the ICT strategy

The interaction of these stages and the activities within them that lead to production of an ICT strategic plan are illustrated in Figure 8.2.

Organisational commitment

Normally the development of an ICT strategic plan is driven by senior management and supported by the organisation's ICT personnel. Commitment from senior management is essential to ensure the plan is based on complete information and has sponsorship when the organisation is ultimately asked to endorse its findings and make the associated investments.

The ICT strategic planning process builds a shared business vision. To ensure success, it must be structured and gain support from personnel at different levels in the organisation, including both management and users. A steering committee that includes senior management, end-user representatives, the CIO and key ICT personnel should oversee the planning process.

The inclusion of health or clinical expertise on the team is particularly important where others on the team may have limited exposure to health issues. On commencing the planning study, senior management should communicate with staff, advising them of the study and its goals and encourage their input.

Figure 8.2: ICT Strategic planning process

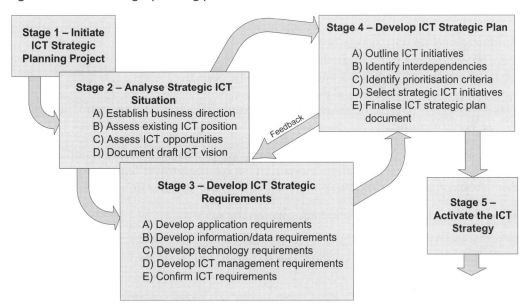

Facilitating the process

While some organisations carry out ICT strategic planning in-house, many engage external consultants to provide assistance ranging from limited external facilitation of user feedback sessions through to having a consulting firm lead and conduct the entire planning process. Irrespective of whether external assistance is obtained, the strategies, initiatives and priorities reflected in the plan must genuinely reflect those of the broader organisation and not those of the consultants, the ICT group or a few key stakeholders.

The principal advantages of using external consultants are their independence from internal politics, their ICT strategic planning experience and tools, and their ability to drive the process and produce a product. However, health is a complex business, and the consultants selected should have sufficient appreciation of the health industry to understand issues arising during consultation.

Carrying out an ICT strategic planning study in-house avoids additional expenditure, but will require the formation of a full-time planning team with requisite skills that can be dedicated to the process, potentially for six months.

Good leadership by senior management can assist in balancing external assistance with internal needs to achieve a shared ICT vision while building skills, confidence and understanding among the internal management team.

Stage 1 – Initiate project

The first step is to set up the project steering committee, which should be chaired by an executive sponsor (from outside ICT) and include the organisation's CIO plus a balance of relevant clinical, administrative and ICT personnel. If a consultant is to be engaged, a consulting brief needs to be written, quotations sought, consultants interviewed and a contract executed with the selected consultant.

At the start of the project proper, the project team should meet with the steering committee and key ICT personnel to confirm:

- project activities and schedule
- the consultation process and persons to be consulted
- the supply of background documentation
- reporting requirements, steering committee meetings, and lines of communication.

On establishment of the project team, executive management should notify staff of the study and invite participation. An early task for the project team is to collect and review background documentation and other relevant information.

Figure 8.3: Checklist of background information for review

1.	Previous ICT strategic plan, other relevant plans, business cases and proposals for new ICT capability.
2.	Recent corporate plans and other statements about strategic directions, including annual reports and financial statements.
3.	Organisation structure and telephone/email contact lists.
4.	Full details of ICT services used and provided by the organisation.
5.	Any enterprise ICT architecture and information on ICT applications, databases, technical infrastructure and standards.
6.	Actual and planned ICT operating and capital expenditures.
7.	Any reviews of ICT activities and systems, including questions arising from annual financial audits.

If the organisation has a health service planning or development unit, the project team should seek to interact with it regularly throughout the process – their input is usually extremely valuable.

Stage 2 – Analyse strategic ICT situation

Analysis of the strategic ICT situation is achieved through four inter-related activities:

- Activity 2A – Establish business direction
- Activity 2B – Assess existing ICT position
- Activity 2C – Assess ICT opportunities
- Activity 2D – Document draft ICT vision

Figure 8.4 below illustrates some of the key questions to be addressed during Stage 2.

Figure 8.4: Key questions for assessing the strategic ICT situation

Stage 2 – Analysing the strategic ICT situation – Key questions		
Activity 2A Business Direction	Activity 2B Existing ICT Position	Activity 2C ICT Opportunities
What are the organisations goals, key result areas, performance targets and the significant reforms it is pursuing? **What** are its 'customer' groups and how may services to each group be improved? **Does** the organisation's capital works program require new ICT services and infrastructure? **What** external drivers, such as government policy or external relationships should the ICT strategic plan address? **What** constraints are there on funds or other factors?	**What** is the status of ICT: — applications? — information and data? — technology infrastructure? — standards? — personnel and services **Are** previous ICT plans being achieved? What new approaches are needed? **What** issues are users raising about ICT systems and services? **Do** personnel have required ICT skills and training? **Does** ICT governance work? **Is** information secure and individual privacy protected?	**Are** there opportunities to share or consolidate ICT activities? **How** can online technology be exploited to better deliver services and information? **Should** new health informatics or ICT standards be implemented? **What** ICT initiatives would: — improve clinical care? — help information handling? — improve information access? — enhance information privacy? — improve information security? — reduce errors? — make it easier to do business with the organisation?

Establishing the business direction (Activity 2A)

The focus of this activity is to identify the structure of the organisation, its business units, the key business goals and issues that should be addressed by the ICT strategic plan. It should draw on information provided by stakeholders during interviews and workshops, as well as the corporate plan and other relevant documentation.

In addressing these issues, health service organisations may face competing business drivers, which need to be captured in an objective, balanced way as part of establishing the business direction.

Assessing the existing ICT position (Activity 2B)

Assessment of the organisation's existing ICT position focuses on the state of the current ICT services, infrastructure and capability.

Current systems of healthcare delivery are inherently fragmented making it hard for them to capture information and deliver it to the right person, in the right place at the right time. Integrating information to support clinical care across a wide variety of disparate settings and using it to track the efficiency and cost of service delivery continue to challenge health organisations. Effective sharing of information particularly depends on having common standards for information interchange, widespread access to electronic networks and communications channels and, for communications with external parties, secure Internet capabilities. Assessment of the existing ICT position needs to understand how effectively the organisation and its ICT infrastructure is addressing these challenges.

As part of this process, a snapshot of the existing ICT position should be prepared for inclusion in the final ICT plan.

Assessing ICT opportunities (Activity 2C)

The assessment of ICT opportunities considers what new, emerging or alternative ICT solutions might be available and how ICT is being used by other similar organisations.

An important part of this activity is to consider whether there are opportunities to change the balance between in-sourcing and outsourcing of various ICT activities, especially where current approaches may not be meeting the expectations of the broader organisation and its stakeholders.

Techniques for analysing strategic situations – SWOT and gap analysis

SWOT analysis and gap analysis are two common techniques for analysing strategic situations. SWOT is short for 'Strengths, Weaknesses, Opportunities, and Threats' and requires strategic factors to be identified and assessed from four separate viewpoints:

- Strengths – internal factors aiding the achievement of objectives
- Weaknesses – internal factors inhibiting the achievement of objectives.
- Opportunities – external factors that can be exploited to achieve objectives
- Threats – external factors that may be barriers to achievement of objectives

Gap Analysis is relatively straightforward – a strategic goal is dissected into subsidiary objectives, each with a desired outcome and these are compared with the actual or projected position. Actions or strategies are then formulated to deal with any 'gaps' that are revealed by the process.

Documenting the draft ICT strategic vision (Activity 2D)

At the conclusion of Stage 2, the draft ICT strategic vision is documented to clearly demonstrate how and why updated ICT activities can benefit the organisation and the achievement of its goals and objectives based on the widespread consultation and review in Stage 2 activities. The document identifies ICT opportunities and high-level ICT requirements in terms of applications, information, technology and actions for management. Specific outcomes and deliverables should also be identified.

Any significant strategic alternatives should be highlighted and discussed, with a view to having the preferred approaches endorsed as the ICT strategic plan develops. The draft ICT vision should also acknowledge practical constraints faced by the organisation and give reasons why any potential opportunities have been deferred to later planning cycles.

The draft ICT vision provides a framework for developing more specific ICT requirements and strategies in Stage 3 and for assessing priorities in Stage 4. The vision may be updated as ICT strategic planning progresses, if challenged by later information on specific initiatives and their likely implications. The final version of the ICT strategic vision provides the basis of the draft ICT strategic plan in the final stages of the planning process.

When the draft ICT strategic vision has been compiled, it should be reviewed by affected stakeholders and accepted by the project steering committee.

Management of consultation processes

Stages 2 and 3 of the ICT strategic planning process are built on a common body of information, which must largely be derived from consultation with stakeholders. To avoid duplication and make best use of stakeholder time, a single integrated consultation process should be used to obtain this information.

Organising consultation for ICT strategic planning

- Interview a small selection of key executives and senior managers to identify the main issues facing the organisation and its ICT function.
- Prepare background papers, workshop agenda and supplementary questionnaire.
- Conduct focus-group workshops for a broad cross-section of stakeholders (in a health service of 6000 persons, over 100 might participate). Each workshop should use a facilitated, participative approach to define and prioritise organisational issues relating to the ICT functions, desired ICT outcomes, requirements and potential strategies for achieving outcomes.
- Obtain input from key external stakeholders (including funding bodies and customer representatives).
- From the broad workshops, select opinion leaders to give input when setting priorities and finalising the ICT strategic plan in Stage 4.
- If necessary, prepare discussion papers on specific issues and conduct follow-up sessions with selected groups of relevant stakeholders.

Stage 3 – Develop ICT requirements

As summarised in the following box, Stage 3 comprises five concurrent activity streams to identify and confirm specific ICT requirements needed to achieve the business outcomes identified in the ICT strategic vision.

- Activity 3A – Develop applications requirements
- Activity 3B – Develop information/data requirements
- Activity 3C – Develop technology requirements
- Activity 3D – Develop ICT management requirements
- Activity 3E – Confirm ICT requirements

During this stage, requirements are identified by gap analysis and described along with a high-level business justification for each requirement and an indication of the ICT initiatives involved to satisfy it. Even though the various activities in this stage are interdependent, the final requirements statements and their supporting initiatives should be well structured with interdependencies clearly identified.

The applications, information/data, technology and management requirements investigated in this stage closely mirror those addressed in enterprise ICT architectures (as discussed in a later section). Where an ICT architecture is available, it should be used and updated by the ICT planning activity to maintain alignment between the organisation's ICT strategic plan and its ICT architecture.

Applications requirements are developed by identifying needs, priorities and service levels for ICT applications arising from potential improvements in current business processes, the impact of new business initiatives and reform projects. Requirements may include the need to introduce new systems, retain, modify or decommission current systems, or to continue, modify or cancel projects or plans.

Information/data requirements are typically developed alongside applications requirements by identifying and documenting the classes of information and data required by different groups of users – clinicians, unit managers, researchers, planners and administrative staff and, also, external stakeholders – consumers, extramural care providers, governments and registries. Information is an important and costly asset that needs to be properly managed, giving rise to considerations about:
- adequacy of processes for managing various classes of information
- balancing the level of detail against the cost of collecting, maintaining and protecting information
- responsibilities for information collection, maintenance and protection
- how the organisation manages confidentiality, integrity and accessibility of information, privacy rights, audit trails and access controls.

Both application and information/data requirements are best identified by formally defining, dissecting and charting high-level business processes and their interactions. Considering the implications of such interactions (for example, where will required information come from? How is access secured? How is its currency ensured?) helps to consolidate application, information/data, technology and management requirements and is an important discipline in the development of a high quality ICT strategic plan.

The development of *technology requirements* normally involves specialist ICT input and considers any gaps in performance, security and availability of: application services, networks, information resources, or voice, data, image or video communications. This activity should focus on the needs identified in the ICT vision (rather than other technology needs) and considers the changes in technology needed to support new applications and systems. In addition to new technology, outcomes may include retaining, upgrading, modifying or decommissioning technology or changing support arrangements. The ICT standards applied within the organisation should also be reviewed and updated.

Today, many health organisations find themselves needing to balance demands for greater information security with those for improved access to information via Internet applications.

ICT governance and management should also be reviewed as part of the planning process with requirements being reflected in the ICT strategic plan. This activity includes an examination of any current ICT organisation, its charter and its capacity and the various means of obtaining ICT capabilities and services, identifying any additional functions or recommended changes in management functions or governance arrangements.

In concluding the activities performed in Stage 3, the ICT requirements should be checked and cross-referenced with the ICT strategic vision to ensure that they are complete and consistent with each other. Finally, the outcomes should be reconfirmed with relevant business managers and presented to the project steering committee.

Stage 4 – Develop ICT strategic plan

In Stage 4 of the planning process, output from the previous stages is consolidated into an ICT strategic plan that defines the most cost-effective manner for the organisation to use ICT in supporting its business direction and goals over the coming years. Development of the ICT strategic plan involves the following five activities:

- Activity 4A – Outline ICT initiatives
- Activity 4B – Identify interdependencies
- Activity 4C – Identify prioritisation criteria
- Activity 4D – Select strategic ICT initiatives
- Activity 4E – Finalise ICT strategic plan document

The broad strategic approaches in the ICT strategic vision and more detailed requirements from Stage 3 need to be developed into a series of specific initiatives, each of which can be undertaken in its own right (or in conjunction with other initiatives).

Each initiative should be summarised along with its benefits, costs and any other impact it may have on the organisation's activities and resources. The summary should also address how the initiative will be implemented, giving critical success factors and strategies for benefits realisation and risk management. Interdependencies between initiatives that may constrain the sequence in which they may be implemented should be identified. As more details of the proposed initiatives become clearer, the ICT strategic vision and ICT requirements may need to be revised (in consultation with relevant stakeholders).

Normally, more candidate initiatives are identified than can be realistically commenced – requiring priorities to be set and some initiatives to be deferred for future consideration. To make this selection in a logical, consistent, transparent way and produce an ICT program that meets organisational needs, prioritisation criteria should be developed and documented based on the ICT strategic vision. Having set the prioritisation criteria, the initiatives to be recommended in the strategic ICT plan are selected by applying the agreed criteria to weigh up the strengths and weaknesses of each initiative.

In concluding the planning process, a final draft of the ICT strategic plan (along with supporting appendices) is prepared and presented to the steering committee for review, comment and acceptance. Review by the steering committee provides an opportunity to secure buy-in from other executives, clinicians and business managers, whose support will be critical to successful implementation of the proposed initiatives and the realisation of benefits.

Stage 5 – Activate the ICT strategic plan

When complete and fully endorsed by the project steering committee, the final draft of the ICT strategic plan is formally presented to executive management (or the organisation's governing body) to obtain final approval for its acceptance, activation and implementation. Once the ICT strategic plan has been approved by the organisation, a summary of its key elements should be prepared and communicated throughout the organisation and to relevant external stakeholders.

Enterprise ICT architectures

Enterprise ICT architectures are designed to formally align the business mission, strategy, and processes of an organisation with its ICT strategy and underlying ICT activities to ensure that they meet broader operational needs and objectives. Contemporary ICT architectures encourage consistent approaches to ICT in an organisation, increasing opportunities for synergies and avoiding duplication and inconsistency.

Formal processes are fundamental to the development of enterprise ICT architectures, which use a series of models and views to depict how the current and future ICT needs of the organisation will be met. An enterprise ICT architecture should be closely aligned with an organisation's ICT strategic plan and may be developed either on its own or as part of the plan, but will usually require dedicated personnel to maintain it.

Interest box

John Zachman first promoted the term 'architecture' in relation to the planning of information systems in 1987. He noted the need for 'some logical construct (or architecture)' to define and control interfaces and integrate information systems and developed a framework for describing many different views of information systems. Use of the term 'architecture' became entrenched through the 1980s and 1990s as it was used widely by the ICT sector to describe any logical organisation of components.

The concept of enterprise ICT architecture (or 'Enterprise Architecture') has evolved from the 1996 Clinger-Cohen Act that required each United States government agency to have an 'Information Technology Architecture' to integrate the agency's IT activities with its strategic goals. In conjunction with these requirements the Federal Chief Information Officers (CIO) Council was established and, in turn, adopted the Federal Enterprise Architecture Framework (FEAF) through the Federal Enterprise Architecture Program Management Office (FEAPMO). Flowing on from these initiatives, various ICT planning consultants and software houses developed tools to support the modelling and reporting required by FEAF. More recently, the US E-Government Act of 2002 (Public Law 107–347) defined 'enterprise architecture' to mean:

> a strategic information asset base, which defines the [business] mission, the information necessary to perform the mission, the technologies necessary to perform the mission, and the transitional processes for implementing new technologies in response to changing needs and includes a baseline architecture, a target architecture and a sequencing plan.

Key components of traditional enterprise ICT architectures have included:
- Business architecture – an accurate representation of the organisation's business environment, strategy and critical success factors, supported by comprehensive documentation of organisation structure, functions and outputs, typically including hierarchical business process models.
- Application architecture (also known as functional architecture or services architecture) – providing views of the application systems and lower-level business services required to support the business mission and information needs of the organisation.
- Information architecture (or data architecture) – defining what information is needed by whom to accomplish the organisation's mission and modelling these information resources.
- Technology architecture – defining the technology services and standards needed to support the application portfolio of the business, and may include enterprise-wide standards and guidelines defining how software, hardware, network and communications products are to be used within the organisation.

The Zachman Framework[1] describes in considerable detail the different levels at which architectural views to support these architectures may be developed.

Continuing work by the Federal CIO Council and others has resulted in ever increasing maturity of enterprise architecture efforts across the commercial and government sector. By 2003, the CIO Council's emphasis had moved from compliance with the FEAF framework towards defining specific architectures for interchangeable service-based components to support government-wide interoperability and identifying initiatives for consolidation and reuse of business processes, systems, and technology.

Business architectures for ICT projects

The concepts used in the creation of an enterprise ICT architecture can also be applied in developing 'business architectures' for major ICT initiatives that cross the boundaries of organisations. An example is a national electronic health records (EHR) program, such as Australia's Health*Connect* Program (Commonwealth of Australia, 2004a).

The primary aim of the business architecture for an ICT project is to communicate the project's business concepts and requirements to various different stakeholder groups that need to understand the project and its impact on their work environments. At the more detailed level, the business architecture elaborates the business requirements through formal business models and an applications architecture, information architecture and technology architecture. These also provide technical specifications that can be used in acquisition and implementation.

The process of developing a business architecture for an ICT project is likely to involve the following types of activities, structured to the needs of the particular project:

- using discussion papers outlining the concepts, scope, benefits and implications of the project as the basis for consultation with stakeholders
- developing a context diagram and outlines describing major business processes and information flows
- identifying key dependencies, principles and policy issues for resolution – including management, legal, financial, socio-political and governance issues
- considering alternative approaches for achieving project outcomes
- identifying governance responsibilities for information resources and business processes during implementation and in production
- developing more detailed architectural models and views to define the project using enterprise ICT architecture principles
- producing an implementation strategy linked to the realisation of benefits.

Once the business requirements and supporting technology requirements have been defined, a high-level engineering design of the technical and systems aspects of the proposed solution (systems architecture) may help to confirm the technical feasibility and implications of the proposed initiatives.

An inherently important part of business architecture development is broad consultation with the stakeholder community before, during and after the preparation of the business architecture documentation.

ICT business cases

Of the various ICT planning artefacts discussed in this chapter, the ICT business case is the most important and certainly the one most commonly encountered in practice.

The business case is a self-contained document that clearly sets out the nature of a proposed ICT initiative and its justification, in order to facilitate approval by senior executives or the governing board of the organisation. Even where potential ICT initiatives have been identified through other ICT planning activities, a separate business case is usually required to authorise the financial investments and other resource commitments associated with the initiative.

While ICT expertise may be needed to define the proposed ICT solution and identify its expected cost, those who will be responsible for securing the benefits from an ICT initiative should endorse it to signify their commitment to achieving the proposed outcomes.

A sample outline of the contents for an ICT business case is presented in Figure 8.5.

Figure 8.5: Sample outline for an ICT business case

---

1. **Executive summary**
   - ✓ Overview of project proposal
   - ✓ Summary of benefits   ✓ Cash flow
   - ✓ Summary of economic analysis and business justification

2. **Business impact of the proposal**
   - ✓ Support for business strategies, directions and policies
   - ✓ Links to other ICT initiatives   ✓ Stakeholder involvement
   - ✓ Capacity to undertake the project
   - ✓ Suitability of proposed ICT directions

3. **Background**
   - ✓ Introduction   ✓ Drivers for change
   - ✓ Overview of current situation
   - ✓ Future trends, service requirements and growth factors
   - ✓ The case for change – status quo vs future vision

4. **Objectives of the proposed ICT initiative**
   - ✓ Purpose and scope   ✓ Objectives, outcomes and benefits

5. **Project implementation responsibilities**
   - ✓ Project management   ✓ Ownership and sponsorship
   - ✓ Implementation plan   ✓ Change management
   - ✓ Monitoring of project outcomes and benefits realisation

6. **Outline of alternative options considered**
   Sets out options considered and describes the relevant differentiating factors. The impact of rejecting the proposed course of action should also be canvassed.

7. **Details of cost/benefit analysis and economic appraisal**
   - ✓ Financial summary (over say 5 years separately identifying operating savings, capital costs, operating costs, returns)
   - ✓ Detailed financial analysis for Option A, Option B etc., including details of cost factors and modelling assumptions.
   - ✓ Other (qualitative) benefits from the initiative

Appendix A – Benefits realisation register

Appendix B – Draft implementation plan

Appendix C – Issues register

Appendix D – Risk management schedule

Many larger organisations have policies regarding the content and presentation of ICT business cases and their timing relative to the organisation's regular budget cycle – where these policies exist, they must be followed.

The hallmark of a successful business case is its ability to communicate clearly and efficiently – it must inform, persuade and not confuse the lay reader. Business cases rarely succeed on the power of their logic and presentation alone – they must also have credibility – and must therefore be thoroughly checked to remove obvious errors and inaccuracies.

ICT business cases should commence with an executive summary succinctly setting out the nature of the proposed ICT initiative, its proposed benefits and the investments required, along with any other significant considerations. The executive summary should not exceed two pages of normal typescript.

The main body of the business case, which should not usually exceed twenty-five pages (excluding appendices), provides more detailed material about the initiative, how the proposed benefits will be realised, the costs and how they were estimated, the principal alternatives considered and the reasons for selecting the proposed approach.

Where investment in an ICT initiative will not pay for itself in direct savings, it is particularly important that the business rationale for making the investment is clearly made out. As a general rule, improvements in productivity may be included in an analysis of economic benefits, but should not be claimed as hard savings unless achievable offsets can definitely be demonstrated.

The business case should also include measures against which the progress and success of the proposed initiative can be measured.

When submitted for approval, particularly if it represents a substantial financial outlay, the business case may be referred to an independent review process, such as a value management study following AS/NZS 4183 (Standards Australia, 1994).

Conclusion

The health informatician has a key role to play in realising the full potential of ICT capabilities in health organisations but needs to understand and be able to exploit sound ICT planning processes as part of this role.

Review questions

1.   You are considering accepting an appointment as the health informatics manager for a health service. What questions might you consider asking about the organisation's ICT plans and architectures?

2.   As a senior health service executive, you have received a stand-alone business case from a major specialist unit seeking to implement a software application widely used in similar units overseas to provide comprehensive patient records and clinical decision support for the specialist unit. What ICT planning and architecture issues are raised by this request? What steps might you take to deal with the situation?

Exercise

Summarise in point form the topics to be covered in consultancy briefs for:

- an ICT Strategic planning study for a major health service

- a business case for a health informatics initiative, and

- a post-implementation review of a electronic health records (EHR) system.

(You may find documents retrieved via web searches helpful.)

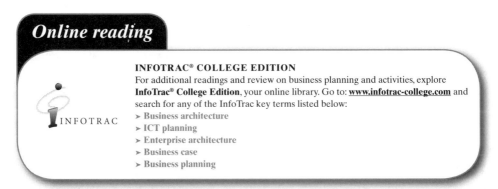

Online reading

INFOTRAC® COLLEGE EDITION
For additional readings and review on business planning and activities, explore **InfoTrac® College Edition**, your online library. Go to: **www.infotrac-college.com** and search for any of the InfoTrac key terms listed below:
- ➤ Business architecture
- ➤ ICT planning
- ➤ Enterprise architecture
- ➤ Business case
- ➤ Business planning

References

Commonwealth of Australia (2004a). *HealthConnect business architecture. Version 1.9*. Canberra. ISBN 0 642 82571 8.

Commonwealth of Australia (2004b). *HealthConnect business architecture Version 1.9: Specification of HealthConnect business requirements*, Canberra. ISBN 0 642 82572 6.

Department of Commerce (2005). *IM&T blueprint*, Government Chief Information Office, New South Wales. Retrieved 2 July 2005 from http://www.gcio.nsw.gov.au/.

New South Wales Premier's Department (1992). *Management of information technology statements of best practice*, Office of Public Management, Sydney.

Standards Australia. (1994). *Australian standard AS/NZS 4183:1994 – value management*, Standards Australia, Sydney.

United States Department of Defense (1999). *Information management (IM) strategic plan: information superiority. Version 2.0*. Retrieved 2 July, 2005, from http://www.defenselink.mil/nii/.

Ward J., Griffiths, P.M. (1996) *Strategic planning for information systems*, John Wiley & Sons, Chichester.

Zachman, J. (1987). A framework for information systems architecture, *IBM Systems Journal* 26(3), 276–92.

Endnote

[1]   Summarised on the website http://www.the-process-improver.com/support-files/zachman-clear.pdf.

9

Project management

Anyes Marsault

'The most successful project managers have perfected the skill of being comfortable being uncomfortable.'

(Anonymous)

Outline

The importance of project management as a function for health informaticians is reflected by the inclusion of project management training in most heath informatics programs offered by Australian universities (Soar, Sara, & Marsault, 2002). This chapter presents essential aspects of the discipline of project management.

Introduction

A large majority of business endeavours and strategies are implemented through projects. The project management approach is relatively modern and originated from the defence and aerospace industries in response to greater complexity in technology. Modern organisations have adopted various structures depending on their particular need to use project management. These include the more traditional structures that organise work around functions, matrix structures where both functional and project work are accommodated, or projectised structures (high project orientation) where all business activities are organised around projects and project managers have a high level of authority.

The anatomy of a project

The Project Management Institute (PMI) offers the following definition, which is widely accepted in the business community: 'A project is a temporary endeavour undertaken to create a unique product or service' (PMI, 2000).

Clarification

Temporary: the project has a beginning and an end. These time boundaries distinguish projects from other operational activities that tend to be ongoing. However, temporary should not be confused for duration. Some projects may be short while others may last several years. Temporary does not mean that the product or service created as a result of the project is temporary. Generally, while the project is temporary, the product may last for a very long time.

Unique: each project will deliver something that has not been done before. Although some projects may be very similar to one another (building a hospital), each project delivers something unique (each hospital is unique and each hospital construction project is unique).

According to the PMI, another feature that characterises and distinguishes projects is that they are 'progressively elaborated' (PMI, 2000) because the product of the service created is unique. This means that not all may be known about the project from the onset and the product or service needs to be progressively elaborated throughout its course. Because of this, projects generally carry risks. For instance, a patient administration system is developed over several months or years, but there is a risk that the new system will not be fully accepted by users. Other characteristics of a project include the need to sequence activities and the limited availability of resources (money and people). Generally in larger organisations undertaking many projects, these are grouped into programs that fit under the organisation's strategic plan.

Programs are defined as a collection of projects managed in a coordinated way to obtain benefits not available from managing them individually. For example, in Australia, Health Online is the national health information strategy. Health*Connect* is a large collection of projects across states and territories and therefore can be considered as a program rather than a project.

Key concepts in project management

The fact that projects have finite resources, most frequently time and budget, is represented through the well-known concept of the triple constraint (see Figure 9.1). The term is used to describe the key project *objectives* that must be simultaneously accomplished – scope, time and budget – while ensuring that customer expectations are met. Changing one of these three elements will impact on at least one if not both of the other items. For instance, increasing the scope of the project (like increasing the number of beds in a hospital) will most likely result in both increased costs and duration.

As projects evolve, trade offs between these three dimensions are almost always necessary and it is the role of the project manager to present options to management to facilitate decision-making about trade offs. Management should set the priority for each of these components, which the project manager uses to plan the project, evaluate the impact of change, and bring the project to completion.

Figure 9.1: The triple constraint

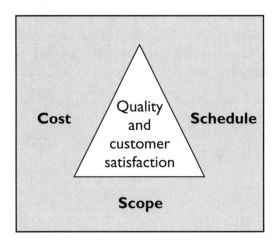

The essence of project management

Project management is the application of knowledge, skills, tools and techniques to project activities to meet project requirements (PMI, 2000). It can be organised around five phases that represent the project life cycle: initiating, planning, executing, controlling and closing. It is important to note that these phases are not discrete and may overlap during the course of the project. Figure 9.2 illustrates the controlling function that continues throughout the project to ensure that it stays on track.

Initiating – the project is officially sanctioned, a project sponsor identified and a project manager assigned; in addition:

- project goals and deliverables are identified
- a budget is defined
- performance criteria are selected
- constraints, assumptions and risks are identified and documented
- resource requirements are sized.

This information is often presented in a key document called the project charter.

Planning – the project objectives, scope, and estimates schedules are refined and the best courses of action to achieve the project's objectives selected (e.g. in house versus procurement):

- the project's control framework is also established
- a key output of this phase is the *project plan*.

The project plan is vital to guide project execution because it facilitates communication among stakeholders and documents the project scope, assumptions, and risks. It also provides a baseline for progress measurement and control.

The project schedule however, should not be confused with the project plan. Instead of the comprehensive document outlined above, the project schedule is only one element developed during the planning phase and incorporated into the project plan. It identifies the project start, completion dates and timeline for accomplishing the work.

Executing – the project manager coordinates people and other resources to implement the project plan. The product or service is created; most of the project budget is generally spent during this stage.

Controlling – measures and monitors the performance of the project to ensure it stays on track. Figure 9.2 demonstrates how controlling activities take place throughout the life of the project at a fairly constant rate. Key aspects of controlling are variance analysis, in particular of time and costs, and the identification of preventative and/or corrective action, as well as change control.

Closing – the final phase of the project life cycle where the client formally accepts and the project is closed from an administrative point of view (for example, when the project information is archived). Documenting the lessons learned is important here because it enables the knowledge and experience gained to be integrated into the planning of future projects.

Figure 9.2: Overlap of process groups during the project life cycle (PMI-PMBOK, 2000)

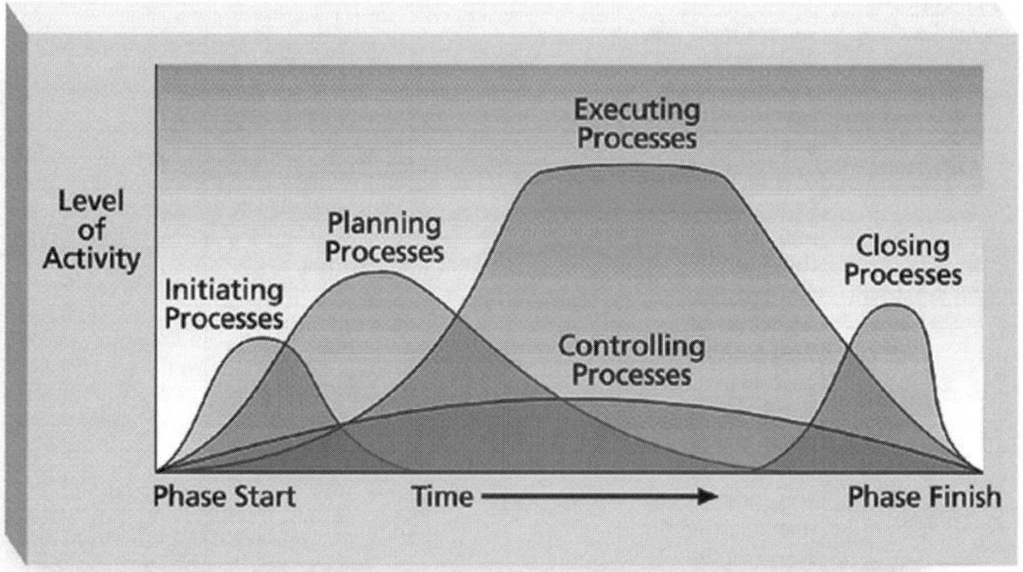

(Reprinted with permission from PMI)

Summarising the project management process

Table 9.1: Project management at a glance – key tasks for each phase

INITIATION (Concept)	PLANNING (Development)	EXECUTION (Implementation)	CONTROL	CLOSE-OUT (Termination) (Finishing)
Select project	Create scope statement and scope management plan	Execute the project plan	Integrated change control	Procurement audits
Determine project objectives	Determine project team	Manage project progress	Project performance reporting	Product verification
Determine high level deliverables, time and cost estimates	Create work breakdown structure	Complete work packages or tasks	Performance reporting	Formal acceptance
Determine high level constraints and assumptions	Finalise the team and create resource management plan	Distribute information	Scope change control	Lessons learned
Determine business need	Create WBS dictionary	Quality assurance	Quality control	Update records
Develop product description				
Define responsibilities of the project manager	Create network diagram	Team development	Risk monitoring and control	Archive records
Determine high-level resource requirements	Estimate time and costs	Progress meetings	Schedule control	Release resources
Finalise project charter	Determine critical path		Cost control	
	Develop schedule and schedule management plan		Scope verification	
	Develop budget		Manage by exception to the project plan	
	Create communications management plan		Ensure compliance with plans	
	Create quality management plan		Reassess plans	
	Risk management planning, identification, qualification, quantification and response planning		Take corrective action	
	Create procurement management plan			
	Create stakeholder management plan			
	Create project control plan			
	Develop formal project plan			
	Gain formal project plan approval			
	Hold kickoff meeting			

The project management framework

The Project Management Institute (PMI) develops practice standards for the project management profession. It has articulated an internationally recognised project management framework that has been endorsed by the Australian Institute of Project Management in consultation with industry. It comes under the auspices of the Australian National Training Authority (ANTA, 2004). The framework identifies the following nine key aspects of project management that take place during the project life cycle.

1. Integration management

Integration management ensures that the elements of the project are properly coordinated and take place throughout the project life cycle. It incorporates, or acts as the glue for, the other processes. The project manager carries out most of the activities involved here because they generally understand the project's 'big picture'. The key activities include the:

- integration of all elements (scope, cost, time, team, quality, control) into a coherent project plan
- coordination between the various teams and elements of the project to create the product
- the management of changes across the project, during its life.

2. Scope management

Scope management describes the activities required to ensure that the project is restricted to the work needed to complete it successfully. This is critical, as scope issues such as incompleteness, inadequacy and superfluousness are common reasons for project failure and rework. The project manager needs to define, control and verify the scope to obtain formal acceptance by the client. Some key activities includes the:

- development of a work breakdown structure (WBS) that takes place during the planning phase. The WBS is a key element of scope management because it organises the total scope of the project in deliverable oriented groupings (see Figure 9.3)
- development of a scope management plan that describes the management of the scope and how scopes changes will be integrated into the project. This is also done in the planning phase
- customer agreeing that the scope is acceptable.

The difference between product and project scope must be clarified. The product scope refers to the features and functions that characterise a product or service, while the project scope is the work required to deliver the product with the specifications and functions required, such as designing, testing and implementing software.

Figure 9. 3: The work breakdown structure

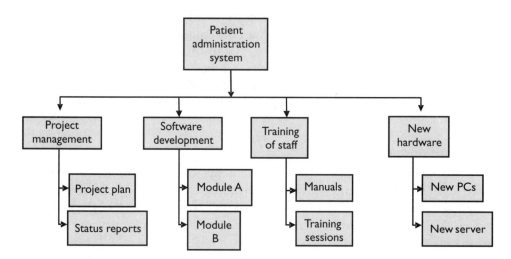

3. Time management

Time management describes the activities necessary to ensure that the project is delivered in a timely fashion. Starting from the WBS, the tasks required to produce the deliverables are identified, sequenced, durations estimated and dependencies incorporated to construct a 'realistic' project schedule. The project manager administers that schedule, measuring progress and managing changes as they arise. Many use some form of scheduling software to assist with these tasks. Key activities of project time management include:

- *Schedule development* – preparing activity lists and network diagrams, preparing time estimates, calculating the critical path, identifying ways to compress the schedule using techniques such as crashing or fast tracking the schedule if the project needs a shorter timeframe.
- *Schedule control* – monitoring schedule progress through performance measurement techniques, ranging from simple variance analysis to more sophisticated earned value management. This is an important activity of project control and is often the largest challenge. Unrealistic schedules are a major cause of project failures.

4. Cost management

Cost management describes the activities necessary to ensure that the project is delivered within the approved budget. This involves:

- *Cost planning*, which deals with planning and costing resources (staff, equipment, internal and external resources) as accurately as possible to develop a 'realistic' project budget while meetings project objectives. Costs include labour, material, third party services, travel, facilities expenses and so forth. Cost planning culminates in the production of a project cost baseline.

- *Cost control* which is concerned with controlling cost variations and managing these changes. Earned value management can be used to predict final project costs. Cost control can be difficult for project managers when projects run significantly over budget due to poor time and cost planning.

Some cost estimation techniques include:
- top-down estimation where a previous, similar project is used as the basis for estimating costs. This is less costly but often less accurate
- bottom-up estimation where individual activities are estimated then aggregated into a total project cost. This technique is more accurate but more costly as it takes longer
- parametric modelling, which involves using some specific quantitative parameters in a mathematical model to predict project costs (e.g., cost of square metre to estimate the costs of building a new hospital).

5. Quality management

Quality management describes the activities necessary to ensure that the project will satisfy the needs for which it was undertaken and the product created conforms to requirements and fitness of use. Achieving quality requires:
- planning for quality from the onset of the project, setting relevant quality standards and determining how to satisfy them. Techniques such as cost/benefit analyses are useful to guide decision about quality.
- conducting quality assurance during the course of the project to ensure that all quality activities are carried out. Quality audits or structured review of quality management activities are commonly used techniques
- undertaking quality control to verify that the work results satisfy the relevant quality standards or to identify necessary rework. Quality control techniques in software development for example, include code walkthroughs, code inspections, testing, control charts, and statistical sampling.

6. Human resource management

Human resource management makes the most effective use of people involved in the project. This involves planning which people to involve, how to secure them and how to develop the team. Clear definitions of roles and responsibilities are important as project structures become more complex, and because this is also a chief complaint of project team members.

A crucial activity to ensure role clarity is the 'kick off meeting', because it is generally the first time the project team meets and it presents the ideal opportunity for the project manager to gain commitment from the team. As part of resource management the project manager exercises many generic management skills such as leading, communicating, negotiating, delegating, motivating, coaching, mentoring, team building, and managing conflicts, to keep the project on course.

7. Communication management

Communication management ensures timely and appropriate generation, collection, dissemination, storage and the ultimate disposition of project information.

Communication is crucial to the project's final outcome. Project managers must keep all stakeholders informed and involved throughout the project, especially during the initiation and planning phases where they can most influence the project. Project communication management involves:
- developing a communication plan that states what information will be communicated, when, how and to whom
- information distribution ensuring that people have the necessary information throughout the project
- effective performance reporting that adheres to specific formats is essential. Project status meetings and reports are key tools to communicate progress of the project.
- administrative closure or archiving project information that must be carefully undertaken to ensure access to lessons learned and other information for use in future projects.

8. Risk management

Risk management is the systematic process of identifying, analysing and responding to project risks to minimising the probability or consequences of adverse events to the project objectives. Managing risk is essential because failure to identify high-level risks and to manage them can have disastrous impacts on the project. Good risk management is rare and is not simply completing a list, as many project managers assume; for this reason Chapter 10 is dedicated to risk management and only a short outline from the PMI is offered here.

The PMI (2000) report the following activities in project risk management:
- management planning that involves deciding how to approach and plan risk management activities
- identifying the risks that might exist
- analysis (qualitative or quantitative) that measures the likelihood of occurrence and consequence if the risk eventuates
- response planning or deciding how to minimise the probability of occurrence (mitigation strategy) or to minimise the impact of the risk (contingency strategy) in the event that it occurs
- monitoring and controls in which risks and risk responses are reviewed throughout the project life cycle.

9. Procurement management

Procurement management describes the processes required to acquire goods and services from outside the organisation. The key processes involved here are:
- procurement planning or what to procure and when
- solicitation planning that identifies requirements and potential sources
- solicitation where quotations, bids, offers, requests for information and so on are sought from potential suppliers
- source selection or selecting a potential supplier
- contract administration where the contract between the supplier and buyer is managed
- contract close-out where the contract is completed and settled.

Roles, skills and standards for practice

Project management in complex settings such as healthcare is a challenge because of numerous stakeholders' views and often, competing interests. The project manager bonds the project and acts as the catalyst for action. An efficient project manager must be multi-skilled and an effective

- *leader* who can establish direction and motivate the team to achieve the vision using team building skills to energise the project team
- *communicator* who can engage with a wide range of stakeholders (client, team members, vendors etc.) with varying formal and informal communication needs
- *negotiator* who can liaise with many different stakeholders who have individual perspectives of the project. It is critical that all stakeholders are involved during the project's planning phase, and that buy-in is achieved to avoid dissatisfaction during subsequent phases, when changes are more difficult to accommodate. Conflict resolution skills are essential to achieve positive outcomes if a conflict arises between the stakeholders
- *problem solver* who can resolve problems to keep the project in good health
- *influencer* who can quickly identify the formal and informal project structures (internal, external) and the 'politics' to influence people for the benefit of the project and increase its ability to meet the desired objectives
- *organiser and administrator* who can coordinate as this is a key aspect as are administrative skills such as budgeting.

While project management principles are applicable across industries, the project manager needs sufficient technical knowledge about the industry. Consider the difficulties in replacing a construction industry project manager with a project manager from the information technology (IT) industry. Wide-ranging skills are required because just as projects vary in size and complexity so does the work of project management. Large complex projects, often the norm in health IT projects, require very highly skilled project managers. These skills are acquired through training and experience over many years.

Project management is an emerging discipline and often IT project managers have no formal project management training. PMI recognised the need for greater professionalism and initiated a project management certification program in 1984 (Ebusiness, 2005). Today the Project Management Professional (PMP®) certification is internationally recognised. In 2004, some 95 187 project managers worldwide were certified PMP® with approximately 300 in Australia (PMI, 2004).

PMI (2000) have also developed standards for project management professionals that focus on the ethical aspects of the profession. These include:

- ensuring individual integrity
- contributing to the project management knowledge base
- enhancing individual competence
- balancing stakeholders' interests
- interacting with team and stakeholders in a professional and cooperative manner.

Other key roles in project management

While PMI stresses that each stakeholder has skills and knowledge that may be useful in developing the project plan some roles are particularly important (PMI, 2000). These include:

- the project *sponsor* who provides financial resources and is the project champion. Many projects fail miserably without a sponsor capable of marketing the project within the organisation.
- the *customer* is the person or organisation for whom the product is made and has a key role during the life of the project. The customer accepts the final product/service as part of the scope verification process and may or may not be the project sponsor.
- the project *team members* are the people most involved with the project and who report either directly or indirectly to the project manager. Their ability to deliver the product is a major influence on the success of the project.

Why projects fail

Statistics on project management are sobering. Most projects fail to meet time and budget goals and many completed projects fall short of fulfilling their business expectations (Shenhar, 2004). A recent study by the Standish Group International estimated that 88 per cent of information technology projects in healthcare and other industries run either over schedule or over budget (Health Data Management, 2003).

There is a plethora of literature in relation to project failure (Charvat, 2003; Heldman, 2005; Kerzner, 2003) and the most frequently cited factors include:

- inadequate project definition and planning (poor scope definition, poor estimate, unrealistic schedule, poor resource requirements)
- lack of project sponsorship
- lack of good project management, not managing the project plan
- failure to understand that a change in scope affects schedule, cost or performance
- failure to involve the project team in planning
- mistaking a project schedule for a project plan
- inexperience in project management
- poor communication in particular with clients or users
- poor risk management
- inadequate change control (scope creep, poor configuration management)
- lack of quality management.

Why projects succeed

Because of relatively poor project outcomes, project managers and researchers identified factors that may influence project success (Kerzner, 2003; Pinto & Rouhiainen, 2001). Success most commonly was due to:

- unequivocal sponsorship and executive management support
- establishing project success criteria
- user involvement
- clear understanding and statement of requirements

- effective planning (making and documenting a realistic plan)
- clear roles and responsibilities
- realistic expectations
- good risk management
- tracking progress
- good change control.

Information box
Rita Mulcahy's (n.d.) Tricks of the trade™
Nine strategies to improve projects –
1. Support the creation of historical records.
2. Provide a project charter with clear goals and objectives.
3. Protect projects from outside influences, changes and resource stealing.
4. Allow teams enough time to properly plan projects.
5. Ensure finalised scope of work before the project starts.
6. Prioritise projects within a company or department.
7. Require proper project management to be done.
8. Do not run at 100 per cent capacity.
9. (Remember) you cannot get something for nothing.

Project management in health informatics

Health IT projects are often characterised by their complexity and large number of stakeholders with differing perspectives and objectives. Modern project management methods appear well suited to these projects and can greatly assist in improving project outcomes. While project management methods can apply across sectors, each sector has its own particularities and healthcare is no different. Dwyer, Stanton and Thiessen, (2004) and Belassi and Tukel (1996) have produced three categories of factors that are specific to healthcare projects.

1. Sector factors

Sector factors set the scene against which projects happen.
- Funding organisations (which are largely public in health) have a major impact on the project portfolios of health organisations because they can dictate which projects are needed. This means that funding bodies may limit the strategic choice of organisations resulting in projects misaligned to the organisation's strategic direction.
- The 'public good ethos' impacts on the ability to make effective decisions as it often translates into projects with commendable but unachievable goals.
- Healthcare has multiple, diverse stakeholders described earlier. This increases the complexity of managing stakeholder groups throughout the life of the project. Health projects are frequently concerned with change (for example in service delivery, roles or work processes) and the ability to manage this and gain acceptance by stakeholders is a challenge generally underestimated.

2. Organisational factors

Organisational factors have a direct impact on the organisation's project management capability and therefore project success or failure. They include:

- Organisational cultures unsupportive of a clear, strong, unified strategic direction as they inhibit the alignment between organisational goals and project goals. Health organisations employ highly skilled and high status professionals who often have vastly differing views on the strategic direction of the organisation.
- Traditional functional structures that do not support modern project management methods. Increased project success has been found in projectised structures where staff are dedicated to the project (Alsene, 1998).
- The ability of organisations to develop a project management culture as it increases the ability for projects to succeed.
- The ability of the organisation to successfully deliver projects as it depends on staff expertise in project management. This may mean developing and training staff as professional project managers.

3. Project factors

Project factors are directly related to the project. Dwyer, Stanton and Thiessen (2004) found similarities between the project success factors in health and those of general project management literature, which suggests that good project management is the key.

Conclusion

The emerging discipline of project management and its application to health informatics is relatively new despite the prevalence of projects in modern health organisations. The project manager significantly increases the likelihood of delivering what the project set out to achieve, by using key project management principles to orchestrate the project life cycle (initiating, planning, execution, controlling and closing). The PMI framework for project management is comprehensive and represents a key foundation for the discipline.

Traditional approaches to project management that have focused on controlling scope, time and budget are being augmented by contemporary approaches that focus on customer satisfaction. This is redefining the project manager function with greater emphasis on the soft skills of people management to deal effectively with customers, staff and other stakeholders. Furthermore, as the business environment is increasing in complexity, projects are also becoming more complex. To carry out project management in these more challenging settings and with the view to increase project success, organisations are now commonly appointing professionally qualified project managers.

Project complexity is evident in the health sector. The initial project start up is often difficult due to large numbers of competing options. Stakeholder management is often highly challenging due to the variety of stakeholders, some with significant power, and their differing perspectives and agendas. Technical complexity is often present due to the complex nature of healthcare delivery. However, sound project management practices supported by appropriate organisational structure and culture can greatly assist improving project outcomes.

Review questions

1. Discuss the human factors in project management.
2. What are the key components of project management?
3. Why is project management so important in health informatics?

Exercise

*   Develop a table of contents for a project plan.

Online reading

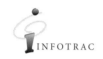

INFOTRAC® COLLEGE EDITION

For additional readings and review on project management, explore **InfoTrac® College Edition**, your online library. Go to: **www.infotrac-college.com** and search for any of the InfoTrac key terms listed below:

➤ Project management
➤ Project framework
➤ Project management roles

References

Alsene, E, (1998). Internal changes in project management structures within enterprises, *International Journal of Project Management* 14(3) 131–6.

Australian National Training Authority (ANTA) (2004). *National competency standards for project management (NCSPM)*. Retrieved 21 February, 2005, from http://www.ntis. gov.au.

Belassi, W. & Tukel, O. (1996). A new framework for determining critical success/failure factors in projects, *International Journal of Project Management* 14(3), 131–6.

Charvat, J. (2003). *Project management methodologies: selecting, implementing, and supporting methodologies and processes for projects*, John Wiley & Sons, New York.

Dwyer, J., Stanton, P. & Thiessen, V. (2004). *Project management in health and community services: getting good ideas to work*, Routledge, London.

Ebusiness (2005). *Project management history*. Retrieved 21 February, 2005, from http:// ebusiness.insightin.com/project_management/history.html.

Health Data Management (2003). *Statistics on project success in health*. Retrieved 15 March, 2005, from http://www.healthdatamanagement.com.

Heldman, K. (2005). *Project manager's spotlight on risk management*, Sybex, San Francisco.

Kerzner, H, (2003). *Project management: a systems approach to planning, scheduling, and controlling*, 8th edn, John Wiley & Sons, Hoboken.

Microsoft (1998). *A history of project management.* Retrieved 10 March, 2005, from http://www.microsoft.com/.

Mulcahy, R, (n.d.). *Tricks of the trade*. Retrieved 2 June, 2005, from http://www.rmcproject.com/.

Pinto, J.K. & Rouhiainen, P.J. (2001). *Building customer-based organizations,* John Wiley & Sons, New York.

Project Management Institute (2000). *A guide to the project management body of knowledge* PMBOK. Retrieved 10 March, 2005, from http://www.pmi.org/.

Project Management Institute (2005). Retrieved 10 March, 2005, from http://www.pmi.org/.

Project Management Institute (2004). *Today statistics.* Retrieved 31 October, 2005, from http://www.pmi.org/.

Shenhar, A. (2004). *Project management evolution: past history and future research directions*, PMI Research Conference, London, UK.

Soar, J., Sara, T. & Marsault, A. (2002). *Health informatics education project*, Commonwealth of Australia, Canberra.

10

Risk management

Malcolm Pradhan

'Risk varies inversely with knowledge'

(Irving Fisher, 1930)

Outline

Health informatics projects and implementations are inherently risky and prone to failure. This chapter discusses some of the factors that contribute to the precarious nature of informatics projects, how to manage these risks and, more importantly, how to manage client expectations to achieve a satisfactory outcome.

Introduction

Healthcare environments exhibit three characteristics that project managers hate: complexity, chaos and culture. Successfully delivering the stated goals of a health informatics project requires the right people, a bit of luck, and a keen understanding of where problems may arise. In other chapters you have learned how to manage a project (Marsault, Chapter 9); you will know by now if you are blessed with the required good fortune. All that is left is to understand how to manage risks in health informatics implementations.

You are about to embark on a health informatics project armed with some great ideas and a careful project plan. What could go wrong? Unfortunately, the odds of success are against you – success being defined as a project delivered on time, on budget and meeting client expectations.

(OASIG, 1995)

Health informatics – a risky business

Health is a difficult industry in which to implement any changes whatsoever, and information technology (IT) projects in particular. There is a long list of common sources of risk for IT and change management projects, including development risks, scope management, configuration management, useability and so on. However, health informatics projects have a few areas of risk that are amplified compared to other industries, and these will be discussed in this section. How to manage the risks will be discussed later in this chapter.

The challenge of requirements

A significant risk in health informatics projects is the problem of requirements. A requirement is a clearly defined specification by users for the functionality of a system. The prevailing view of IT project management is that the correct requirements generate the correct solution, and consequently changing requirements after a project is underway is a major project risk.

The bad news for health informatics implementations is that, in health, generating a final set of requirements is very difficult – particularly in clinical projects that interface with multiple clinical staff. Experience in developing and implementing software in healthcare has shown that *clinical staff generally do not know what they want, but they certainly know what they do not like*. This is not due to any conscious duplicity by clinical staff, but a manifestation of the fact that it is very hard for clinical staff to fully envision the impact of a future IT system on a complex and chaotic work environment.

The changing nature of healthcare almost ensures that a system specified today will require modifications in the future. Examples of factors that make healthcare a dynamic environment include (a) faster uptake of new medical knowledge as a consequence of evidence-based medicine, (b) the introduction of new medical technology such as bedside testing, new treatments and imaging modalities, (c) business process redesign in hospitals aimed at improving patient flows, and (d) increasing interactions between GPs, community service providers, and hospitals to provide more care outside of the hospital system.

Culture and workforce restrictions

The strong influence of 'culture' within healthcare is often discussed. 'Culture' in this context is used to describe prevailing attitudes within a work environment. Examples of cultural factors may include attitudes between disciplines (for example, nurses and doctors), views on compliance to management directives, and attitudes to information technology. Cultural issues can be a significant barrier if it is not recognised that implementations have to be sensitive to these factors and the presentation of the project must be sensitive to the local culture.

A related challenge is the issue of workforce restrictions, which are essentially bad attitudes enshrined in a workplace agreement. Managing workforce restrictions is often a case of avoiding the problem by providing enough benefits to the target users.

Infrastructure variations, reliability and access

Healthcare suffers a chronic under-investment in IT. This has resulted in a heterogenous and often unreliable IT infrastructure throughout the healthcare system. In recent years certain standards have become adopted widely, such as HL7 in the hospital system. However, because of the lack of funding and support each hospital has had to implement the standard in their often unique IT systems. Consequently, many hospitals have slightly different implementations of HL7. It is worth keeping in mind that most of the healthcare infrastructure was designed to duplicate paper processes and not necessarily facilitate communication between heterogenous systems. These aspects of healthcare IT infrastructure increase significantly the *integration risk* of the project.

General practice has received practice incentive programs (or PIPs as they are affectionately known) to purchase IT systems, but often these have not been enough to generate market competition in general practice IT, and hence innovation in IT systems has been low. The reliability of IT in health is another symptom of the general under-funding of infrastructure. IT infrastructure in hospitals and GP practice are simply not designed to be fault-tolerant, high reliability 24 x 7 systems. Numerous states in Australia, such as New South Wales, Victoria and Western Australia, are beginning to invest in centralised infrastructures for core data systems for each of their public hospital systems.

These efforts will result in improvements in standards compliance and reliability, but increased centralisation can potentially result in greater administrative barriers to innovative health informatics projects that integrate with the infrastructure; this has been the case in South Australia where five years after deployment, there is yet to be a single non-government project that uses the state's centralised IT data system.

Opportunities for training and change

In most industries staff training and change management are an integral part of IT implementations, and in most industries it is possible to schedule downtime or to remove workers from their environment for training. Training and change management are more problematic in healthcare – it is not easy to close a hospital or even a unit for training sessions or team building exercises for every new project. Consequently, healthcare relies on informal channels for change management and training. In hospitals, the situation is further exacerbated by the high turnover rate of clinical staff; in a large emergency department, for example, there may be as many as 150 doctors and students that move through the department in a twelve-month period. This is in stark contrast with non-health industries that have a relatively stable workforce.

Risk management principles

While risks in a project can be managed using ad hoc methods it is prudent to use established methods so we can take advantage of pre-existing work in the area, but also because it is important to manage projects in a way that is accepted in the industry. The frameworks available for risk management are useful tools for research projects, but in commercial projects a formal and documented approach to risk management also reduces the opportunities for conflict between the implementers and the customer.

In risk management a risk is defined as being an event that may cause a loss. This may be directly financial but may encompass any harm to the objectives of the project. Risk has two components:

1. What is the chance that the event will occur (the likelihood)?
2. What would be the loss if the event did occur (consequence)?

Formally, the likelihood is expressed in terms of *probability* and the consequence in some form of *utility* that may include money, quality of life, or some other real-valued measure of value (Keeney, 1996). Risks can be ranked by the *expected loss*, that is, the probability of the event in question multiplied by the loss. As we will see shortly, this numeric approach is unnecessarily complex for most projects and is rarely applied in risk management. Commonly, qualitative approaches to ranking risks are used as short cuts to applying risk management principles.

The Australian/New Zealand risk management framework

One of the most widely used frameworks for risk management is based on the Australian and New Zealand Risk Management Standard (Standards Australia and Standards New Zealand, 2004). This document states that 'Risk management involves managing to achieve an appropriate balance between realising opportunities for gains while minimising losses. It is an integral part of good management practice, an essential element of good corporate governance'.

The steps outlined in the Risk Management Standard (or 4360:2004 as it is affectionately known in the risk management community) can be summarised as follows:

- Establish the *context* of the project and identify the potential risks.
- *Analyse* the risks. For each risk identified estimate how likely it is to occur, what would be the consequences, what controls there are in place to mitigate the risk.
- *Evaluate* the risks and form a ranking. The ranked risks and their details are sometimes stored in a risk register (a database or spreadsheet) for all stakeholders to see and comment on.
- *Plan and control* for the risks. Put into place measures that will mitigate the risks if they arise, and communicate the risks to the stakeholders of the project.
- *Monitor and review*. As a project develops, the risks will change. The review process will keep the risk register up to date.

It is important to understand that the exercise of risk management is not simply a cataloguing process, but rather a process that should facilitate communication between the project team and stakeholders. The risk management process should lead to a greater understanding of how different stakeholders value particular aspects of the project.

For example, in a health informatics project the risk of software failure resulting in printing problems will require double entry of data; once in the computer to keep the IT system up to date, and then on paper for immediate reference. Consultants and senior staff may not find this to be a major issue, but for junior staff who are under significant time pressure, the extra work required for double entry may put them off engaging with the system completely. Different staff will often have significantly different values on potential outcomes.

What about risks that you cannot predict? Does the risk management framework just give us a false sense of security? Remember, risk management does not offer protection from risks; it helps to communicate potential risks and assists in managing them. Reading through a complete and accurate risk register of what could go wrong in a project generally increases stress rather than lulling the reader into a sense of security.

It is not possible to define accurately all possible risks for a project. The accuracy and completeness of risk identification will improve with experience in health informatics, and implies that lessons will be learned the hard way. If an unforseen event arises, then Step 2 of the risk management framework can commence: analyse, evaluate, plan and monitor. The risk management framework will assist in putting the new situation into perspective, communicating the problem to the stakeholders, identifying the ranking of the new problem, and developing a plan to reduce losses. The plan may also involve rescheduling the project plan.

Ranking risks

Potentially the most complex part of the risk management framework is the evaluation of risks required to create a priority ranking. It is not easy to establish a figure for the probability of an event, nor is it always easy to quantify the consequences of a possible event. To ease the evaluation process, the Risk Management Standard uses a qualitative risk grid as a fast method for evaluating risks. The risk grid comprises a table that maps the likelihood of an event against the magnitude of the consequences if that event were to occur (see Figure 10.1).

Figure 10.1: Risk grid (Standard Australia and Standard NZ, 2004)

Expected Consequences ▶					
Likelihood ▼	Insignificant	Minor	Moderate	Major	Catastrophic
Almost certain	High	High	Extreme	Extreme	Extreme
Likely	Moderate	High	High	Extreme	Extreme
Moderate	Low	Moderate	High	Extreme	Extreme
Unlikely	Low	Low	Moderate	High	Extreme
Rare	Low	Low	Moderate	High	High

Extreme	Extreme risk	Immediate action required
High	High risk	Senior management attention needed
Moderate	Moderate risk	Management responsibility must be specified
Low	Low risk	Manage by routine procedures

The danger of using qualitative terms to describe probabilities has long been documented (Wallsten, Budescu, Rapoport, Zwick & Forsyth, 1986), however the caveats of this approach are outweighed by the convenience of avoiding formal probability assessments. Once the risks have been assigned a priority, they can be ranked and addressed. In many projects the risks may require additional resources to manage, or some preliminary work to assess the true state of the risk. For example, because integration with existing IT systems is such a high risk in health informatics projects, some preliminary work may be done to assess the state of existing systems and their consistency before the project. Running workshops with the target intervention group before the project proposal is completed will enable a better understanding of the resource requirements to improve the project's acceptance.

Contingency

Many large commercial projects have a 'contingency' budget, usually 10–20 per cent of the implementation cost that can be used to mitigate risks during the project. It is not always possible to obtain a contingency budget in a grant situation; using a risk management framework and elaborating the risks in detail will assist in convincing other sources that a contingency is important, and that the budget will be tied into managing specific risks. The contingency budget is usually only used with the agreement of the project steering committee and is not part of the general implementation budget. Ideally, the project should not have to use the contingency budget. Keep in mind also that you cannot always buy your way out of a problem. Some events may require specific skills that cannot be easily scaled on demand, or rely on third parties' deliverables.

The conception-reality gap

While the risk management framework helps to identify and manage risks during a project implementation, it does not assist to determine if the project is simply too risky to start at all. Inspired by the high failure rate of IT projects in healthcare, the Institute for Development Policy and Management in the United Kingdom developed a method for determining the gap between the current state of a workplace, the 'reality', and the goals of the health informatics project, the 'conception'. The framework they propose is called ITPOSMO after the acronym that describes 'dimensions' that are used to measure the gap (Heeks, Mundy & Salazar, 1999). The dimensions described in this approach are:

- *information* needs that are to be met
- *technology* that must be introduced in the project compared to the existing technology in use
- *processes* that require change
- *objectives and values* of the users and the impact of the system upon these
- *staffing and skills* required to run the proposed system
- *management and structures* – will the project fit into the existing organisational structure?
- *other factors* such as maintenance and support.

The exact definitions of the dimensions are not of primary importance as they are really meant as prompts to consider a variety of factors involved in the success of a project. The ITPOSMO framework provides a method to quantify the gap and suggests that certain scores are high-risk projects that should not go ahead without modification. This approach is useful as a general risk management assessment without having to elaborate on specific risks for the project. If the gap between conception and reality is too high, then a project should be broken down into smaller, lower risk increments.

Managing specific risks in health informatics implementations

This section deals with the approaches that may be useful in managing specific risks that arise in health informatics implementations. Some of the background for the topics that are fundamental to implementations, such as project management, are presented in dedicated chapters.

Project structures and sponsors

Several authors in other chapters have used their preferred structures for health informatics projects. The one used here as ideal for risk management in health informatics projects comprises (a) a senior clinical sponsor who can drive the project through the layers of management, (b) a ground-level clinical champion, (c) a management sponsor, and (d) an IT champion and the necessity for this is reinforced in other chapters.

While the senior clinical sponsor is important to get the project underway, the clinical champion is pivotal to risk management providing key information on culture, attitudes, and expectations of the end users. The management sponsor is required to ensure the benefits of the project reach the appropriate people in the organisations, and that the business needs of the organisation have been addressed. Finally, an IT champion is someone who can get the system working within the healthcare infrastructure that is being targeted.

Stakeholder analysis and workflow analysis

Perhaps one of the most important risk reduction steps is a stakeholder analysis. This process requires a clear understanding of what each potential user of the system expects, and defines what benefits they will receive. The most important concern of staff in healthcare is time. If a system will incur more work for any group of users then they will fight against the project.

It is usually acceptable if the health informatics system requires more time for some tasks if the *benefits of time are realised by the same group of users* within a short period. In other words, if nurses are expected to enter data to save time for doctors, then the system will not be well received. Similarly, if a doctor does additional data entry to receive a time-win three days later on discharge, compliance may also be low. Benefits to the patient are only relevant to the patient. Other classes of users receive their own benefits from a system and these are often in decreased time to do existing work because workloads are a major problem in health. The problem is easy to quantify in general practice, where even small increases in time per patient result in fewer patients seen and therefore reduced income.

Understanding how to achieve benefits for stakeholders is closely related to understanding their workflow and identifying low-risk intervention points within the workflow. This may be as simple as placing an IT system in the right place where it will be convenient to use, or it may involve acknowledging that paper is a good technology to use in certain parts of the workflow (unlike computers, paper does not break when you drop it). Formal methods for workflow mapping (Pradhan, Edmonds & Runciman, 2001) may be useful to clearly understand the opportunities for delivering user benefits.

Requirements and project estimation

There has been a significant amount of research into why IT projects fail. A lengthy, but very readable summary of this work can be found in McConnell (1996). Research into project budget and time estimation has revealed, not surprisingly, that the more refined the requirements the better the estimation of the project time and budget (Laranjeira, 1990). Defining clearly the specification and requirements in health informatics is notoriously hard. If time estimates are out then it is likely the project will be behind schedule from an early stage. Related research has shown that programmers are very bad at estimating times for completion, and both output quality and estimation accuracy suffer as projects start to fail (Jones, 1994). So how do we avoid this spiral?

The only factor that can be controlled in a fixed budget and fixed level of quality is the number of features in the system, also known as project scope. Unfortunately, a common response to delayed projects is to promise more features as a way of compensation, which sets off another spiral of delays and poor quality.

A *feature register* is a method for controlling project scope when the requirements may change. The feature register should document each requirement as it arises, the importance of the feature to the users, which group of stakeholders it applies to, the risk of implementation (including inter-dependencies between software components), and the marginal cost of implementation. This technique requires a good relationship with the users and good communication to manage expectations. The feature register will present the implementers and the users with a ranked priority of features. It is an explicit way of trading-off features in the project while attempting to stay within budget, and allows the users to target additional funds to specific features if they fall below the cut-off for implementation.

Implementation and integration

The way in which projects are implemented can make a significant difference to whether the project succeeds or fails. In healthcare traditional methods of development, including the Rational Unified Process, are not ideally suited to refinement during the project. Newer development methodologies such as Extreme Programming (Beck, 1999) and Agile Development (Martin, 2002) present some interesting ideas on how to manage the development process in a *highly iterative* manner that is essential in health informatics projects.

Perhaps the most important design decision for projects is to use a *loosely coupled architecture* for software systems. Loosely coupled systems use standard methods of communication between software components, such as XML and Web Services. In a loosely coupled architecture, components communicate using XML messages to request *what* they want done, whereas tightly coupled systems must know *how* they want tasks completed using a series of method calls. The significant benefit of a loosely coupled architecture is that changes in one component do not cause instability through multiple other components, so changes are lower risk compared to tightly coupled systems.

An additional benefit to using XML and Web Services is that the XML family of standards provides highly efficient technologies to handle data mapping and validation, which are important when dealing with the variable data standards in healthcare. Integration with existing health IT infrastructure, such as HL7 messages and database queries, should be done well in advance of the final project plan to clearly identify the risks involved. There are a number of commercial and freely available tools that provide integration capabilities, and they each have their advantages and quirks.

Within the same hospital or healthcare organisation there may be different sources of data using different semantics within their systems, or interpreting standard terms in different ways. For example, often pathology systems and radiology systems use certain HL7 codes in different ways because these systems come from different vendors and the information was never designed to be integrated. It is best not to assume that a healthcare organisation's data systems are standardised or even compatible; it is best to conduct a risk assessment on each system individually and if possible access data on each system to test the data reliability, structure and speed.

Asking vendors to upgrade their tools to support a specific health informatics project can be expensive and can be a source of significant delays. These are risks that should be identified and managed prior to an implementation. Managerial champions and clout may be required to expedite the requests.

Clutching defeat from the jaws of victory

You have completed the project, the budget was only slightly over, the users love it – or at least they do not hate it – it is deemed a success, and all thanks to the skills you have learned in this chapter! Unfortunately there are some final risks that need to be managed when steering a project from pilot into full production.

Many of the post-implementation risks should be handled earlier in the project, but they are often ignored, particularly in research projects. The risks for the ongoing maintenance of a system should be defined clearly before the project starts. This can be an uncomfortable process because it may inspire managers to calculate the lifetime cost of the project, say over five years, rather than just the implementation cost, and the lifetime costs are always higher than everyone expects. The skills required to maintain the system over time may be specific and result in a risk for the organisation unless the system has been designed to be maintainable.

System reliability is also a significant concern that is not often addressed in pilot projects. Full testing and profiling take skill, time and effort and are often forgotten in a busy project. The costs for testing and bulletproofing a system may be quite significant compared to an initial prototype and often this is not part of the budget.

Finally, responsibilities for liability should be agreed with the healthcare organisation. If they require the project to be indemnified independently then the project cost may easily blow out. It is important to negotiate these factors prior to the project otherwise it may easily be assumed that the project is carrying complete indemnity.

Conclusion

The AS/NZS 4360:2004 Risk Management Framework is a well-accepted method for risk management and is understood by most government agencies in Australia and overseas. Creating and maintaining a good relationship with clients and users of a system is of utmost importance in health informatics because these projects are inherently multi-disciplinary and complex. Approaching projects as a team with explicit assumptions and clear communications is the only way to successfully navigate the many potential perils in health informatics implementations. If the team works well it can actually be enjoyable and rewarding.

Review questions

1.   Identify the steps in conducting a risk assessment.
2.   List and summarise each potential risk in health informatics implementations related to human factors.
3.   Identify the number of potential electronic data sources in a general practice, and in a hospital.

Exercises

- Use the AS/NZS 4360 framework to generate a risk register. Use the risk management grid (Figure 10.1) and outline mitigation strategies for each risk.
- Attend a clinical workplace and identify the workflow (movements, information requirements) of each type of profession working in the environment. Where are the points of interaction between professions? Are information needs made in a static location (by a desk) or when mobile (during a ward round or in an examination room)?

Online reading

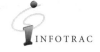

INFOTRAC® COLLEGE EDITION

For additional readings and review on risk management, explore **InfoTrac® College Edition**, your online library. Go to: **www.infotrac-college.com** and search for any of the InfoTrac key terms listed below:

➤ Risk
➤ Risk management
➤ Risk assessment
➤ Workflow analysis

References

Beck, K. (1999). *Extreme programming explained*, Reading, Addison-Wesley, MA.

Heeks, R., Mundy, D., & Salazar, A. (1999). *Why healthcare information systems succeed or fail*, Unpublished manuscript.

HL7 Working Group (2003). *HL7 2.4 Standard*.

Jones, C. (1994). *Assessment and control of software project management*, Yourdon Press, Englewood Cliffs.

Keeney, R. (1996). *Value focused thinking*. Harvard Press, Boston.

Laranjeira, L. (1990). Software size estimation of object oriented systems, IEEE *Transactions on Software Engineering* 16(5).

Martin, R. (2002). *Agile software development, principles, patterns, and practices*, Prentice Hall, New Jersey.

McConnell, S. (1996). *Rapid development*, Microsoft Press, Redmond.

OASIG (1995). *Why do IT projects so often fail?* University of Sheffield, Sheffield.

Pradhan, M., Edmonds, M. & Runciman, W. (2001). Quality in healthcare: process, *Best Practice and Research Clinical Anaesthesiology*, 15(4), 555–71.

Standards Australia and Standards New Zealand (2004). *AS/NZA 4360:2004 Risk Management*, Standards Australia, Sydney.

Vanderbeek, J., Ulrich, D., Jaworski, R., Werner, L., Hergert, D., Beery, T. et al. (1994). Bringing nursing informatics into the undergraduate curriculum, *Computers in Nursing*, 12(5), 227–31.

Wallsten, T.S., Budescu, D.V., Rapoport, A., Zwick, R. & Forsyth, B. (1986). Measuring the vague meanings of probability terms, *Journal of Experimental Psychology*, General, 115(4), 348–65.

11

Change management

Rodney Gapp

> 'People/organisations are like rivers, they take the easiest course.'
> Anonymous

Outline

The way individuals and organisations approach their day-to-day activities is summarised in the quote above. Within this context, it is easy to see why change programs often fail or fall short of their projected outcomes. This chapter mostly uses classic change management theory to discuss the individual's owning of the change process in an environment of knowledge development and information sharing, so that the final outcome is effective because it has become a natural course of action for those involved.

Introduction

A torrent of water that has chosen its path engulfs or pushes past incomplete obstacles put in its way. The organisation and its people are no different. Managing change with an incomplete strategy is no more effective than sandbags trying to contain the Amazon. Not surprisingly, there are thousands of studies on resistance to change, many focusing on individuals and the lower levels of Maslow's Hierarchy of Needs. These factors include overcoming habituated behaviour (habits), threats to the individual's security, financial and economic implications, and fear of the unknown.

The concept of change

Broadly speaking organisational change is any response to internal or external pressure or force by the organisation, from the whole of the organisation or any of its parts. It occurs regularly, is planned or unplanned, and only the scale and level of planning differs in each case. The amount of coordination, understanding and communication regarding the need for the change, combined with appropriate and timely provision of skills, resources and leadership, dictates the level of acceptance or rejection. Given these factors, change will always develop stress. The critical issue is not this stress, but managing it to obtain an optimum and productive level for the change required.

Seeing quality as fundamental to successful organisational transformation, Ackerman (1986) reported three levels of change (1) developmental change, (2) transitional change and (3) transformational change. Developmental change represents the simplest approach of fine-tuning or improving existing processes. It is based on skills development and acquisition and the evaluation of existing situations with the view to improving them. This simple stepwise progression is the least stressful and demanding on individuals, management and the organisation in general (Ackerman, 1986).

Transitional change is the intermediate stage and is larger in scale than developmental change. It involves a change in thinking or the introduction of new technologies. The approach starts with evaluating the existing system, then the development, introduction, piloting and re-evaluation of the new system, implementation and training, followed by a complete departure from the old and reliance on the new system.

Ackerman's (1986, p.7) transformational change is 'akin to letting go of one trapeze in mid-air before a new one swings into view'. At this complex level, there is less available knowledge and therefore less control and limited initial information for planning. This type of change is forced on an organisation due to extreme financial or external pressures. Because transformational change requires higher order innovation, it is often more difficult to manage. Many organisations react to the situation rather than address it through strategic processes. Transformational change is the most dependent on extensive managerial capability, knowledge and effective leadership ability.

An adaptation of Ackerman's (1986) three dimensions of change is presented as Figure 11.1. This model demonstrates that the most simple, quick and therefore easiest to manage approach to change is the provision of knowledge via training and/or communication. However, providing knowledge does not translate to new values or behaviours, making it akin to developmental change. This falls far short of the necessary levels of transitions or transformational change. Most organisations and their managers focus on knowledge, because the complexity of identifying and developing the appropriate type and level of values and behaviours is too difficult. Therefore, attitudinal shifts do not occur and neither does long-term higher level change.

Figure 11.1: The time and difficulty involved in internalising change (adapted from Ackerman, 1968)

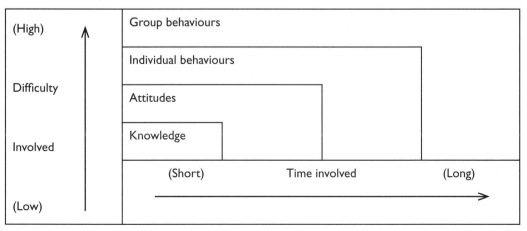

This simplistic approach results in a competitive and defensive stance described as *Model 1*. Organisations and their management 'maximise eliciting negative feelings and are focused on being rational at the cost of emotionality' (Argyris, 1982, p.86). This defensive mindset protects and defends the actor(s) or supra individual unities. The primary reasoning processes include testing the assumption using self-referential logic; that is, testing a claim by using the same logic that was used to create it. For example, a person declaring 'trust me, I know this organisation' assumes that others should use the same reasoning as themselves. Transparency is avoided and self-deception is denied by cover-up. For the cover-up to work it too must be covered up and the strategy here is to make both undiscussable. Undiscussablity is protected by making the undiscussablity undiscussable (Argyris, 2003).

Lower order change creates 'organisational dynamics that include quasi-resolution of conflict, uncertainty, avoidance, mistrust, conformity, face saving, inter-group rivalry, invalid information for important problems and valid information for unimportant problems, misperceptions, miscommunication, and parochial interests' (Argyris, 1985, p.85). This is single-loop learning and results from a focus on superficial learning that treats the underlying assumptions as fixed.

'Most people hold micro theories of effective action that are relatively effective in changing routines (single-loop) and relatively ineffective in making more fundamental changes in the status quo (double-loop)' (Argyris, 2003, p.1184). Double-loop learning challenges the appropriateness of existing approaches. It addresses the values and norms of an organisation and provides the basis for moving from the knowledge level of Figure 11.1 to the higher levels of attitudes, individual and group behaviours. 'In single-loop learning, we learn to maintain the field of constancy by learning to design actions that satisfy existing governing values. In double-loop learning, we learn to change the field of constancy itself' (Argyris & Schon, 1974, p.19).

In a double-loop environment, each individual's self-satisfying governing values overlap substantially with the corporate culture. This type of organisation is termed a Model 2 organisation and works on 'valid information, free and informed choice and internal commitment to the choice and constant monitoring of the implementations' (Argyris, 1982, p.102). Organisations that manage change at higher levels are typically more collaborative, less defensive and allow more substantial learning by fully testing assumptions.

Although Model 2 organisations are superior to Model 1, the Model 2 approach is more difficult and is not typical of most organisations because it requires an understanding of people and the development of new values and behaviours. There is a need for greater openness about beliefs and feelings and consensus must be achieved at all levels of the organisation. Generally speaking, it goes counter to many of the implicit rules followed in traditional organisations. It demands that managers be well versed in human psychology and the technical and functional demands of the organisation.

While these concepts are important to the success of change management programs, they represent a very complex starting point. Argyris and Schon (1974) provide a simpler approach to understanding where the organisation is situated in relation to these two models. The approach is based on:

- espoused theory, the view of the world and values and beliefs a person believes they follow in their normal behaviour (what people say)
- theory-in-use, the view of the world and values and beliefs implied by the individual's actual behaviour and actions (what people actually do).

The difference between espoused theory and theory-in-use leads to dissonance that in change management is the feeling of discomfort, which arises from inconsistency. It occurs when individuals test the words spoken by the actions taken. For example, management requests input, however when individuals provide valid input that questions the proposed strategy, management ignores or worse criticises the input, without testing its validity. This reinforces *Model 1* behaviour.

The relationship between espoused theory and theory-in-use produces a gap between what we think and what we do. Most people are generally blind to this gap, while others may perceive it but are reluctant to admit to this, let alone draw attention to it. Therefore, understanding and managing the size and nature of this gap within our own behaviour, then taking this to the organisational level is the essence of truly effective change management (the amount of dissonance is the issue, not its existence). Defensive reactions result if this is not accomplished. Effectiveness consists of being congruent, that is, bringing behaviour more in line with espoused values and providing a platform for trust, a key to any change program (Argyris, 2003).

Dialogue box 1: Fear of the more powerful other

Technology has become more and more embedded in daily work life. This sits comfortably when the process is seamless and the outcome is non-threatening, however technology is often rapidly introduced or even imposed. This can create a perceived threat, which can be even more pronounced in the health environment where human interaction is seen as caring and technological intervention may be seen as dehumanising. When individuals feel threatened or even intimidated by the technology, resistance occurs. This resistance relates to a long-held psychological view of the 'more powerful other', where the individual loses a sense of internal control due to the imposition of a perceived greater or more dominant external force that assumes control. For these individuals this perceived situation leads to a phobic response where a persistent fear far outweighs the actual threat.

The concept of 'the more powerful other' becomes a major threat to the introduction of informatics to front line health providers. This can often occur as a result of not being involved and therefore understanding the reason and value of the change to them personally. This important issue is why this chapter will focus on the implementation of change through the use of inclusive and participative processes.

Starting the change management process

Hersey, Blanchard and Johnson (2001) stress two characteristics for the successful delivery of organisational change. These are organisational diagnosis and

implementation methods and strategies. Organisational diagnosis provides answers to the following:
- What is actually happening now?
- What is likely to be happening?
- What would people ideally like to occur?
- What are the blocks or restraints to the ideal?

The three components of diagnosis are: (1) the point of view; (2) identification of the problem; and (3) analysis. This approach considers the organisation to be an integrated system within a complex external environment or the big picture, looking through the eyes of all concerned and where possible using outside consultants to obtain a different perspective. Problem identification starts with insight into the difference between what is really happening, the point of view of all involved, and the ideal outcome. It attempts to reduce discrepancies between the real (actual) and the ideal by the use of a theoretically based framework. A clearly defined and accurate problem is often the most difficult yet most essential component of any change program; without a clear identification of the problem any analysis is flawed. Analysis provides a link between problem-solving and implementation, through the identification of discrepancies between the end-result and intervening variables such as leadership or management style, organisational structure and organisational objectives (Hersey, Blanchard & Johnson, 2001).

Implementation requires the translation of diagnostic data into implementation plans, strategies and procedures. This requires an understanding of the capabilities of the organisation and its people to identify the optimal level for change. It also prioritises the adaptive and resistant forces associated with the change, providing meaning to the following:
- What is the nature of the organisation's leadership, decision-making and problem-solving skills and ability?
- What is the motivation, communication, and commitment to the objectives and climate within the organisation?
- What is the readiness level?
- Are individuals willing and able to take significant responsibility?
- What need level seems to be most important for people right now?
- What are the hygiene and motivation factors (Hersey, Blanchard & Johnson, 2001, p.379)?

Small amounts of change can be handled internally, however, managing complex change is a different question. While management has a ligament role, its extensive use creates a number of issues including the following:
- its authority and role can create resistance, miscommunication or over-commitment
- it tends to be out-of-date on emerging knowledge and change techniques
- it tends to overplay a specific idea or approach
- it lacks time for following through
- it must maintain the organisation's balance between stability and change. (Mink, Schultz & Mink, 1986, p.82)

The use of highly skilled and independent change agents or change specialists is an effective method of balancing the role of internal management. According to Walton (1969, p.150) these experts have the following characteristics:

- high professional expertise regarding social processes
- low power over fate of principals
- high control over confrontation setting and processes
- moderate knowledge about principles, issues, and background factors
- neutrality or balance with respect to substantive outcome, personal relationships and conflict resolution methodology.

Not only is the use of effective and competent external change agents important, their inclusion in the early planning stages, prior to the intervention stage, is a necessary consideration. This early inclusion increases the validity and reliability of the process.

The intervention stage

Intervention in a change management context has a different meaning from the normal understanding of the word. 'To intervene is to enter into an ongoing system of relationships, to come between or among persons, groups of objects for the purpose of helping them' (Argyris, 1970, p.17). Therefore, change agents or managers of change must see themselves in the roles of both advisor and counsellor. The intervention signifies to those involved that the move from the old to the new has commenced.

As in counselling situations, the process requires clear and well-defined boundaries between the client undergoing the change and the change agent or intervenor. The change agent must remember that the client (the organisation and its people), not the agent, has an obligated accountability and responsibility for the change. The change agent's role is to assist with the diagnosis and implementation of the change program.

An effective participative intervention, based on Model 2 behaviours, has three basic requirements:

1. the provision and use of valid and useful information
2. free and informed choice
3. internal commitment.

(Argyris, 1970, p.18)

> 'A statement devoid of rational prediction does not convey knowledge … information, no matter how complete and speedy, is not knowledge.'
>
> (Deming, 2000, pp.104–6)

Valid information is not isolated fact, it holds up under the test of logic, is applicable, and provides insight into the interrelationships throughout the organisation. Knowledge derived from valid information can predict and have control over phenomena. Tests for organisational validity include repeated diagnosis that produces consistent meaning, predictions that are confirmed by factual outcomes, and information that provides systemic changes organisation-wide. Information that does not provide insight or relevance to the intervention should be made redundant, as its inclusion will increase dissonance and increase mistrust (Argyris, 1970; Hersey, Blanchard & Johnson, 2001).

Valid information allows participants to make free and informed choices leading to a shared and clear cognitive map. The participants are then able to explore and select alternatives central to their needs. These alternatives can range from commitment to the change through to the decision to leave the organisation. One of the quickest ways to reduce commitment and empowerment is to remove accountability and responsibility in the actions and activities that constitute the individual's day-to-day work (Argyris, 2003). Free choice and valid information allows for interaction and review of the process by those involved in the change so that adjustments required to improve the process can occur. The best-planned changes start with a limited knowledge base, the greater the involvement the more relevant the information, the better the redefined program. This approach is the basis for action research, an important component of the management and success of change (Mumford, 2001; Avison, Lau, Myers & Nielson, 1999).

High internal commitment sees individuals readily taking up new values allowing them to lead aspects of the change themselves. This does not imply the need for less leadership, but an evolved leadership, aligned with double-loop learning and Model 2 concepts. There are examples in the development of effective self-managed teams where change agents and the organisation's leadership had great difficulty keeping up with those involved in the change. These individuals sought and developed valid information, implemented their own improvement strategies, and demanded new and advanced skills and training, creating the knowledge to drive the change successfully themselves (Gapp, 2003, 2004).

Dialogue box 2: Beginning with the end in mind

When discussing initial issues of technology implementation, many clinicians indicate that when the interface with the technology is difficult and frustrating, the issues of 'the more powerful other' occur more readily. In analysing the relationship between systems designers and the end users, an important issue was the difference in the thinking or logic used in the development of the technology and the requirements for application or use (for example, theoretically the most secure software system is one that denies access, which removes its function). This knowledge gap increases tension, as the new system seems less effective than the old to the practitioner. Many clinicians feel stressed and comment: 'I hate it, I don't trust it, and we have lost control.' They feel threatened, as their performance suffers, increasing already existing levels of anxiety and pressure to perform. These words are very important cues to those managing the introduction of systems. A start on the solution is to begin with the end in mind and at this point the change management agent needs to create dialogue between the designers and the end users so that all benefit and gain insight from the process.

Creating readiness for change

Schein (1979, p.144) found that the 'reason so many change efforts run into resistance or outright failure is usually directly traceable to them not providing for an effective unfreezing process before attempting the change'. Organisational readiness is an insightful approach aligned to intervention (Armenakis & Harries, 2002). Readiness refines Lewin's (1951) pioneering work on unfreezing because the language of unfreezing delivers a feeling of disconnectedness. It generates the sense of being acted upon rather than being involved in the change process. Readiness on the other hand is seen as 'the *cognitive* precursor to the behaviours of either resistance to, or support for, the change effort' (Armenakis, Harries & Mosholder, 1993, p.681) and provides an understanding of the need and capability for change.

The readiness approach consists of the message, interpersonal and social dynamics, influencing strategies, change agent attributes, and a typology for change. It is based on participation decreasing resistance and improving the performance and outcomes of the change program's and work on cognitive change (Bartlem and Locke, 1981; Bandura, 1986).

Managers need to be seen in terms of mentors and coaches as well as leaders and planners to create readiness. On average, 50 per cent of managers find the transition from controlling to coaching extremely difficult. It means fully addressing issues raised by Argyris in moving from *Model 1* to *Model 2* values. Managers are often forgotten and receive little support and development; if this is not addressed they will block any attempt for readiness (Gapp, 2003).

The message communicated should clearly define the change (from existing to desired state), how change will occur, how the success of the change will be measured, and the reasons for the change. It contains two parts, 'the discrepancy between the desired end state (which must be appropriate for the organisation) and the present state, and the individual and collective efficacy (that is, people's perceived ability for change) of parties affected by the change effort' (Armenakis, Harries & Mosholder, 1993, p.683).

The interpersonal and social dynamics of the organisation provides the change agent with an understanding of the differences between individual and group efficacy. The challenge is to harness these collective and individual capabilities to improve the readiness for the change. Providing individuals with an understanding of people's individual differences and temperaments provides clarity as to why certain people react differently to the same situation and how best to support and develop each other through the change process.

Identifying and monitoring increases in efficacy and decreases in discrepancy can influence the change. Conflict will be a natural result if changes in efficacy and discrepancy are not directed to the stated end goals throughout the whole process. This will require qualitative and quantitative feedback at the individual, group, department and organisational level at regular intervals that demonstrates an integration and alignment in the implementation process. The final source of influence is to observe and understand the leadership involvement during the process, to prevent the threat of defensive organisational routines, and to ensure the congruence between process and outcomes (Armenakis & Harries, 2002; Argyris, 1999, 2003; Gapp, 2003).

Three practical methods for influencing and maintaining change strategies are:

1. Persuasive communication presented in any form. The key is the motivational nature of the communication.
2. Active participation in the form of:
   - enactive mastery, the gradual building of efficacy through involvement and practice
   - learning from others (vicarious learning)
   - direct involvement in decision-making.
3. The management of information; this encompasses the direct use of both internal and external information.

Internal information provides direct feedback on the organisational environment and its requirements. External information provides external validity for those undergoing the change through material such as articles, case studies and world trends, and other factors impacting on the organisation (Armenakis & Harries, 2002).

The readiness approach places emphasis on the role of the change agent and organisational leaders. As interventionists these people must display 'credibility, trustworthiness, sincerity and expertise' (Armenakis, Harries & Mosholder, 1993, p.681) to those undergoing the change. When such attributes are not seen as core to the change agent, then the chance for change is reduced dramatically.

The last component is a typology of readiness, which is based on an understanding of employee readiness and the urgency for change. There are four types of change programs:

1. 'An aggressive program' is used when employee readiness and urgency for change are both low. It requires persuasive communication, active participation, external information and change agent attributes.
2. 'A crisis program' is relevant when employee readiness is low and urgency high. Here the ability of the change agent is very important, along with persuasive communication.
3. High readiness and low urgency leads to 'a maintenance program', which uses persuasive communication, active participation and external information.
4. Finally, high readiness and high urgency leads to 'a quick response program'; the primary approach here is persuasive communication (Armenakis, Harries & Mosholder, 1993; Armenakis & Harries, 2002).

Continued assessment of the change program and the interplay between discrepancy and efficacy must be constantly assessed at this point, with these assessments used to inform the program, the participants and improve the change processes.

> ## Case study: The drop-in chat room
>
> The following presents a summary of the effective use of information technology in assisting individuals during a change management process. As a method of empowering the individuals involved and opening lines of communication, a major health provider made available to its staff a secure online chat room. An independent organisation provided a website with two functions; the first was an area where staff could log on anonymously and discuss issues with one another as a method to assist in coping with the change. The second anonymous area provided access for staff to raise issues, difficulties or concerns related to the change process with senior management. Responses to the second area were then posted by the most relevant people for all to read and review.
>
> This system provided a number of benefits for all involved. (1) The chat room provided a caring and sharing forum, which became important as it granted access to different work areas and shifts allowing individuals to see that they were not alone in their concerns. This approach also addressed issues of communication for those who did not have physical contact with other staff. (2) The use of technology was also seen as a way of encouraging and expanding the day-to-day exposure of staff to the Internet and other useful technologies. (3) The direct questions on the change program provided an assessment tool from which the change agents gained greater understanding of the acceptance and resistance to the change. (4) Creating the feedback mechanism enabled direct communication between relevant management and staff. (5) The system assisted in improving the organisation's ability to implement change and assisted staff in the acceptance and use of new technologies.

Maintaining and improving change through vision and cultural climate

The message component of organisational readiness can be expanded by a series of three organisational visions that develop in complexity over time. This approach is found to maintain momentum and motivation while enhancing the change program (Nutt & Backoff, 1997). In Vision 1 a comprehensive trigger identifies the first moves made in a radical change and reinforces the importance of a threat or environmental turbulence as a key motivator by explaining their impact on the sustainability of the organisation. Vision 2 expands Vision 1 by incorporating the ideas of key insiders. Vision 3 includes inputs from diverse stakeholders with varied opinions and dissimilar interests and increases the chance of success. These visions will be 'challenging, inspirational, value adding, and energy releasing' for maximum effect (Nutt & Backoff, 1997, p.491). An essential message within all three types of vision is crafting win-win outcomes that create something of value for each interested group.

This strong approach provides a clear message, however Argyris (1998, p.98) provides the following warning:

> It has been said that no vision, no strategy can be achieved without able and empowered employees. Top-level executives accept their responsibilities to try to develop empowered employees. Human resource professionals devise impressive theories of internal motivation and experts teach change management, while executives launch change programs. But little of it works. There has been little growth in empowerment over the last 30 years. Empowerment remains very much like the emperor's new clothes: it is praised loudly in public, but privately we ask ourselves why we cannot see it.

Reduced empowerment is addressed by Allen and Craft (1982). They see organisations as having two clear and distinct parts, the first being the conscious organisation that consists of physical attributes, including structure, rules, policies, procedures and manuals; it is expressed in stated goals. The second, the unconscious organisation, represents aspects of efficacy and expands to include social behaviour and normative practices. This invisible organisational characteristic lies quietly under the surface and plays a dramatic role in determining long-term outcomes. In many organisational change programs, the unconscious is not even acknowledged let alone addressed. Change that does not address the unconscious organisation appears to succeed, then gradually the unconscious forces grind it down and the process then fails.

Identifying the dynamic social factors that influence us is achieved through understanding cultural norms within an organisation. A positive cultural climate is able to maintain the change process through the use of cultural norming and humanising work practices. According to Allen and Kraft (1986), norms provide effective building blocks for change through:
- rewards and recognition
- modelling behaviour
- confrontation
- communication and information systems
- interactions and relationships
- training and development
- orientations
- commitment and allocation of resources.

Gapp (1999) agrees with Allen and Kraft (1986) that the work practices that humanise the change program include:
- involving people in the problems and programs affecting them
- refraining from blaming people
- having clarity of goals, objectives, purpose and task
- focusing on results, both short and long-term
- working from a sound database
- being systematic and using multilevel change strategies
- emphasising sustained cultural change.

Summary box

The following steps create a change program:
- isolate people from single-loop learning and taboos of the existing culture that develop and maintain *Model 1* behaviour
- generate a supportive environment, building trust through involvement and informed understanding
- enable the dissonance-arousing mismatch between espoused and in-use practices to become apparent, provide effective feedback on this behaviour through the use of inventions that build trust
- through the use of valid information, link information to application and identify and manage any discrepancies
- escape the conventional organisational taboos through the use of organisational readiness and the development of internal efficacy
- link information given with *Model 2* behaviour through freedom of choice and internal commitment
- encourage feedback and clarification in *all* communications.

(Argyris, 1985; Dick & Dalmau, 1990)

Strategies to enhance this process:
- open communication based on a non-defensive interpersonal style is essential
- developing systems and structures where openness and non-defensiveness are easily achieved and encouraged
- change actions without controlling them, address issues as issues and not sources of blame
- develop environments that encourage participation, joint problem-solving and openness
- make provision for ongoing monitoring whenever plans are being developed or decisions made, use action research and make the findings freely available
- set up organisations, groups or programs as self-improving systems, by ensuring that the most relevant performance feedback is available, without threat to those who can best use it to change their performance.

(Argyris, 1985, 2003)

Conclusion

It is clear that change management is complex, requiring an approach that is not just managed but more importantly led, that socio-cultural issues are understood and addressed, and that the organisational members are involved. The ability to undertake effective organisational diagnosis, which includes change agents for both their independent perspective and knowledge, is the initial starting point. Effective change is seen when the organisation and its members take on Model 2 behaviours. The implementation phase consists of intervention followed by organisational readiness, then the development and use of vision and cultural climate activities and the continuous improvement of the process through feedback and interaction.

Change is not something to be done to a person or an organisation, it is the process of having those who make up the organisation understand the need for change and empowering them to achieve the outcome. This embeds the change as it allows for the development of the values and beliefs required for the change. It may take more time but it is often far quicker in the long-term than change driven without a clear purpose and method.

Review questions

1. How has health informatics driven change for health professionals?
    *   Has this been done well?
    *   Place yourself in the position of a change agent implementing large-scale change being driven by the use of informatics. What would be your major considerations to assist health professionals with the change?
2. Many organisations fail in their desire to change because of the internal resistance seen as organisational defensive routines. How do you recognise this defensiveness? What approaches can be used to overcome this resistance? What considerations do you need to have in order to prevent them from recurring?

Exercise

*   Take an organisation that you are familiar with and design a change program for implementing a health informatics system. In not more than five pages include the concepts discussed in this chapter. Methods that provide feedback to all involved over time and the selection and role of change agents in the program should also be discussed.

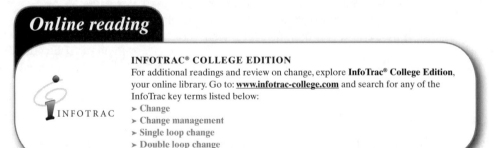

Online reading

INFOTRAC® COLLEGE EDITION
For additional readings and review on change, explore **InfoTrac® College Edition**, your online library. Go to: **www.infotrac-college.com** and search for any of the InfoTrac key terms listed below:
➤ Change
➤ Change management
➤ Single loop change
➤ Double loop change

INFOTRAC

References

Ackerman, L. (1986). Development, transition or transformation: the question of change in organisations, *OD Practitioner, December*, 1–8.

Allan, R.F & Kraft, C. (1982). *The organisational unconscious*, Prentice-Hall, Englewood Cliffs, NJ.

Allan, R.F & Kraft, C. (1984). Transformations that last: a cultural approach, in J.D. Adams (ed.), *Transforming Work* (36–54), Miles River Press, Alexandria, Virginia.

Argyris, C. (1970). *Intervention theory and method: a behavioral science view*, Addison-Wesley, Reading, MA.

Argyris, C. (1982). *Reasoning, learning, and action: individual and organisational*, 1st edn, Jossey-Bass, San Francisco.

Argyris, C. (1985). *Strategy, change and defensive routines*, Ballenger Publishing, Cambridge.

Argyris, C. (1998). The emperor's new clothes, *Harvard Business Review, 76*(3), 98–105.

Argyris, C. (1999). *On organisational learning*, 2nd edn, Blackwell Business, Malden, MA.

Argyris, C. (2003). A life full of learning, *organisational studies, 27*(7), 1178–92.

Argyris, C. & Schon, D.A. (1974). *Theory in practice: increasing professional effectiveness*, 1st edn, Jossey-Bass Publishers, San Francisco.

Armenakis, A.A. & Harris, S.G. (2002). Crafting a change message to create transformational readiness, *Journal of Organisational Change Management, 15*(2), 169.

Armenakis, A.A., Harris, S.G. & Mossholder, K.W. (1993). Creating readiness for organisational change, *Human Relations, 46*(6), 681.

Avison, D., Lau, F., Myers, M. & Nielsen, P.A. (1999). 'Action research', *Communications of the ACM, 42*(1), 94.

Bandura, A. (1986). *Social foundations of thought and action: a social-cognitive view*, Prentice Hall, Englewood Cliffs, NJ.

Bartlem, C. & Locke, E. (1981). 'The Coch and French study: a critique and reinterpretation', *Human Relations, 34*(7), 555–66.

Deming, W.E. (2000). *The new economics: for industry, government, education*, 2nd edn, MIT Press, Cambridge, MA.

Dick, B. & Dalmau, T. (1990). *Values in action: applying the ideas of Argyris and Schon*, Interchange, Brisbane.

Gapp, R. (2003). The influence the system of profound knowledge has on the development of leadership and management within an organisation, *Managerial Auditing Journal, 17*(5), 338–42.

Gapp, R. (2004). The risk to organisational excellence by processes that limit managerial knowledge and perception, *Manufacturing Technology Management, 15*(5), 387–93.

Gapp, R.P. (1999). *Leadership, learning styles, and dealing with individual difference: keys to quality management in a learning environment*. Paper presented at the Third International and Sixth National Research Conference on Quality Research, Melbourne.

Hersey, P. & Blanchard, K.H. (2001). *Management of organisational behaviour: utilizing human resources*, 8th edn, Prentice Hall, Englewood Cliffs, NJ.

Lewin, K. (1951). *Field Theory in Social Science*, Harper & Row, New York.

Mink, O.G, Shultz, J.M. & Mink, B.P. (1979). *Developing and managing open organisations*, OHRD Associates, Inc., Texas.

Mumford, E. (2001). Advice for an action researcher, *Information Technology and People, 14*(1), 12–27.

Nutt, P.C. & Backoff, R.W. (1997). Facilitating transformational change, *Journal of Applied Behavioural Science, 33*(4), 490–505.

Schien, E. (1979). Personal change through interpersonal relationships, in J.V.M.W. Bennis, E. Schein and F. Steele (eds.), *Essays in interpersonal dynamics,* The Dorsey Press, Homewood, IL, pp.129–62.

Walton, R. (1969). *Interpersonal peacemaker: confrontation and third party consultation,* Addison-Wesley, Reading, MA.

12

Health economics

Ian Edwards

> 'The more we have, the more we want, and the more we want, the less we have.'
>
> (Josh Billings, 1818–85)

Outline

Health economics is a branch of economics concerned with the analysis of costs, benefits, management and consequences of healthcare. Information and data are frequently drawn from epidemiological studies and biostatistics to support the analysis, enabling informed decision-making. This chapter introduces the principles of health economics and issues of economics in health informatics.

Introduction

Economics is a very broad subject ranging from the behaviour of governments and organisations to individuals. It is the study of the allocation and use of scarce resources using various measuring techniques and is concerned with the analysis of the factors of production and consumption of goods and services.

The subject can be broadly divided into two main topics, macroeconomics and microeconomics. Macroeconomics is concerned with the economy in total, with particular focus on resource allocation, factors of production and competition. Microeconomics focuses more on individuals, households, businesses and organisations.

While there are many definitions of economics, it is usually described as the relationship between scarcity, opportunity cost and choice. Within an economic context it is frequently stated that human wants are unlimited and that the resources to satisfy those wants are limited. Therefore, individuals and societies have to make decisions about resource allocation and which wants will remain unsatisfied.

The case study below is typical of the dilemma faced in the public (and private) healthcare systems where various departments compete for limited public funding. Applying an appropriate economic method can greatly assist in the decision-making process.

Case study 1

As part of the government's strategy for the management of scarce and expensive healthcare resources, the need for a new hospital information system has been recognised. It is hoped that the new system will further facilitate the integration of acute (hospital) and community care as it has the ability to store clinical patient information from both settings. This is a significant advantage in comparison to the current stand-alone systems. The new system will also enable unique patient records to be established allowing clinicians to view integrated patient history and the care provided regardless of the setting. Once installed, this system will play a major role in establishing a new standard of clinical management of patients.

The cost of the new system is significant with approximately $200m required for the initial implementation. Ultimately the system will extend to the General Practitioner setting further supporting integrated clinical care. Funding for the new system is competing with other projects from various government departments.

A basic economic problem for healthcare is the allocation or use of limited resources to enable the wants and desires of people to be as fully satisfied as possible. This needs to be relative to the availability of scarce resources, which can be used to satisfy these desires. Given that the total wants within a society exceed the scarce resources available to satisfy them, choices have to be made. Economic theory is basic to this debate and for that reason it is pertinent to discuss it here in some detail.

The basis of economic theory

In a clinical context, decisions are made every day regarding choices. For example, if a decision is reached to introduce a new drug in a hospital, data are gathered from the clinical information systems to gauge the impact of the new drug given the clinical protocols for its administration. Either an increase in budget is required or similar savings need to be identified to enable the drug to be introduced. The implementation of information technology (IT) competes for funding in the same environment and with direct clinical care issues.

Although advances in clinical consumables and drugs frequently correlates to higher costs, their effectiveness is usually well demonstrated through clinical trials. The introduction of IT does not always have a direct clinical outcome and can be problematic to evaluate. Simply, a choice has to be made on how the scarce resource (budget) is used.

What is an economy?

An economy can be defined as a mechanism that allocates scarce resources among alternative uses. The economy is said to determine what goods and services will be produced, in what quantities, how, when and where the goods and services will be produced, and who will consume the goods. Given that resources are scarce, how are resources allocated and rationed and who makes the decisions?

It is generally considered that there are three groups of decision-makers in the market consisting of:

- households – individuals and groups of people
- firms/companies – organisations that utilise resources to produce goods and services
- governments – organisations that redistribute income and wealth, and produce goods and services.

A market is any arrangement or mechanism that assists trading, which includes goods and services as well as 'factors of production'. There are three types of factors of production:

1. land – all natural resources
2. labour – human resources
3. capital – in economic terms, all plant, equipment and buildings. This category also includes human capital, which is the knowledge and skill of human beings.

All three factors of production are traded in a market and are generally coordinated in two different ways. Firstly, by market forces through the supply and demand for products and services that influences the costs and decisions of buyers and sellers. This is achieved through the constant adjustment of prices. The second way is through government intervention, where government decides what, how, when, where and for whom the goods and services are produced. This is best viewed as a continuum with no economy being at either of the extremes.

The individual decisions made in a market that are reacting to constant price adjustments assume consumer sovereignty, where consumers are assumed to be the best judge of how to use their resources. How they choose to spend their money, together with the cost of producing those goods, determines the variety and quality of the goods and services being produced. Consumers must have full knowledge and information regarding the products or services they wish to purchase for this to occur. Within a healthcare setting, this is quite often not the case due to the level of specialist clinical knowledge required to make informed decisions. However, with the amount of information that is available on the Internet, many healthcare consumers are starting to question the care that is being recommended.

Supply and demand

The wants and choices of millions of individual decision-makers are coordinated within the market or economy through the process of supply and demand. This process constantly adjusts prices in accordance with how much decision-makers are prepared to pay relative to how much is available. The increase in application and use of information technology has made information regarding prices, availability and product specification readily available and easily obtained. The interaction of supply and demand is dependent on information that enables both consumers and producers to make informed decisions about their resource allocation.

The concept of consumer wants and choices is the demand for products and services. Demand is the quantity of a particular good or service that consumers are willing to buy at a particular price. The higher the price the less people are willing or able to buy. Conversely, the lower the price the more they will be willing and able to purchase (see figure 12.1).

Figure 12.1: The demand curve

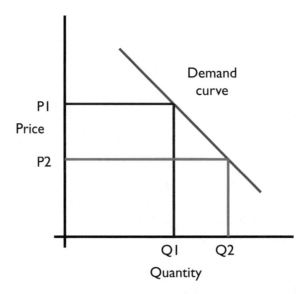

Figure 12.2: The supply curve

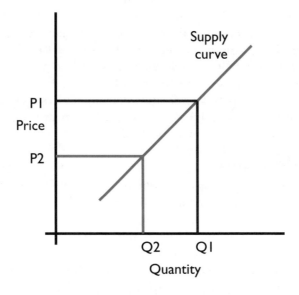

Supply simply refers to the quantity of particular products or services available for purchase. It is the relationship between the price of a product or service and the quantity that suppliers are collectively prepared to make available on the market. Suppliers can choose among alternative activities and do so as the benefits and costs change. The higher the price for any particular item, the more attractive it is for supplies to provide this item (see Figure 12. 2).

Elasticity

Elasticity is a measure of supply and demand responsiveness to changes in price and any other factors that affect demand or supply. It is useful to be able to understand and measure how much the quantity demanded or supplied will change with a movement in price or costs, for example a 10 per cent increase in the price of an item may result in a 15 per cent reduction in demand.

The change in demand also varies for different types of products or services. For example, a small percentage increase in a luxury service may have a significant decrease in the level of demand for the product. Alternatively, a large increase in the price of an essential item such as a prosthetic device or drug may have little impact on the level of demand, particularly when there is often only one manufacturer of the item.

There are four main factors that influence the elasticity of demand:

1. If there are a number of *close substitutes* for the product, demand will tend to be very responsive to price change.
2. If the product is a *luxury* consumers will tend to go without if the price rises.
3. If the *proportion of income* spent on a product is very small, consumers are not likely to be very sensitive to price changes.
4. The *time period* involved in rearrange spending patterns – a price change may have little influence in the short term, but may have a larger consequence on demand in the long term.

> The concept of elasticity is useful in answering questions such as 'Will a decrease in the price result in an increase on the total amount spent'.

The majority of healthcare in Australia is relatively insensitive to price change from a consumer or patient point of view. This is due to the majority of healthcare being either publicly provided or, if private, a large proportion of costs covered by private health insurance. Similarly, from a healthcare provider's point of view, they are frequently faced with little choice other than to purchase the item. This is particularly the case in highly specialised prosthetic devices and drugs or with highly specialised healthcare software programs such as clinical costing, nurse rostering or drug dispensing systems.

The interaction of supply and demand

Market systems are composed of individual decision makers that influence the demand and supply of products and services. When supply equals demand the market is said to be in equilibrium. The market price is such that the quantity supplied equals the quantity demanded (see Figure 12.3).

Figure 12. 3: Supply and demand

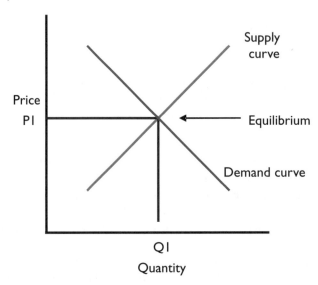

While economic theory can clearly depict relationships between supply and demand, the above example assumes **perfect competition** that is dependent on the willingness and ability to pay by informed decision-makers. A perfect competitive market is the most competitive of all the theoretical market structures. Economists often use it as a benchmark for comparing other market structures. Perfect competitive markets are unlikely to exist in practice. The four characteristics of a perfect competitive market are that:
1. There must be a large number of buyers and sellers so one individual buyer or seller cannot influence the market
2. The products sold by the sellers must be homogeneous
3. There are no barriers to entry or exit from the industry
4. There must be full information to all buyers and sellers about price and cost conditions.

When a comparison is made between the Australian market for healthcare and a perfect competition market, it is apparent that there are significant differences.
- Healthcare providers are limited through barriers to entry, for example, limited number of university places, medical colleges and registration.
- Healthcare products or services are not considered homogeneous.
- The market price of healthcare usually does not represent the true cost.
- There is an imbalance of information between producers of products or services and consumers. The consumer usually relies on the producer for advice and information. This situation is often referred to as supplier induced demand.
- Some healthcare providers have the ability to set the price.

The majority of countries usually have some level of government intervention with healthcare free at the point of delivery, but supported through general taxation of the population. Healthcare is provided for the good of the general population with a trade-off between the provision of equitable services and efficient systems.

Market failure

There are various situations in which the market system may fail to allocate resources efficiently. For example, this can happen when competition is reduced due to a monopoly or where there is collusion between producers. Market imperfections give incorrect signals to both buyers and sellers resulting in resources not being allocated efficiently.

Markets may completely fail to produce particular goods and services termed 'public goods'. When the market fails to allocate resources efficiently, there exists a role for government intervention. While the provision of publicly funded healthcare enables a degree of equity of access to medical services within Australia, it removes the direct costs from the consumers. Therefore, the costs that healthcare consumers pay do not reflect the true costs. The supply and demand equilibrium and efficient allocations of scarce resources (as within a perfect market), fails. Even in a private healthcare system, market failure still exists. How then can resources be allocated to ensure that the health needs of the population are met?

Understanding costs

Marginal analysis

Marginal analysis is the evaluation of the costs and benefits of producing an additional unit of activity. In order to understand marginal analysis, it is important to first understand the various economic components in producing goods. Table 12.1 below illustrates the various relationships and different costs in producing goods and an explanation of the various costs follows the table.

Table 12.1: Marginal analysis

Number of units	Fixed cost	Variable cost	Total cost	Marginal cost
0	50	0	50	
1	50	50	100	50
2	50	78	128	28
3	50	98	148	20
4	50	112	162	14
5	50	130	180	18
6	50	150	200	20
7	50	175	225	25
8	50	204	254	29
9	50	242	292	38
10	50	300	350	58

Fixed costs

Fixed costs represent a portion of the costs that do not change as the number of items produced increases or decreases. For example, the infrastructure and staff costs of the IT department in a hospital would probably not be affected by changes in the number of patients being treated.

Variable costs

Variable costs are the expenses that change in proportion to the number of items produced. For example, expenditure on drugs is highly likely to be proportional to the number of patients being treated. Although variable healthcare costs are unlikely to be influenced by information technology, but within a broader context, technology such as patient CT and MRI scans can, in some diseases, be a significant variable cost.

Total costs

Total costs are the sum of both the fixed and variable costs.

Marginal costs

The marginal cost of production is the difference in total costs for providing or reducing one unit of production. It can be seen from Table 12.1 that the marginal cost of increasing the number of units of production from five to six is $20 (200 – 180 = 20).

If the unit was a service such as an extra theatre case, the relationship between performing the additional case and the increased costs incurred in doing this involves marginal analysis. In understanding the cost implications of providing this additional theatre case, an informed decision can be made about whether it is provided given the income or additional budget that is available. If the cost of providing the additional case is higher than the income or budget, from an economic point of view it does not make sense to undertake it. This type of information is now frequently available in larger public hospitals in Australia with the introduction of complex clinical costing systems.

While various clinical costing systems have been introduced in hospitals within Australia, they perform similar functions. These systems supply information by gathering data from various information systems within the hospital, for example, finance, payroll and patient records. They provide detailed patient information and individual patient costs for the clinical care that has been provided. This powerful tool is able to assist both clinicians and medical administrators in understanding the cost of healthcare and the implications of various changes, including marginal analysis.

The benefit for a healthcare organisation (public or private) in providing a unit of care or a service is usually the revenue generated from the procedure. Therefore, **marginal revenue** is the difference or additional revenue generated as a consequence of providing the one extra procedure. While marginal revenue is sometimes thought of as being constant, many factors cause it to eventually decrease. One obvious factor is that as supply increases so does an expectation of lower charges, as eventually their demand is fully satisfied. It could be reasonably expected then if all cardiac services are produced in a dedicated hospital a government could expect that costs could be reduced.

Marginal analysis is the evaluation of the costs and benefits of adding or subtracting an additional unit of activity. Therefore, it is the relationship between marginal costs and marginal revenue. From a financial perspective, the point where the marginal costs crosses marginal revenue is the equilibrium point at which the quantity of services supplied to purchasers equals the quantity they want to purchase at a mutually agreeable price. This is illustrated in Figure 12.4.

Figure 12.4: Marginal analysis

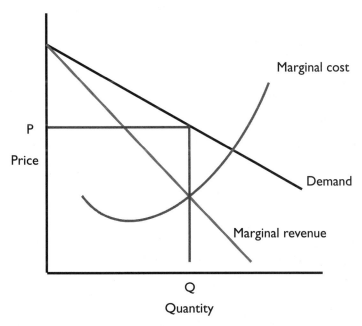

In the figure above, it is evident that if the organisation produced more services than the equilibrium point, the marginal cost would be higher than marginal revenue. Simply, the services in excess of the equilibrium would cost more to produce than the additional revenue they would generate. Conversely, if they were less than the equilibrium point the company would not be maximising their potential profit. Providing services up to the equilibrium point would generate more marginal revenue than the marginal costs that would be incurred and maximise profit.

Economic evaluation

Economic evaluation techniques are methods that aim to improve the efficient use of resources. The various techniques that can be used given different situations assist the decision-making process by providing a numeric analysis of the relative costs and consequences of alternative uses of resources. Evaluating proposed healthcare information systems requires identifying the initial implementation costs together with training, support and ongoing maintenance. In addition to the costs, the benefits that the system will realise need to be identified and costed.

Economic evaluation techniques are concerned with the maximisation of social welfare. This implies that they take into account all of the costs and benefits in relation to the resource allocation decision, regardless of who incurs the cost, and who obtains the benefit. The interest in cost and benefits relates not only to the present, but also to the future. Economic evaluation techniques take a 'wide' view of all the benefits and costs together with a 'long' view over a period of time.

An important characteristic of economic evaluation techniques is that they utilise value judgements. In particular, cost–benefit analysis involves the application of the Kaldor-Hicks (also referred to as Potential Pareto or Hypothetical Compensation) test of efficiency.

The Kaldor-Hicks (1939) criterion states that any change in resource allocation, in principle, is worthwhile if those who gain from the change outweigh those who may lose. Therefore a change is warranted from an economic perspective if the net social benefit is positive. The Kaldor-Hicks criterion is based on a utilitarian notion of welfare maximisation and is not concerned with the identification or discrimination between those who have gained and those who have lost. When the Kaldor-Hicks test is applied, all costs and benefits count equally, regardless of whether they are incurred or enjoyed by the 'rich' or the 'poor', or any other group in society.

Considerations of the effects of change on specific societal groups, that is, the rich, the poor, the infirm, the healthy, the young, the elderly, and so on, are important; and, in reality, these groups are not always treated as equals by decision-makers for moral, philosophical, political, or other reasons. It is important to understand that utilitarian notions, on which economic evaluation techniques are based, may not be consistent with the goals of the relevant policy-makers.

The methods of Cost Benefit Analysis (CBA), Cost Effectiveness Analysis (CEA) and Cost Utility Analysis (CUA) help decision-makers to make direct comparisons of alternative resource allocations based on established economic principles. These various techniques can be used as planning devices, providing a methodical way of comparing the costs and consequences of allocating scarce resources. They provide the means of ensuring that the limited resources available to any decision-maker are used to produce the greatest benefit possible.

All organisations and governments have to choose between various activities as the resources available are limited. They must decide what products to produce, and how to produce them. The two questions that need to be asked are:

1. Is it worthwhile to produce a service?
2. How should the service be produced or provided?

The first of these questions can be answered by applying Cost Benefit Analysis (CBA), while the second would usually require Cost Effectiveness Analysis.

Cost–benefit analysis

In asking the question, *is it worthwhile* to produce some health service or introduce new technology, it is necessary to compare the benefits and costs of the various proposals in present value terms enabling direct comparison in dollar terms. In simple terms, a benefit:

- is an outcome that an organisation considers to be attractive (for example it achieves a positive contribution to a strategic goal)
- can have a value ascribed to it, which in some cases can be difficult to quantify (for example placing a value on life or pain and suffering)
- is the reason why an organisation decides to make an investment or undertake an initiative.

(Commonwealth of Australia, 2004, p.20)

The CBA method is the most powerful and demanding of the economic evaluation techniques. While this is where the strength of the method lies, it is also where the difficulties are. CBA determines whether or not it is worthwhile from a society's point of view to proceed with a single investment or project. In taking a whole of society perspective, all costs and benefits that result from the proposal need to be included in the analysis, including all the externalities that can result. It is this broad perspective that is the strength of performing a CBA; it is also where the difficulties lie in determining and evaluating the externalities.

Externalities are when a proposal has cost and benefit implications for sectors of society other than the main group contained in the proposal. For example, when a child receives a vaccination they directly benefit, however the remaining unvaccinated children also benefit as they are less likely to become infected from children who have been vaccinated.

CBA could be used to help determine if a telehealth program would be economically worthwhile. It would involve the estimation of all the benefits and costs of the program and estimates of other costs such as the distress caused by having to leave one's community for care. This would include the fiscal benefits of being treated at home, family support and so on.

There are three different ways by which the benefits or health outcomes from programs are usually valued:

1. Human capital

The 'human capital' approach places a value on the total time gained from implementing the proposal. This method places a monetary value on the healthy time gained using market wage rates. The value of the program is assessed in terms of the present value of future earnings.

Case study 2

This type of analysis is appropriate to understand the benefits of integrating an Internet-based self-management system for diabetic patients into a clinical system. If exception-reporting basis for patient blood sugar levels and other information was implemented it may reduce the frequency of General Practitioner or outpatient visits saving the patient and the health system time and money.

2. Revealed preference

This approach involves estimating the benefit people place on improvements in health, or a reduction in health risk, by observing their actual consumption choices. An estimate of the value consumers place on health benefits can be derived by observing how consumers trade off the consumption of 'health' and 'non-health' commodities.

3. Willingness to pay

This method involves a consumer survey where consumers are asked to indicate the maximum amount they would be willing to pay to improve, or maintain, their health status.

The application of CBA to IT can be problematic, but not unfeasible. The idea that IT can be evaluated in the same way as other clinical adoptions can be misplaced, because techniques such as randomised control trials are often inappropriate. Although the IT system can have a direct patient outcome, this is not always the case.

Previous cost benefit studies have concluded that computers and IT have resulted in a reduced cost and/or improved patient outcomes. These include disease management with electronic clinical pathways and protocols; increased immunisation and dental check-up rates with systems that generate patient reminders, and reduced number of patient pathology tests with the introduction of a computerised system (Commonwealth of Australia, 2004; Donaldson, 2004). They can also have indirect benefits. For example, in the primary prevention of diabetes it is thought that Health*Connect* (The Australian National summary Electronic Health Record) will contribute by:

- the empowerment of consumers to be more responsible for their own health record
- the effective transfer of up-to-date guidelines (to consumers and practitioners)
- or the treatment, management and diagnosis of diabetes (Commonwealth of Australia, 2004).

Cost effectiveness analysis

Cost Effectiveness Analysis (CEA) is similar to CBA, but assumes that the objectives have been decided and seeks to determine the most cost efficient method of achieving them. This type of analysis can either identify the maximum benefit from a fixed budget or provide a defined goal for the least cost.

While CBA can provide an indication of whether or not the social benefits of an investment exceed its social costs, the information provided from cost effectiveness analysis (CEA) can only be used to compare different investments that have the same or similar characteristics. The costs of the project are measured in a similar manner to CBA and the health benefits are measured in units that are most appropriate given the proposal, for example, lives saved or years of life gained.

CEA may be used to assess the efficiency of alternative methods or investments, provided the objectives are identical. For example, CEA has been used to compare the costs related to the various methods of issuing prescriptions and their affect on the cost of drugs dispensed. This has revealed that the introduction of a computerised prescription system was more cost effective and had a decision support facility that reduced error and drug interactions (Commonwealth of Australia, 2004).

Cost utility analysis

Cost utility analysis is a variation of cost effectiveness analysis and attempts to define outcomes of health interventions through measurements in changes of life expectancy adjusted for the quality of life experienced. This technique assumes that healthy life is more highly valued than disability or morbidity. Effectiveness is expressed in terms of Quality Adjusted Life Years (QALYs) gained.

QALYs can be calculated in a variety of ways. One method involves asking people to rate disease states along a scale with death at one end and healthy life at the other. Another method involves questionaries designed to give a health profile of the individual before and after the healthcare intervention. The focus of QALYs is on the effect that symptoms or treatments have on a person's life, rather on the symptoms or treatment itself.

Case study 3

If new technology became available to increase the accuracy of an area requiring radiation treatment in melanoma smaller doses may be possible. This would possibly reduce the impact of the treatment on the patient and improve their quality of life. Cost utility analysis (CUA) would be an appropriate economic evaluation technique in comparing healthcare interventions that result in different consequences and impact on quality of life of the patient.

Discounting

The effects of various investment proposals are usually spread over an extended period of time. The future value of costs and benefits are likely to have a lower value in today's terms, due partly to the uncertainty of the future and the view that benefits available now may be invested to produce further benefits for the future. To enable a comparative analysis of the proposals, it is necessary to discount the costs and benefits back to the net present value. This enables a comparison of different investment proposals without the distortion of time.

The procedure of discounting requires the application of a discount factor to future cash flows and benefits. The discount factor (d_n) is calculated as follows:

- $d_n = 1/(1+i)^n$
- d_n is the discount factor for time period
- n is the time period
- i is the discount or 'interest' rate.

For example, the discount factor for three years, with a discount or 'interest' rate of 5 per cent is as follows:

- $d3 = 1/(1+0.05)3 = 1/(1.1576) = 0.8638$

This means that the net present value of $1 in three years' time is $0.86 based on a discount of five per cent per annum or, alternatively, if you invested $0.86 at five per cent interest per annum, its value in three years' time would be $1.00.

Once the benefits and costs of a proposal are discounted and measured in present-value monetary units, they can be compared. Proposals with a social marginal benefit greater than social marginal costs are considered economically worthwhile. Alternatively, projects with marginal costs greater than marginal benefits are considered inefficient.

The discount rate that is used depends, to some extent, on whether the proposal is in the private or public sector. The usual rate within the public sector is the long-term bond rate (that is a 10-year bond rate). Conversely, the private sector frequently uses a discount rate that reflects the cost of borrowing the money for the proposal plus an allowance for risk. Discount rates of at least 15 per cent are common within the private sector.

Evaluating the costs, the healthcare information system (Case study 1) would require the identification of the initial implementation costs, for example, hardware, software and installation. In addition to this, the system is likely to require training, support and ongoing maintenance. It is the long-term costs of implementing a new system that would require to be discounted to the present value to enable an appropriate cost comparison of different systems.

Sensitivity analysis

Sensitivity analysis provides an understanding of the relationship between the assumptions and the overall conclusion. Conclusions can be compared allowing for a greater understanding of the importance of different assumptions by changing some of the assumptions. One of the most common forms of sensitivity analysis involves varying the rate of discount.

Conclusion

It is frequently argued that economics has no place in understanding and analysing healthcare as healthcare is a basic right and should not be subject to the detached numeric analysis of health economics. However, there is a place for health economics in assisting individuals, clinicians and governments in understanding the cost of providing healthcare and how the use of limited healthcare resources can be maximised.

The role of IT in healthcare has expanded considerably over the past two decades and has assisted health professionals to understand the relationship between costs, clinical care and clinical outcomes. The challenge for clinical informatics is defining its role and ensuring that appropriate techniques are applied when evaluating information technology.

The efficient use of healthcare resources is important to ensure that the maximum number of individuals benefit from appropriate healthcare. Economics can assist to answer questions about the types of services that should be produced with the available resources and how they should be provided.

While various economic techniques can be used to gain insight in to these questions from a resource use perspective, epidemiological and biostatistics information is frequently required to gain a deeper understanding. The application and use of this type of information requires accurate clinical data, which is dependent on health informatics systems and the data entry standards and protocols.

Review questions

1. What are the principles of supply and demand and how are these applied to technology in healthcare?
2. What is cost benefit analysis?
3. In cost benefit analysis how are the benefits and outcomes valued and how are these applied to information technology?

Exercise

Using Case study 1 and a health economic framework, identify which analysis methodology would be appropriate in this exercise and develop a list of possible benefits, externalities and costs.

Online reading

INFOTRAC® COLLEGE EDITION
For additional readings and review on health economics, explore **InfoTrac® College Edition**, your online library. Go to: **www.infotrac-college.com** and search for any of the InfoTrac key terms listed below:
➤ Health economics
➤ Cost benefit analysis
➤ Cosy effectiveness analysis
➤ Marginal analysis

INFOTRAC

References

Clewer, A. & Perkins, D. (1998). *Economics for healthcare management,* Prentice Hall, London.

Commonwealth of Australia (2004). *Indicative Benefits Report.* Retrieved 22 February, 2005, from http://www.healthconnect.gov.au/research/.

Culyer, A.J. (2001). Equity – some theory and its policy implications, *Journal of Medical Ethics*, 27, 275–84.

Donaldson, P. & Conrick, M. (2004). *The effectiveness of using a patient dependency system to Develop and Audit Clinical Pathways*, Paper presented at the HIC2004, Brisbane.

Fuchs, V.R. (1998). *Problems and choices in Who shall live?: Health, economics and social choice.* World Scientific Publishing Co Pty Ltd., Singapore.

Getzen, T.E. (2004). *Health economics: fundamentals and flow of funds*. John Wiley and Sons, Inc., New York.

Harvey, P. (2003). Managing healthcare in Australia: Steps on the healthcare roundabout?, *Australian Journal of Primary Health*, 9(2 and 3), 105–8.

Heyne, P., Boettke, P.J. & Prychitko, D.L. (2003). *The economic way of thinking*, 10th edn, Prentice Hall.

Hicks J.R. (1939). The foundations of welfare economics, *Economic Journal*, 49: 696–710.

Kaldor-Hicks, N. (1939). Welfare propositions and interpersonal comparisons of utility, *Economic Journal*, 49: 542–9.

Mitchell, E. & Sullivan, F. (2001). A descriptive feast but an evaluative famine, *BMJ* 2001 322: 279–82.

Musgrove, P. (2004). *Health economics in development*. The World Bank, Washington.

Penner, S.J. (2004). *Introduction to healthcare economics and financial management*. Lippincott Williams and Wilkins, Philadelphia.

Part 4

Health information systems

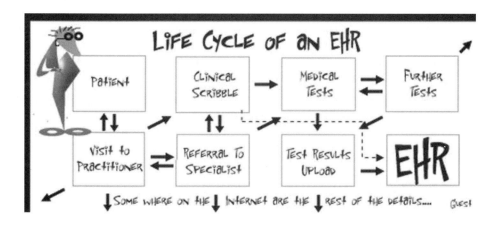

13

Systems development

Michael Strachan

> If the car was like a computer, occasionally, for no reason whatsoever, it would lock you out and refuse to let you in until you simultaneously lifted the door handle, turned the key, and grabbed hold of the radio antenna.
>
> (Rich Cook, General Motors)

Outline

Whether building a small or large-scale system, it is critical to use information systems development methodologies to reach the optimal design. In the same way as an architect's floor plans provide the requirements for the builder to construct a house, systems development methodologies provide the architectural plans to build healthcare information systems with solid foundations that support healthcare processes. This chapter discusses the systems development life cycle and healthcare information systems development. It integrates case studies and activities to reinforce the issues being discussed.

Introduction

Systems development is critical to the successful implementation of healthcare information systems. Systems development in its purest form is the combination of hardware, software, data, processes and people to form an information system. The challenge is to successfully document the design requirements that meet the needs of the healthcare individual or team. This can be a complex exercise depending on the size of the system.

Systems development life cycle

The systems development life cycle (SDLC) is a commonly known methodology used to develop information systems. It typically involves five major phases: planning, analysis, design, implementation and operation/support (Shelly, Cashman & Rosenblatt, 1998). The following definition encapsulates the purpose of the SDLC:

System Development Life Cycle (SDLC) is the overall process of developing information systems through a multi-step process from investigation of initial requirements through analysis, design, implementation and maintenance. There are many different models and methodologies, but each generally consists of a series of defined steps or stages (Computerworld, 2002, p.1).

The SDLC is an iterative process designed to ensure that changing system requirements are incorporated into the ongoing development of information systems. A number of models have been developed to enhance the practical utilisation of the SDLC in developing information systems (see Table 13.1). The most common was the Waterfall model developed in the 1980s that is now widely recognised to be out of date when managing modern complex system development projects.

Table 13.1 Systems development life cycle models

Fountain model	Recognises that there is a considerable overlap of activities throughout the development cycle.
Spiral model	Emphasises the need to go back and reiterate earlier stages like a series of short waterfall cycles, each producing an early prototype representing a part of the entire project.
Build and fix model	Writes some programming code; keeps modifying it until the customer is happy. Without planning, this is very open-ended and risky.
Rapid prototyping model	Emphasis is on creating a prototype that looks and acts like the desired product in order to test its usefulness. Once the prototype is approved, it is discarded and the 'real' software is written.
Incremental model	Divides the product into builds, where sections of the project are created and tested separately.
Synchronize and stabilise model	Combines the advantages of the spiral model with technology for overseeing and managing source code. This method allows many teams to work efficiently in parallel. It was defined by David Yoffie of Harvard University and Michael Cusumano of Massachusetts Institute of Technology (MIT), who studied how Microsoft Corporation developed Internet Explorer and how the Netscape Communications Corporation developed Communicator, finding common threads in the ways the two companies worked.

Project management methodologies

While information system developments are predominantly about providing a software/hardware solution for a business requirement, equally important are the people factors, such as training, change management and business re-engineering associated with a development project. Successful information system developments require effective application of sound project management methods, such as the Project Management Body of Knowledge (PMBOK®), which is just one of many frameworks that project managers can use to ensure successful project completion (Project Management Institute, 2005). Well-managed information technology projects will incorporate best practice project management methodologies discussed by Marsault in Chapter 9 and the principles of SDLC.

Healthcare information systems have very complex development requirements and the strategy for developing an information system will be dictated by the complexity of user requirements. To illustrate this, two case study examples are included in this chapter to demonstrated development options and alternatives.

Healthcare information systems development

General Practitioners (GPs) lead the way with the adoption of healthcare information systems within their practices. However, the hospital sector is predominantly reliant on inefficient cumbersome paper information systems and an expansive number of isolated departmental healthcare information system developments. Larger scale systems development in the hospital sector within Australia has historically focused on Patient Administrative Systems (PAS) as the user requirements have a higher level of maturity in comparison to Clinical Information Systems (CIS).

The healthcare sector has been slower than other industries to adopt information systems technologies to innovate business processes. The business case for mainstream information system developments such as financial, payroll or point of sales tends to have a positive economic return on investment (ROI) over a period of time. Healthcare information systems do not have the same demonstrable economic benefit to the organisation's bottom line. In more recent times, a body of literature has reported evidence of the benefits of implementing clinical information systems as improving patient safety, quality of care and healthcare efficiency (Westbrook & Gosling, 2002). This is changing the landscape and paving the way for new and exciting healthcare information system developments for organisations with the vision to see past economic returns and realise the significant benefits for patients.

Planning

The demand for information system developments within any organisation will originate from any number of sources including users, executive management, the information systems department and external factors. The prioritisation of information system developments should be determined by an organisation's strategic or business planning processes (Shelly et al., 1998). An information systems strategic plan (ISSP) is a key activity undertaken to determine which information systems developments are required to support the organisational goals and objectives.

The ISSP within a healthcare organisation must incorporate healthcare information systems development as a key priority given that the core business is providing healthcare to patients. Healthcare organisations must engage clinicians and patients to prioritise healthcare information system developments, which will have maximum benefit to patient safety.

A request for information system development could entail a replacement or small modification to an existing or a totally new system development. Determining the feasibility of information system development is an important first step for evaluating a system development request. This involves understanding the nature and scope of the problem and recommending whether the project is worthwhile pursuing. This stage is often referred to as the initiation of the system development project.

Case studies

The following case studies illustrate the levels of complexity within CIS developments and will form the basis for discussion in the remainder of this chapter. These studies are peppered with jargon commonly used within IT projects, some is explained, and some is not. It is up to the readers to gain an understanding of the context of the jargon. Why? Successful involvement with information technology (IT) projects relies on a sound understanding of IT jargon. This can be achieved by simply searching the Internet or asking IT professionals if in a situation to do so.

Case study A: Operating room management information system

The operating theatre department of a 350-bed hospital has had a 15-year-old legacy theatre management system for many years based on a Unix platform. It is a mainframe system that was originally designed to aid management of administrative theatre functions, such as inventory management and basic theatre scheduling. The software maintenance company has decided to sunset the product, mandating a need to replace the current system.

In addition to the replacement of the basic administrative theatre management functions, the Director of Surgery believes it is the ideal opportunity to acquire a system that will become the surgical clinical information system. The system needs to fulfil the requirements for production of all theatre documentation, including operation notes and surgical audit, which is currently undertaken within a local Microsoft Access database developed by the IT department.

A project manager is appointed to undertake planning for the operating room management system (ORMIS) replacement project within the surgical department. Fifty medical and 100 nursing staff with surgical backgrounds will be users of the system. A proposal for the best replacement strategy for the current theatre management system is required for the Director of Surgery who is the project sponsor.

Case study B: Enterprise clinical information system (CIS)

A 500-bed teaching acute hospital, including medical, surgical, paediatrics, obstetric, emergency specialities, outpatient and day surgery departments, uses a paper medical record to access information relating to its patients. There are issues with missing records, delayed access to information for clinical appointments, information missing from the record, and the list goes on.

The burgeoning and inefficient paper record system was highlighted when undertaking the organisation's ISSP process that recommended the development of a plan for implementing an enterprise CIS. While the paper record system is less than satisfactory, the medical and nursing staff perceives that a CIS is an unrealistic aspiration. Comments with respect to the cost and the increase in time away from the patients are key drivers behind the attitudes of medical and nursing staff.

A project manager is appointed to investigate the best way forward for the implementation of an enterprise CIS that meets the needs of the 200 medical staff, 900 nursing staff, and 120 allied health professionals within the hospital. The key outcome from the initial phase of the project must include a business case that recommends the preferred option to the organisation's board of directors.

At the end of the planning stage of systems development, a feasibility report or the like will usually need to be produced to seek authorisation to proceed. Depending on the size and complexity of the system development, a more detailed system analysis may need to be undertaken as part of developing the business case for approval.

Systems analysis

Systems analysis is the next logical step in the SDLC, which includes the determination and analysis of system requirements. Determining the system requirements involves undertaking a factual assessment of the current system inputs, outputs and processes. This involves undertaking fact-finding techniques, including interviews, user focus groups, questionnaires and review of any other documentation relating to the current system. Once a thorough review of current system requirements has been completed, analysis of system requirements can be undertaken (Shelly et al., 1998).

One of the common failures of healthcare information systems occurs when clinicians are not sufficiently engaged in the determination of system requirements. In 2002, Cedars Sinai Hospital in Los Angeles had a well published multi-million dollar failure of a Computerised Physician Order Entry (CPOE) due to lack of involvement of clinicians and poor consideration of the impact on clinical workflow (McGee, 2005).

Healthcare information systems must incorporate clinical workflow analysis as a key feature for the determination and analysis of system requirements. Workflow analysis is recognised as a key determinant to project success at Intermountain Healthcare, which has been implementing healthcare information systems for the past thirty-five years. The importance of workflow analysis is summarised by Gardner (in Rhodes & Costin, 2005) at Intermountain Healthcare:

> Medical informatics is very much a social science. The success of a project is 80 per cent dependent on the development of social and political interaction skills and 20 per cent or less on the implementation of the hardware and software technology!

Structured systems analysis tools must be used to accurately document healthcare information system requirements. Process and data modelling tools should be used in combination to effectively analyse and document system requirements. For example, a complete review of relationships between data may be undertaken using entity relationship (ER) models. Process analysis tools, such as data flow diagrams, data dictionary and narrative process descriptions should also be undertaken.

It is important to recognise the impact that the highly specialised nature of medicine has on the complexity of system requirements. For example, Case study A illustrates clinical users who all have surgical backgrounds and therefore consistent system requirements. The clinical users also have experience with the current legacy system and a clear understanding of their system requirements. The determination and analysis of system requirements are a straightforward proposition for Case study A.

Case study B has clinical users with many and varied clinical speciality backgrounds and with little or no experience with healthcare information systems. The task of determining and analysing system requirements in Case study B is a greater and more complex undertaking.

The final stage of systems analysis is to evaluate the best strategy for software alternatives. There are generally three basic alternatives for software acquisition, which include developing an in-house system, purchasing an off-the-shelf software package, or customising a package. The most appropriate software alternative depends on the ability of the various options to meet system requirements. The documentation of system requirements should be used to evaluate all possibilities and alternatives for software and hardware acquisition (Shelly et al., 1998).

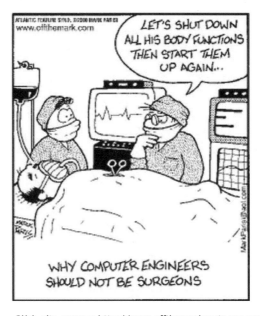

(Web site source: http://www.offthemarkcartoons.com/cartoons/2000-09-28.gif)

The project manager in Case study A has completed determining and analysing system requirements for the ORMIS replacement project. It has been decided that the nature of the system requirements is quite complex and not suited to an in-house development. Due to the very specific nature of the system requirement, there are only a handful of software vendors in the marketplace potentially capable of meeting the system requirements. Because of this, the tender process will differ slightly from the method used in Chapter 15.

A Request for Proposal (RFP) document is developed and sent out to the vendors as a closed tender process. An RFP is a formal document used to engage potential vendors, which includes a written list of system specifications. Vendors will respond to the RFP if they feel that their product meets the specifications outlined. Once the responses to the RFP are received, the software solutions are evaluated in a similar manner to that described in Chapter 15. The final decision as to the best product is based on functionality, flexibility, initial and ongoing costs and overall system architecture. An implementation planning study (IPS) is undertaken and a business case developed. This process is described in detail by Dixon-Hughes (Chapter 8).

Design

This phase involves the design of the physical information system based on the documentation produced in the analysis phase. It includes the detailed design of system input, output, data, software, hardware and people. The following table (13.2) provides sample design questions that could be asked of each design component of an information system. However, it should be realised that, as samples, these are not totally inclusive.

In Case study B a software vendor was selected to implement its CIS software solution, which would be customised to meet the system requirements of hospital clinical users. The configuration of hardware, software and processing methods for the CIS is referred to as the 'system architecture'. The selected software is a web-based product that can easily be distributed across the hospital's intranet as a thin client. A thin client is the main software program, which resides on a web server that performs all of the processing, and the client (personal computer or input device for the clinical user) only requires an Internet browser to use the product. Therefore, the computer devices utilised by clinicians' only need to run an Internet browser as the back end web server performs the processing functions. It also makes the IT department's ability to administer the system easier. A web-based CIS can be accessible via secure access across the Internet.

Conversely, a fat client relies on installation of the software on every individual personal computer (PC). This system architecture would not be appropriate for use in Case study B due to the significant overheads involved with administering the system. However, in Case study A, a fat client system architecture may be appropriate due to the smaller size and scope of the system.

Table 13.2: Sample design questions for each of the components of an information system

Component	Sample design questions
Output	• Will the screen outputs use a Graphical User Interface (GUI)? • How much screen real estate will be used and what is the impact on data entry efficiency? • What reports need to be developed for system go-live? How will future reports be developed and maintained?
Input	• How will users enter data into the system? • Will data collection be free text or highly structured? How can input screens be designed to facilitate efficient data entry? • What sort of validity checks, mandatory fields and rules could be incorporated into input design to improve the accuracy of data collection?
Data	• What type of database design is the most appropriate for the system? For example, a relational or object oriented database design? • What type of propriety database will be utilised? For example, Microsoft, Oracle, etc.
Software	• What operating system or platform is required to run the software? For example, MS Windows XP? Linux? Other? • Does the software code need to be written from the ground up? • Does the software from a vendor need to be configured or customised to suit the system requirements?
Hardware	• What is the system architecture to support the system? • What type of network will be best to distribute the product? For example, client server structure or a web-based system design? • How many and what type of input devices are required?
People	• What is the best training strategy for the type of system, users and organisation? • What impact will the system have on business process or workflows? • What change management strategies need to be in place to ensure successful implementation?

The selected CIS product has a centralised clinical data repository and it will need to interface with the hospital Patient Administration System (PAS) via Health Level 7 (HL7) messages. The PAS incorporates the hospital Patient Master Index (PMI), which includes a single unique identifier and demographics for all patients who attend the facility. Interfaces to hospital pathology and radiology systems also need to be undertaken. Interfacing is critical for reducing duplication of data entry and provides a patient-centric view within the CIS. Interfacing between clinical systems is a key design consideration for an enterprise CIS as all information relating to a patient needs to be incorporated into a patient-centric view.

Implementation

This phase includes application development and deployment of the product into the live production environment. A rigorous process of testing the application and establishing system documentation must be undertaken, irrespective of the application development strategy. Once the product has been constructed, it will be released into a test environment for end user acceptance testing. On completion of end user testing, the product is ready for deployment into a live production environment. Training of system users must then occur before 'go-live' of the product with system users (Centre for Medical Informatics, 2000).

In Case study B, the vendor's CIS software needs to undergo what is commonly referred to in the industry as a 'software build' to meet the specific hospital's system requirements. CIS software must be highly configurable to enable customisation to meet the requirements of hospital clinical workflow.

Implementations of CIS are not like a typical information system project. Re-engineering of clinical processes and workflow must be the key impetus for adopting CIS (PricewaterhouseCoopers, 2005). The implementation of a CIS in the production environment will typically not occur as a 'big bang' approach. Big bang refers to going live with all system functionality on day one of installation into the production environment. A 'slow and grow' implementation approach within CIS projects is very common due to the complexities associated with re-engineering clinical workflow practices (Amatayakul, 2004). For example, a staged approach in Case study B will be undertaken with first implementing the diagnostic results reporting component of the CIS.

Training is a key implementation issue, particularly in the hospital environment where the release of medical, nursing and allied health staff for training away from clinical duties is a major challenge. A creative approach to training is required to minimise the clinical users time away from their duties. Sites that have implemented CIS have used nursing staff to buddy up with medical staff for training in system functionality on the job. Clinical champions in medical and nursing positions are standard practice for hospitals that have successfully implemented CIS.

A data migration strategy for legacy systems that interface to other systems is a key implementation requirement that must not be underestimated in terms of size and complexity (Chapter 15 deals with these further). Case study A will focus on migration of data from the legacy theatre management system to ensure continuity in the new system installation. Case study B will focus on data migration from the PAS and other interfaced systems into the CIS data repository.

Operation/support

Once the system is operational, it will be important to ensure system users' expectations have been met. A post-implementation review can be undertaken to ascertain if system requirements have been met by engaging system users. In this phase the system must be properly supported and mechanisms for further enhancements, fixes and developments must be available to system users.

CIS implementations are staged over a long period of time and require vendor products, which are highly configurable to meet ongoing changing clinical user requirements. This is a key factor for consideration in the acquisition of CIS so that hospitals are not at the mercy of ongoing costs associated with further developments from software companies (Handler, 2003).

Conclusion

Traditional information system development methodologies are valuable tools for application within the health industry. Widespread application of healthcare information systems remains in the minority in Australia and internationally. However, patient safety benefits have escalated the priority of healthcare information systems implementations worldwide.

Healthcare information systems are not typical information system projects because they are primarily tools for reengineering clinical workflow. Healthcare information system software solutions must be highly configurable to facilitate improved clinical workflows. The key challenge for healthcare information systems is not the technology; it is the significant leadership commitment at all levels to enact change of clinical workflow practices.

Review questions

1. Describe the main phases of the Systems Development Life Cycle.
2. What are the key activities required to successfully evaluate the most appropriate software strategy?
3. Discuss a scenario where a 'Big Bang' implementation approach would be appropriate for a healthcare information system implementation?
4. What is the most common reason for healthcare information system failures?

Exercises

- Perform a search on the Internet for an RFP document. Review two or three different RFP formats to become familiar with the type of content usually included in an RFP.

- The next time you visit the hospital or your general practitioner, either in a work capacity or as a patient, ask whether the healthcare facility maintains one patient index or one unique number for indexing and retrieving patient medical records. Outline the benefits associated with maintaining a unique index for patients attending a healthcare service provider.

Online reading

INFOTRAC® COLLEGE EDITION
For additional readings and review on systems development, explore **InfoTrac® College Edition**, your online library. Go to: **www.infotrac-college.com** and search for any of the InfoTrac key terms listed below:
- ➤ Systems development
- ➤ Systems development lifecycle
- ➤ Systems analysis

References

Amatayakul, M. (2004). *Electronic health records – a practical guide for professionals and organisations*, 2nd edn, American Health Information Management Association (AHIMA).

Centre for Medical Informatics, Monash University (2000). *Graduate Certificate in Health Informatics*, Multimedia Dynamics, Melbourne.

Computerworld (2002). *Systems development lifecycle definition*. Retrieved 14 May, 2002, from http://www.computerworld.com/.

Handler, T. (2003). *Steps to take when selecting a new clinical system– article series*, Gartner Research. Retrieved 2 June, 2005, from http://www.gartner.com.

McGee, M (2005). Computerized systems can cause new medical mistakes, *Information Week*. Retrieved 27 June, 2005, from http://informationweek.com.

PricewaterhouseCoopers (2005). *Reactive to adaptive: transforming hospitals with digital technology*, Global Technology Centre, Health Research Institute, Delaware.

Project Management Institute (2005). *Project management body of knowledge (PMBOK®), definition*. Retrieved 14 April, 2005, from http://www.pmi.org/.

Rhodes, M. & Costin, M.Y. (2005). *Achieving success with physicians and the ehr*. Paper presented at the Towards Electronic Patient Record (TEPR) proceedings May 2005, Medical Record Institute (MRI).

Shelly, G., Cashman, T. & Rosenblatt, H. (1998). *Systems analysis and design*, International Thomson Publishing Company (ITP), Cambridge, MA.

Westbrook, J. & Gosling, S. (2002). *The impact of point of care clinical systems on health care: a review of the evidence and a framework for evaluation*, Centre of Health Informatics, Sydney.

14

Health information systems

Dianne Ayres, Jeffrey Soar and Moya Conrick

> 'If builders built buildings the way programmers wrote programs, the first woodpecker that came along would destroy civilization.'
>
> Anonymous (with no offence intended)

Outline

Healthcare is an information-intensive industry in which quality and timely information is a critical resource. There is a wide range of information systems in health that perform different functions and all are involved in the management of data and information. This chapter provides an overview of health information systems and their use in supporting healthcare.

Introduction

Health information systems collect data as part of the patient care process. These data can be used across a number of systems for many different purposes and, as with all patient data, they must be subject to confidentiality and security safeguards. Patient data must integrate with data from other facilities; and it must meet the needs of various professional groups. Health information systems generally comprise several different applications that support organisations' needs, but they need to integrate well for the system to function efficiently. Central to health information systems are the electronic health records systems that deal with patient-specific information.

To allay confusion with the numerous terms frequently used to describe electronic records, the term 'Electronic Patient Record' will refer to the hospital-held record in this chapter.

Health records systems

Curiously, clinical information systems and electronic health records (EHR) have been the last areas automated, although it seems that this is the area in which most good and real saving can be made. The silos in health data have led to a plethora of problems from inadequate and missing data to duplication and so on. Many health entities still exchange information using paper-based records with all of the attendant problems.

In the past, health information systems have been deployed using different software applications hosted on a variety of platforms with little consistency in data or technology standards. Fortunately these situations are changing and are influenced by numerous factors including:

- a critical need to improve quality and safety and reduce the number of adverse events that result in death and disability, costing the health system an estimated AUD $4billion a year (Wilson, Harrison, Gibberd & Hamilton, 1999)
- the need for data, information and technology standards to improve interoperability between the many health information systems
- the Australian national summary Electronic Health Record (Health*Connect*), which is a policy directive arising from the National Health Information Action Plan (Commonwealth of Australia, 2001).

To be a credible and reliable source of health information, an EHR like Health*Connect* needs to be populated from source systems such as a hospital Electronic Patient Record (EPR), general practice, allied health systems and other private sector sources of health information.

Purpose of health information systems

A computer-based information system provides an organisation with data processing capabilities, and knowledge workers with the information required to make better quality, more informed decisions (Long & Long 2005).

Health information systems support all functions of an organisation, such as patient billing and finance; staff rostering and human resource management; departmental management such as pathology, medical imaging and pharmacy; clinical business functions including order management and results reporting; and clinical documentation and knowledge resources for decision support. Ideally a health information system enables the sharing of information with speed and accuracy that contributes to quality patient care.

There are also external uses for the data, including to:

- meet funding requirements
- meet reporting requirements
- assess and plan for accrediting bodies
- demonstrate compliance with standards
- project and redirect demand in the use of health services
- advance research.

Benefits

Access to quality information from health information systems across the continuum of care should have benefits for clinicians, management, patients and health consumers. Some of these benefits are specific to health records, others are more general attributes of health information systems. It must be remembered however, that a good deal of research is required before the extent of these benefits can be fully determined.

Patients/consumers

Autonomy in health is something that we hear in relation to patients and consumers in the digitalisation of healthcare. The other phrase is 'patients taking responsibility for their own health'. Until now, with the paper record locked within organisational and jurisdictional boundaries, this was impossible. Electronic records will change this so that patients and consumers have improved access to the health system and to their care details.

They will be able to annotate their record to keep it current, check for incorrect data such as an out-of-date medications list and to monitor the security of their information by checking that only those people authorised have accessed their record. A current record will reduce the dependency on memory about their health history and enable better sharing of information between care providers across the continuum of care. Consumers will have more confidence in a system that appears to be efficient and that provides a better experience for them free from duplication, error and lengthy delays due to the unavailability of data.

Clinicians

Access to quality information when and where it is needed has been at the forefront of the development of systems for clinical use. The use of fragmented data and inadequate information, on which life-changing decisions are made, has little place in a modern health system. Automation will not only enable timely access to clean data and information, it will enable clinicians to use evidence-based practice to underpin decisions and will assist in reducing medical error and improve patient safety. It will also save clinicians time in accessing the information.

When information systems (IS) are integrated and interfaced, the rhetoric about continuity of care can become a reality. Systems will support this by improving the coordination of information sharing between clinicians, patients and clinicians, services, and across all care settings.

Management

The health system has many challenges, for example, supplying quality timely information to health services with reduced funding, a mobile and changing workforce and an increasingly ageing population. Health information systems enable management policy functions to better support research and education, and facilitate a learning culture that will assist in building a best practice evidence-based health system. They can better plan clinical services and population health and enable better forecasting and management of demand.

Although the picture above is exciting and paints a 'rosy' picture of the future in a digitalised health system, it is tempered with some spectacular glitches along the way. The analysis of the Australian New South Wales Precision Alternative experience (case study below) gives an insight into these.

Case study

In 1995, the New South Wales Health Department terminated the pilot trials of The Precision Alternative (TPA) Point-of-Care Clinical System and Patient Administration System, the central components of its information technology strategy. While pilot terminations are valid options in such programs, this one did represent a substantial loss in committed resources, in strategy development, and in frustrated expectations. In the light of this, a study was undertaken to find out what happened and why. While the strategy was based on a rational plan implementing a proven system, there was a range of organisational aspects, which thwarted its effective implementation in New South Wales. These aspects are analysed in terms of the transfer of proven technology from another environment, and the diffusion of the technology through the large, divisionalised structure of the New South Wales health system. The major problems identified were the differences in organisational environment from where the system had been proven, and in the inappropriate consideration of organisational aspects in the diffusion strategy.

(Southon, Sauer & Dampney, 1997, 1999)

Hospital information systems (HIS) environment

A HIS environment is vast, and the diagram (see Figure 14.1) demonstrates this by depicting the variety of information systems that would typically support just one hospital or Area Health Service/Region. Note that the number of users and the cost and complexity of the systems increase to support direct patient care.

The diagram illustrates the dominant information source that the EPR has become. Also noteworthy is the concept of separate information systems to support the various business functions of the hospital. All departmental systems will need to be closely interfaced (preferably integrated) with the EPR while Enterprise Management systems have a less direct link to them. However, the distinction being made here is between Health*Connect* (discussed below) and a hospital-based electronic record. The difference between the two is apparent in Table 14.1.

HealthConnect

Health records at multiple sites pose problems from a clinical, health services planning and research perspective. Health*Connect* is based on an information and technology architecture, information and data standards, and a security and privacy framework that is sensitive to issues across Australia.

The Australian Government (2000), defines the Electronic Health Record as an electronic longitudinal collection of personal health information usually based on the individual, entered or accepted by healthcare providers, which can be distributed over a number of sites or aggregated at a particular source. The information is organised primarily to support continuing, efficient and quality healthcare. The record is under the control of the consumer and is stored and transmitted securely.

Figure 14.1: A typical HIS environment

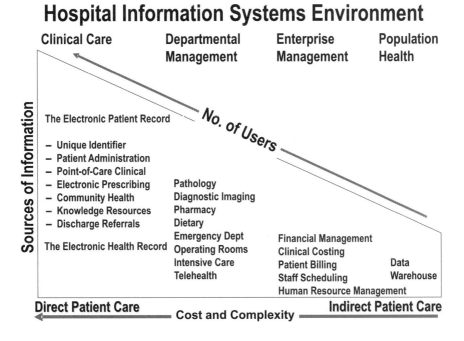

Hospital Information Systems Environment

Clinical Care   Departmental   Enterprise   Population
                     Management   Management   Health

Sources of Information

No. of Users

The Electronic Patient Record

– Unique Identifier
– Patient Administration
– Point-of-Care Clinical
– Electronic Prescribing   Pathology
– Community Health   Diagnostic Imaging
– Knowledge Resources   Pharmacy
– Discharge Referrals   Dietary
                               Emergency Dept
The Electronic Health Record   Operating Rooms   Financial Management
                               Intensive Care   Clinical Costing
                               Telehealth   Patient Billing   Data
                                                      Staff Scheduling   Warehouse
                                                      Human Resource Management

Direct Patient Care   Indirect Patient Care
                        Cost and Complexity

HealthConnect has undergone trials of its various components and is now being implemented in Tasmania, South Australia and the Northern Territory. New South Wales is trialling a Child Health Information Network and a Chronic Disease Management System, which are scheduled to 'go live' by the end of 2005. Trials to test the systems architecture are ongoing in Queensland as are peri-operative care trials. However, the current Health Minister has stressed that he would like the system implemented nationally in the next twelve months (Abbott, personal communication, 20 June 2005). This seems very ambitious given the paucity of electronic records systems that can provide source data to HealthConnect and the other info- and infrastructure needs of the sector.

In the 2004–2005 budget, the Australian Government provided $128.3 million over the next four years to fund the implementation of HealthConnect as a major platform for reforming healthcare delivery in Australia. The implementation of HealthConnect will include the integration of MediConnect to form the medicines component of HealthConnect.

General Practice is more advanced than many hospitals in computerising patient records, but then again General Practice is far less complex. The intensity and complexity of information is vastly different, there are fewer care providers interacting with the General Practitioner's electronic record, and the integration and interfacing needs with multiple systems are minimal. Add to this the freedom from the politics and bureaucracy of large organisations, which often impede timely progress.

Table 14.1: Differences between the EPR and the EHR

Electronic patient record (EPR)	**Health***Connect* Electronic health record system (EHR)
All patients who enter hospital will have an EPR – it is not an option.	Opt-in model (Opt-out in NSW) Consumers' consent for information to be sent to the Health*Connect* repository.
The EPR is a dynamic 24 X 7 record of all observations, interventions and outcomes entered by many health professional who have a direct or indirect relationship with the patient. Patients do not have access to the EPR.	A passive record of information received from multiple sources including hospitals, community centres, general practices and pharmacies across the public and private sectors. Patients/clients may annotate information into the EHR but cannot write to it.
The hospital EPR is not generally accessible to external sources in the private sector because of security and privacy requirements. Computer viruses from external sources are a real threat to hospital information systems.	The EHR is accessible to authorised users from any health sector with the consent of the patient/client. Consumers can influence what information is recorded, viewed etc and by whom.
All information generated about a patient is captured in the EPR and is available online to authorised providers.	Summarised information from each encounter is sent to the EHR repository. This includes current medications lists.
Integral to an EPR is real time decision support at multiple levels, e.g., rules, alerts, prompts, embedded links to reference databases and knowledge sources.	No real time clinical decision support capabilities. Timely, current information will be useful for management decisions across the continuum of care.
All authorised care providers that have a direct or indirect relationship with the patient will be able to access some or all of the information in the EPR according to security access level.	Clinicians have access to the EHR (with the patient's consent) and populate/update the EPR with past medical history and other relevant data.

From p.8199, *General Practice*.

The EPRs are the key information system support of direct patient care. In most organisations they comprise a number of disparate systems (often legacy systems) that interface with the core modules of the record. These are the point-of-care clinical system and the patient administration system. The following is a functional overview of the systems that typically comprise an electronic patient record.

Patient administration system and unique patient identifiers

The patient administration system (PAS) is the administrative foundation of the EPR, which is also required for all other information systems that require patient-specific information. Most healthcare organisations will have a system to manage the registration, admission, transfer and discharge of patients.

The role of the unique patient identifier (UPI) is to ensure that, whenever information is received about a patient, it can be reliably linked to the correct patient record. The UPI system provides a mechanism to link patient demographic information from a variety of sources and allocate a unique identifying number that is then stored by various source systems to allow authorised information exchange on a reliable basis.

The PAS supports the following functions:

- patient master index including demographic information, that is, name, address, date of birth, next of kin, financial status, national health service and/or health insurance number
- allocation of encounter/episode number and medical record number
- storage of the area and health service unique identifier
- waiting list and pre-admission management to book patients into hospital
- inpatient management, including admission, transfer and separation
- bed management, including bed census, ward/bed transfers and closures
- patient location history – present and past episodes of care
- appointment and resource scheduling
- coding and classification
- medical record management, including record request and tracking
- reporting.

Systems for clinical care

Only a brief outline of the components of clinical and clinical decision support systems is offered here because they are fundamental to the digital transformation of health and, accordingly, they are dealt with at length in dedicated chapters.

A *point-of-care* clinical system is the clinical foundation of the EPR. It provides access to information and clinical decision support tools to support the care process. It must be integrated with a number of clinical support systems, including the emergency department, pharmacy, dietary, pathology, medical imaging and other clinical specialty systems to provide a comprehensive EPR. This will provide critical summary information from inpatient episodes of care to Health*Connect*.

Electronic prescribing decision support systems

A strategy to reduce medication error is to implement electronic prescribing decision support systems (EPDS). In a clinical business context, EPDS should be a core function of a point-of-care clinical system, but software vendors tend to develop it as either a stand-alone system or an additional module to a point-of-care clinical system.

In a General Practitioner's surgery, stand-alone systems can work well because there is one prescriber interacting with one software system and the activity is generally only to prescribe. However, in a hospital environment prescribing is only one part of the medication management loop. To automate only this aspect, and not dispensing and administering, causes discontinuity in the medication management process that may lead to errors and omissions. EPDS therefore should be built on to the point-of-care clinical system as there is an interdependency with order management, clinical documentation, results reporting and knowledge resources, for example, MIMS, to address all aspects of the medication loop.

Decision support systems

Decision support systems (DSS) are those that use forms of logic to analyse data and suggest courses of action to clinicians and other professionals. In addition to EPDS, another example is a system that presents diagnostic test results back to the ordering clinician, as well as the potential diagnoses. DSS might also suggest appropriate tests and treatments on the basis of initial diagnoses saving time for clinicians entering orders.

In the 1970s there were expectations that Artificial Intelligence systems would assist clinicians making diagnoses. These have not been widely accepted and instead there is an expectation that systems that provide support for doctors to make diagnoses and other decisions will be more accepted in the complex environment of healthcare.

Community health information system

A number of Australian states contributed to the development of a Community Health Information System to provide a case management focused system for community-based health workers. The aim was to improve service delivery, outcome measures and productivity through improved capture and management of information generated in the community-based services. This system supports the following functions:
- client assessment tools
- appointment scheduling
- management plans
- client outcomes and management reports.

In New South Wales community health information systems will be phased out as the integrated EPR being implemented in hospitals is extended to community health centres. (*Note*: In New South Wales, the EPR is known as the electronic medical record (EMR). Although some professions might find this disenfranchising, it will be interesting to see if this is an Australia-wide trend.)

Electronic discharge referral systems

An integral component of a point-of-care clinical system is the electronic discharge referral system (eDRS). These have been implemented to meet an urgent need for information to be transferred from hospitals to general practitioners, community nursing services, nursing homes and other care settings, as well as to provide event summary information for Health*Connect*.

eDRS is an information system that supports clinical staff in the production of timely, accurate and clinically useful hospital discharge referrals. These discharge referrals are summaries of the hospital episode, include advice to community-based providers and, where appropriate, advice to the consumer on their immediate self-care. The National Health Transition Authority (NeHTA) in consultation with major stakeholders has standardised this by developing the requirements for discharge referral summaries and the data groups they should contain.

Knowledge resource systems

Most Australian states have programs and systems that provide a great variety of knowledge resources to support informed clinical decision-making. Integration of specific databases with point-of-care clinical systems is a future goal as these become more established throughout health.

The Internet/Intranet is also used to disseminate locally developed knowledge sources such as clinical protocols, clinical practice guidelines and clinical pathways in most digitalised organisations. The World Wide Web also enables documents to be shared to assist in the ongoing development of protocols and guidelines to promote best practice.

Interest box

In 1997, New South Wales Health established the Clinical Information Access Program (CIAP) to provide clinicians and other health professionals in the public health system as well as rural General Practitioners with access to knowledge resources via the Internet and Health Intranets (Ayers & Wensley, 1999). The aim was to provide 24-hour access to information to aid decision-making and promote evidence-based practice. Information included citation databases; full text journals; drug reference databases such as MIMS, Micromedex; Therapeutic Guidelines and Australian Medicines Handbook; decision support databases and much more.

Departmental management systems

Pathology management information systems

Pathology services were one of the first areas to computerise and now make extensive use of robotics and other automated systems for processing specimens. Pathology test results are critical to diagnosis, often requiring a fast turnaround time for results reports to initiate treatment. Pathology results reporting should be integrated with order management and CIS as the EPR is deployed to provide timely access and faster turnaround time for results reports.

Pathology information systems support the following functions:
- receive orders and provide results
- specimen management
- scheduling
- biosurveillance
- inventory/stock management
- billing and reporting.

Radiology information systems

The radiology information system (RIS) manages information relating to the order or request for service for a patient, the procedures applied, reporting on images by a radiologist and the communication of results back to the requesting clinician. Picture archiving and communication systems (PACS) manage electronic communication of the images. PACS systems allow for film images to be digitised for communication to requesting clinicians.

These film-less systems allow images to be taken directly to digital media. However, one of these images can be around a gigabyte in size and it is not difficult to imagine the storage and infrastructure required to accommodate this. PACS cannot work as a stand-alone system and requires integration with clinical and radiological information systems.

The typical RIS provides the following functions:
- patient registration
- scheduling
- patient tracking
- film library management
- results reporting
- department management.

Pharmacy

Retail pharmacy was a leading innovator in information systems to support its businesses. Pharmacy information systems manage the receipt of prescriptions, dispensing of medications and printing of labels. They also check for drug interactions, but only within the records held at that particular pharmacy. These systems may also manage pharmacy stock, including reorder levels and checking for use-by dates. Hospitals also have pharmacy systems with similar functionality.

Pharmacy systems typically support the following functions:
- drug dispensing and interaction checking
- imprest supply
- stock management
- drug purchasing.

Unfortunately pharmacy has been stifled by legislation that does not permit the transmission of electronic signatures on scripts and hopefully the work in progress now will resolve this issue. Currently pharmacists receive and process orders for medications on paper and transcribe the data into their system.

As the electronic patient records continue to be deployed, the pharmacy network will receive orders directly transmitted to their pharmacy systems. This was trialled in the MediConnect project that linked patients, doctors, pharmacists and hospitals to enable the sharing of medications information. In this trial, consumers became active participants in their medication management and it enabled doctors and pharmacists – with patient consent – to make prescribing and dispensing decisions based on knowledge of previous prescriptions, the current medications regime and previous medication reactions.

The trial demonstrated the potential to lead to significant and genuine improvements in health outcomes (DMR Consulting, 2004). Great gains are expected at the hospital interface, where quick access to a patient's medication record could be life saving.

Dietary management systems

The aim of a dietary management system is to improve the efficiency of the food services and support nutritional services through reduced costs and wastage of food and better nutrition therapy, and to improve the timeliness of communication between wards and food services to reduce errors in the delivery of meals to patients. The dietary system supports the following functions:

- food services and diet office management
- menu management
- inventory management
- bedside menu entry
- nutritional analysis
- nutritional accounting.

Clinicians who may need to alter patients' diets from their ward or unit can also access these systems through the EPR.

Emergency department information systems

The Emergency Department (ED) is often referred to as the 'front door of the hospital', as this is the place where up to 50 per cent of admitted patients become inpatients. An emergency department information system (EDIS) assists clinicians to manage patient information flows.

Most EDISs include functions that capture triage information, clinical data, admission and transfer details, daily activity census, and patient tracking. An EDIS provides a variety of reports to local management, area management, and the Department of Health, including the volume of presentations, waiting times for each triage category, access block, and benchmarking information. This data enables Health Departments to compare the performance of EDs and predict the demand for ED services. EDIS support the following functions:

- emergency department registrations
- triage categories
- clinical data on presentation
- collection data for injury surveillance and biosurveillance
- healthcare standards trauma indicators
- reports, such as 24-hour activity report and daily attendance register – outlining details of each presentation and its outcome for a selected date.

These systems can also be interfaced more widely to the general clinical systems and, in some countries, to the ambulance service and other emergency services. Field data such as observations and measurements can be downloaded to the EDIS for specialist assessment before the patient arrives to the ED.

Administrative systems

Healthcare uses systems common to many other organisations to manage finance, assets, payroll, billing, purchasing, inventory and other 'back-office' administrative functions. Some of these have features specific to healthcare, but they all need to exchange information with clinical information systems that manage patient health information.

Financial systems

Financial systems assist with managing the processes of setting and monitoring budgets that may be devolved to individual departments; placing orders for supply of goods and services from suppliers; matching invoices with orders; printing of cheques; managing bank accounts; managing staff expense claims; asset and inventory management; and other financial and accounting functions. Modules of a financial software system might include:

- accounts payable
- accounts receivable
- purchasing
- inventory or stores management – managing the process of goods in and any issues from the hospital warehouse to departments and wards
- processing payroll with information received from Human Resources
- assets management – registering and tracking all assets above a certain specified value.

The current trend is for most organisations to purchase a ready-made financial management system and it is increasingly rare for financial systems to be developed by in-house programmers. Well-known names of suppliers of financial systems include Oracle, PeopleSoft, JD Edwards and SAP.

Human resources

The Human Resources (HR) Department typically uses software to assist in core functions of recruitment; staff classifications; salary and other entitlements; leave records and managing staff records. HR in healthcare is more complex than many other industries owing to the wide range of disciplines involved. These can include medical classifications covering all the specialties; a wide range of nursing skills and classifications; diagnostic services specialists, scientists and technicians; allied health practitioners; administration staff; catering; grounds and maintenance staff; and many other categories. An HR information system might include the following modules:

- recruitment
- personnel records
- training
- rosters
- staff time recording.

Resource scheduling

Resource scheduling is a function that is frequently a separate module or function of an HIS that optimises the use of key and expensive resources such as CT-scanners and MRIs (Medical Resonance Imaging).

Appointment scheduling

Appointment scheduling, as the name suggests, manages the appointment times for patients at outpatients and other clinics. In primary cases most General Practitioners will use a practice management system. This manages appointments, patient medical histories, drafting and printing of pharmacy prescriptions, and checking for drug interactions.

Executive information systems

Specialised systems that interact with other systems and present summary information to executives are known as executive information systems (EIS). These will interface to financial and other operational systems to find key data to present to executives often in a graphic format to enable them to quickly identify trends and issues.

These systems also supply data for decision-making and policy development, supporting activities such as cost-benefit analysis and other economic analyses of data.

Data warehouse

A data warehouse integrates data from multiple information systems including from most of those described in this chapter. Although not a primary source of information for clinical purposes and not always accessible in real time, the data is primarily used for health services planning.

Conclusion

Health information systems should form the backbone of an integrated, cost effective and efficient health system. However, to realise this, significant work and resources must be injected into the sector. The resources are not all fiscal; it depends on the goodwill of all sectors of health and all health workers. If this is harnessed, consumers and patients will at last be the 'winners' in their health system.

Review questions

1. What has led to the disintegration of health data?
2. What is the purpose of a health information system?
3. Why are electronic health records said to be central to electronic health information systems?
4. What are the benefits of automated systems to a) clinicians b) consumers and c) the health system?

Exercises

- Discuss the reasons why there are so many failures in implementing information systems and investigate an example in the health environment.

- Select one of the health information systems outlined in this chapter and investigate how it can improve a clinician's/health professional's working life. Discuss the benefits and the impact on the organisational culture.

- Discuss the barriers to the implementation of health information systems addressing the issues from a political, organisational and individual perspective. How can these barriers be overcome?

- What would be the advantages and disadvantages of a National Electronic Health Record from a patient/client perspective?

Online reading

INFOTRAC® COLLEGE EDITION

For additional readings and review on health information systems, explore **InfoTrac® College Edition**, your online library. Go to: **www.infotrac-college.com** and search for any of the InfoTrac key terms listed below:

➤ Health information systems
➤ Hospital information systems
➤ Health records

References

Australian Council for Safety and Quality in Healthcare (2002), *Second national report on patient safety: improving medication safety.* Australian Government Publishing Service, Canberra.

Ayers, D. & Wensley, M. (1999). The clinical information access project, *The Medical Journal of Australia*, 171, 544–6.

Bates, D., Cohen M., Leape, L., Overhage, J., Shabot, M. & Sheridan, T. (2001). Reducing the frequency of errors in medicine using information technology, *Journal of the American Medical Informatics Association*. 8(4). 299–308.

Commonwealth of Australia (2001). Health Online: a health information action plan for Australia. National Health Information Management Advisory Council, Canberra.

DMR Consulting. (2004). *Indicative benefits report*. Retrieved 2 February, 2004, from http://www.healthconnect.gov.au/research/benefits.htm.

Long, L. & Long, N. (2005). *Computers*, 12th edn, Prentice Hall, Sydney.

National Electronic Health Records Taskforce (2001). *A health information network for Australia*, Department of Health and Ageing, Canberra.

Southon, G., Sauer, C. & Dampney, K. (1997). *Central IT policy: analysis of the NSW precision alternative experience*. Presented to HIANSW'97, The Sixth Health Informatics Association of New South Wales, Pokolbin.

Southon, G., Sauer, C. & Dampney, K. (1999). Lessons from a failed information systems initiative: issues for complex organisations, *Int J Med Inform* 55(1), 33–46.

Wilson, R., Harrison, B., Gibberd, R. & Hamilton, J. (1999). An analysis of the causes of adverse events from the quality in Australian healthcare study, *Medical Journal of Australia*, 170, 411–5.

15

Software management

Jeffrey Soar and Moya Conrick

'Act in haste and repent at leisure; Code too soon and debug forever.'
(Raymond Kennington)

Outline

In healthcare there is a range of software systems used in information management. These software systems include those common to most businesses as well as the ones specific to healthcare. This chapter discusses software and software engineering in the context of the healthcare system.

Introduction

'No matter how sophisticated the computer system, software is necessary to tell the hardware what to do and when to do it.'
(Conrick, 2001)

Computer software is a set of instructions written in a programming language that the computer can understand. When a computer switches on, it loads the software required for it to operate. While many people use software packages on their personal computers such as MSWord, behind the scenes the operating system software will control communications, printers, disk and other storage devices, the display on the monitor screens and other aspects of the computer. This software is developed and supported by systems programmers.

Most users however, will only ever interact with applications software that is either purchased as a ready-made package or developed in-house by programmers or by computer users themselves. Table 15.1 outlines major software groups; as these are the subject of dedicated books, many of which cater for beginners to advanced users, a more detailed description will not be pursued here.

Table 15.1: Major applications software groups used in healthcare (adapted from Conrick, 2004)

Software type	Use/Description
Data processing	*Databases* – data storage, manipulation and structured output (see Chapter 5).
Desktop publishing	Communication via good quality documents.
Educational	Bibliography packages, statistical packages, library catalogues, drug calculation. Simulation and virtual reality enables laboratory practice that is close to reality (see Chapter 26).
Games	Proven platform for engaging both adults and children in health education.
Graphics	'A picture tells a thousand tales.' Animated graphics add visual appeal if used sparingly.
Multimedia	Use of more than one medium – text, video, audio full motion video and so forth.
Office automation	*Word processing* – general typing of text documents. *Spreadsheets* – complex calculation operations; or many variable elements or parameters such as financial calculations, rosters.
Presentation	Replacing overheads as a vehicle for enhancing presentations and communications. Can be used in information kiosks.
Security	Virus checkers, worms, spyware and so forth.
Communication	Connecting dispersed healthcare providers and patients (see Chapter 19).
Voice recognition	Captures data using a microphone – effective in areas with routines, e.g. pathology reporting.
Workgroup	Business software that combines electronic scheduling, email, address book.

In the past, health systems software was developed and maintained by in-house Information Technology (IT) departments. In the government sector, Departments of Health had large IT sections that developed and supported a suite of health or hospital information systems (HIS). Increasingly there has been a move away from developing software or customising packages and towards purchasing ready-made packages.

Systems development methodologies

Software development is the process of producing software systems, but over the years these projects have had a reputation for being behind schedule, over budget and not satisfying user needs (McNurlin & Sprague, 2006). However, system development methodologies (SDMs) have evolved over the past forty years and these have addressed many of the challenges of software development. They have also led to greater project rigour, control, monitoring and improved communication between users and developers. As the approaches to software development have evolved it has become known as software engineering.

Systems development life cycle

Software projects, whether developed or off-the-shelf purchase, should be planned and follow a project development model. Although there are some less structured methods used such as prototyping where a system is developed as a prototype or model and presented to users to confirm requirements. Refinement of this system is achieved through iterations of the prototype. Prototyping can produce smaller systems more rapidly than the more formal approach like the systems development life cycle (SDLC).

The SDLC sets out a formal process that steps the development team through the development process (Laudon & Laudon, 2006). These steps consist of:
1. requirements analysis – defining the requirements
2. technical requirements – translating these into technical specifications
3. systems design
4. systems development – developing the code or writing the software using an appropriate language
5. testing
6. implementation
7. maintenance.

1. Requirements engineering

Deriving and documenting users' requirements for a system is one of the first steps in software development. This step should produce a Statement of Requirements that should be signed-off by executive management in the area of the organisation requesting the new system. This presumes that the project has gained executive approval to proceed and has been allocated resources. It may also involve the development of a Business Case.

A Business Case (as discussed in Chapter 8) should provide an Executive Summary detailing the nature of the problem. A cost benefit analysis should be undertaken (for more detail refer to Chapter 12). Essentially this determines what the benefits will be and what the opportunity cost is of not proceeding, that is, what the costs and other impacts are of not having the software. The Business Case will report on the alternative courses of action and why software development is the preferred approach.

Requirements engineering is a critical step. Getting this step right will help reduce problems elsewhere in a software project. Project failures can be reduced through improved communications and better management of expectations. Users may not appreciate the time it takes to develop systems or the practical limitations of software. Consequently, they may become frustrated after participating in workshops to develop the requirements for the system because it seems to be a long time before the software is available.

Requirements engineering involves determining users' needs, documenting them and receiving management sign-off to confirm them. This may involve workshops with users, obtaining copies of all the forms used in current processes, modelling data and processes and developing a document describing requirements for the new system.

Process improvement and business process engineering

When analysts and users meet to develop a User Requirements Specification for a new software system, it is important to avoid automating existing processes that might be inefficient. Instead both analysts and users should look for ways to improve processes and reduce unnecessary steps. Business Process Engineering involves setting radical targets for process improvement and can streamline processes.

2. Technical requirements

The User Requirements feed into a document that will guide programmers in the task of writing the programs, or code, that will deliver the required functionality and support clinical and business operations. This technical specification document should be an indisputable and comprehensive blueprint of the design of the program.

3. Systems design

The system needs to be designed before the coding phase commences. This will include the design of the user interface and how the data will be stored and managed.

Software development is often undertaken because a package is not readily available for purchase. There are advantages and disadvantages in purchasing an already developed package. Generally industry has moved towards purchasing packages because software implementation projects themselves can be problematic and lengthy. When this is added to the time required for developing software then it might be a very long time before the organisation can reap any benefits.

4. Systems development

Systems development is the coding phase, which in larger projects is undertaken by teams of programmers working from the systems design and technical specifications. This phase will incorporate its own quality assurance processes to ensure that every module developed will perform as expected.

Software development languages

There has been an evolution of languages used for writing software. Older languages such as COBOL and FORTRAN often involved long lines of code. The software was often difficult to maintain as the people who originally designed or added to the code may have moved on from an organisation and new staff often struggled to understand all the components, how they interacted, and what the impact of making a change might be elsewhere in the system. Adding to the problem is that programmers may not always provide sufficient documentation within the code to remind themselves or others of what it does, of any changes made, and a record of its links and impacts.

5. Data transfer

An essential component of projects, which occasionally is not included in the initial scoping phase, is the transfer of data from an old system to the new. If the previous system was manual then there may be years of historic data.

It is not always possible to leave the old system for reference and in health it is a common requirement for the old data to be moved across to the new system. This may be a challenge as the old data may have many errors, duplicate records or incomplete data. Tidying this data is called Data Scrubbing.

However, the structure of the data in the old system may be different from the new system. For example, the new system may have separate fields for street and suburb whereas the old system stored the data in one field. Therefore, data transfer often involves writing another program that will take the old data, check for errors and duplicates, and will store it in the new system according to the new data structures.

6. Testing

There are several stages of testing and this includes testing individual modules and the total system. Stress testing is an important undertaking; it detects problems in the system and is used to evaluate the system's readiness for implementation. In this process, the system is given a heavy processing load to test whether its performance is acceptable. Test data that are both routine and unusual are also entered to see if the system can detect when unacceptable data is entered. Users will be involved in the later stages of testing and need to develop Test Scripts. Any problems found are reported back to the developers.

Testing is essential for both software development and ready-made off-the-shelf systems. When a project is at this stage, there is often a strong desire to have the system implemented and testing can be cut short. This temptation should be resisted as undetected errors can cause problems later and a poorly tested system should never be put into production use.

7. Implementation

An Implementation Planning Study that identifies all the resources necessary to successfully implement the system needs to be undertaken. This will include backfilling so that all staff on all shifts can attend training. Once the system has passed through testing without major errors or with identified minor errors, a schedule for correction is established and the system is ready for implementation.

8. Maintenance

Software development is an ongoing process in that once a system has been implemented maintenance and support arrangements need to be in place. In the case of ready-made packages there will usually be a support contract with the supplier for an annual fee. This may give users access to a Call Centre for telephone support and cover access to bug fixes and to new releases of the software.

> 'It's not a bug – it's an undocumented feature.'
>
> Anonymous

Project governance

Effective communications are critical to successful projects. Establishing a steering committee for the software project is important for both communications and good governance. Without constant, consistent communications, users may be unaware of the developers' work and the developers may have incorrectly interpreted the user requirements.

A Project Steering Committee should meet regularly to receive reports on the project from the project manager and other key participants. These should be made available to other stakeholders as appropriate. The chairperson for the Project Steering Committee should be the project sponsor and should be the most senior executive from the department or business unit within the organisation requesting the software.

Project ownership

Engaging the most senior executive helps to encourage user engagement at each step of the process. Too often when users request software there is inadequate attention paid to this and when the system is delivered, developers often find that they have interpreted specifications differently from the way users expected. Users need to be constantly consulted during the project and have a sense of ownership of the process. Each project needs to consider ways to achieve this.

Projects office

A projects office provides a central point for support across the project. This will assist with methods, templates for business cases, progress monitoring, risk management and quality assurance. It can also help to keep the project on schedule. Its role of monitoring progress across multiple projects will include early warnings of delays or other problems to enable executives to take action to avoid project failure.

Purchasing software

When software is purchased rather than developed there is still a need for a rigour, adherence to a methodology and competent project management. Quality processes will provide a sound basis for purchase decisions, enhancing the chances of overall project success and the realisation of the benefits. This is especially the case in public organisations where files are discoverable through Freedom of Information legislation because unsuccessful suppliers may wish to satisfy themselves that appropriate processes were followed.

Templates are available to assist in the process of specification, calling for tenders, evaluation and contract negotiation and many government departments and larger corporations have their own processes. Consulting firms also have methods that their staff follow when assisting clients in software acquisition.

Call for tender processes

As with software development, the first steps in software acquisition involve the development and approval of a business case and requirements engineering. Rather than moving on to development, the next step involves developing a Request for

Tender document. This will include the requirements definition and any technical specifications such as the technical environment and standards. A method of evaluation needs to be developed to guide the selection panel that will be charged with reviewing tenders and selecting preferred products and suppliers.

Some large acquisition processes might involve massive effort both on the part of IT suppliers in preparing their tenders and on the part of the purchaser organisation in evaluating tenders. In these cases it is good practice to follow a two-step process with an Expression of Interest (EOI) stage before the Call for Tenders. The response to an EOI is less costly for both parties. The outcome of the EOI stage will be an Invitation to Tender for those suppliers who have been selected through the EOI stage. The EOI responses will be used to evaluate those companies that meet minimum criteria. It helps avoid waste of time and effort on the part of suppliers that will have little chance of success.

Increasingly selection criteria and even the evaluation method are made available to potential suppliers to assist them in compiling their tenders. To negate any bias based on pricing, a sound approach is to require tenderers to submit their costs in a separate envelope. It is advisable to open the envelope only at the final stages of selection. That way the selection will initially be made on the product functionality and fit with requirements. It will minimise the influence of cost upon the decision-making processes. When the short-list is reduced to two or three potential suppliers it is reasonable to open the proposals of the short-listed suppliers to assist in finalising decision-making.

Selection panel

A selection panel should be composed of key users as well as IT technical specialists. Once the receipt of tenders has closed, this panel will receive the submission. It may initial key pages of documents submitted to limit possibilities for later tampering. It will perform the initial cull of the tenders based upon criteria that should be specified in an evaluation method agreed earlier.

The criterion for initial cull involves matters that would make tenders unacceptable and this produces a shorter list of tenders for more detailed analysis and comparison. The selection panel reports on the rejected or preferred products and suppliers based upon the selection criteria to the Project Steering Committee.

Integration

Whether a software system has been developed or purchased off-the-shelf, there will be a need for its integration with other systems as few software systems function in isolation. Most systems need to link with other systems to send and receive information, using the same databases. The linkages between systems (interfaces) are also software that either need to be developed or are purchased with a new software package.

In the 1980s and early 1990s there were expectations that fully integrated Hospital Information System (HIS) packages would become available and reduce the need for interfacing with its attendant complexities and costs. This architecture placed the HIS at the centre of the system, within an ever expanding range of integrated modules extending across the hospital and to outside organisations.

In the early 1990s it became apparent that the availability of a fully integrated system would be some time off, if ever. While some vendors have broadened the range of modules in their HIS packages, it is often a challenge to convince a hospital department to accept a module of an integrated HIS package when department staff may be aware of a specialised best of breed package for their particular speciality.

Integrated packages were expected to obviate the need for multiple interfaces, at least between the various modules of patient information systems. Consequently, initial HIS implementations of the early 1990s were sometimes under-funded for integration. It became apparent that the cost of building complex interfaces was expensive. While interfaces to financial and billing systems could be less expensive, batch transfers of information, interfaces between HIS modules needed to be real-time for effective patient care. This was more complex, and so more expensive.

Integration of best of breed packages, and messaging between them, will be around for some time and it may be beyond the capacity of individual vendors to build and maintain these within integrated packages. Standards are essential for effective messaging, to avoid miscommunication that might lead to patient adverse health events, to enable interfacing between applications, and to minimise costs of interface development and support.

Software versioning

It is reasonable to expect that after purchasing software the business environment will constantly change and even during the development process there will be a need to change software specification. A Variation Control process is required to register changes, to scope their impacts including cost, and to reach agreement between the user and the developer on incorporating a change. Many software projects become unstable if there is not a formal and tightly controlled process to manage this. In the past developers agreed to incorporate changes that were requested sometimes without thinking about the impacts on the schedule, the cost and the impacts that any change might have on other components of the system.

During the process of software development all documents should be identified with a unique version number. Similarly releases of software including fixes to problems (bug fixes or patches) should be numbered and these should be made available as software problems are identified. It is reasonable to expect a new release of a major software package annually. New releases normally contain new functionality to keep the software up-to-date and perhaps incorporate new features to assist users.

The processes for agreeing upon new functionality to be included vary by vendor and developer. For in-house use, the software developers might be more responsive as the facility might be the only users. Where large vendors have thousands or even millions of customers across the world, a formal process of prioritisation is needed so that a change requested by one customer does not disadvantage another.

User Groups are one method of providing prioritised lists of requested enhancements for software to a developer. Ballots are another means where users can vote either directly or through User Groups to indicate their support and the priority for proposed enhancements to software. User Groups are also a good means for users to communicate with developers or suppliers. Often users do not make full use of the functionality of systems and problems can sometimes be resolved through explanation from developers.

Generally is it important to keep software up-to-date. It is difficult for suppliers to support multiple versions of software, however some vendors do not support software that is two to three versions behind the current release.

Conclusion

As computer software becomes more sophisticated and complex, it becomes more expensive, therefore its optimal use is essential. Software systems design must involve users and identifying champions early in the design process as this impacts on the effectiveness and effacement use of the software. This translates into efficient clinical and administrative process and improved outcomes of care.

Review questions

1. What are the major risks in software development and how can these be managed?
2. What are the advantages and disadvantages of purchasing ready-made 'off-the-shelf' software packages compared with software development?
3. Compile a table of software packages that you are aware of currently in use in healthcare along with the supplier and the modules or key functions that the package provides.
4. Why is testing so important? What different types of software testing are there?

Exercises

- Requirements engineering is a crucial step in software acquisition. Discuss this statement.

- Analyse the information needs in your place of work or home office. Develop a list of software requirements to deal with these needs. Justify your choice.

- Develop a plan for implementing a new software system into a clinical area.

Online reading

INFOTRAC® COLLEGE EDITION

For additional readings and review on software management, explore **InfoTrac® College Edition**, your online library. Go to: **www.infotrac-college.com** and search for any of the InfoTrac key terms listed below:

➤ **Applications software**
➤ **Operating systems software**
➤ **Software systems life cycle**
➤ **Software architecture**
➤ **Software engineering**

References

Conrick, M. (2005). Nursing informatics, in R. Funnell, G. Koutoukidis and K. Lawrence (eds.), *Tabbner's Nursing Care*, 4th edn, Elsivier Churchill Livingstone, Melbourne.

Conrick, M. (2001). *Rethinking Chalk and Talk: Using Technology in Education*. Paper presented at the Education and Employment Conference, Brisbane.

Kennington, R. (n.d.). Retrieved 8 August, 2004, from http://www.softwarequotes.com/.

Laudon, K. & Laudon, J. (2006). *Management information systems: managing the digital firm*, 9th edn, Pearson Prentice Hall, New Jersey.

McNurlin, B. & Sprague, R. (2006). *Information systems management in practice*, 7th edn, Pearson Prentice Hall, New Jersey.

16

Electronic health records

Sam Heard

'I don't know the key to success, but the key to failure is trying to please everybody.'

Bill Cosby

Outline

Electronic health records are a massive change from current paper-based practice. The promise of benefit to all from sharing information that can be displayed and automatically processed has not yet been realised as it requires shared concepts, terminology, models and architectures. Systems that can deliver in this evolving environment require complex engineering solutions, with shared models. Two of these – HL7 and *open*EHR – are also discussed in this chapter.

Introduction

The electronic health record (EHR) is a relatively new entity that has deep roots in the world of bulging and ragged paper medical and nursing records. At the beginning of the twentieth century health records were universally organised as a diary or statement of work for the clinician. As such, patterns of presentation over time were easier to recognise and monitoring the work of the clinician relatively straightforward. After the First World War, the innovation of keeping records organised within a patient folder – the so called 'unit record' – was developed at St Mary's Hospital London, and became a 'hit' in the new world, quickly becoming the norm.

This made the individual patient the focus of care, and enabled clinicians to share the responsibility of healthcare efficiently within an organisation. The monitoring of work and performance of clinicians became far more difficult as a consequence. Weed's efforts to organise the unit record generated considerable interest in the latter part of the twentieth century (Weed, 1968) as paper records grew to multi-volume tomes. His 'problem oriented record' required recording of the problems that needed management and then linking these problems to the information in the record and hence to the healthcare offered.

With the advent of computing in medicine in the 1970s, the EHR promised the advantages of all three historical recording paradigms (the clinician or provider worksheet, the unit record, and the problem-oriented record) while adding two more: the distributed record, working for the patient as they move around a more complex health system, and automatic processing. Just as the problem-oriented record aimed to bring organisation and structure to the growing and increasingly chaotic unit record, the EHR aims, through decision support and knowledge bases, to go beyond what the clinician can read (and even know) to enhance patient safety and quality of care. There have been many innovations in the development of the EHR with isolated examples of achieving major healthcare benefits, but on the whole the realisation of the promise has been slow and even elusive.

The paperless office

The advent of technology to capture paper documents and provide a typewriter interface for word-processing has enabled systems to create an EHR that is a collection of images, facsimiles or documents. Transcription is a common source of this 'digital paper' form of the EHR, which incidentally remains the form with which many people feel comfortable. A familiar records format is tangible in a medico-legal sense and this familiarity has been expressed in a range of requirements in standards documents (CEN, n.d.; Dolan, 2005). It can also be seen in the need to sign (or attest to) an image of entries in a health record.

Even the most comprehensive of EHR architectures, *open*EHR, provides a means of associating an image with a digital signature to appease those who are not comfortable with anything else (*open*EHR, 2005). The advantages of this EHR over the paper record are largely in storage and retrieval; the 'paperless office' offers benefits that are well documented, but often underestimated (Audit Commission, 1995). The enhancement of workflow is considerable but time limited, particularly in a larger organisation. Once the number of documents grows, the ability to search and find the information required for patient care diminishes.

In parallel and from the outset, builders of EHR systems have aimed to do more than render the record on the screen in a form suitable for human reading: they have sought to maintain the information in a form that allows automatic processing. This approach aims to make the life of the clinician easier and to add functionality that cannot be supported when the record entries are images or word processing documents. To be successful in this endeavour, EHR systems have to use other tools to attach meaning to specific information. This has usually been done using programming languages to generate forms on the screen, which are then associated with relational databases behind the scenes. Users are required to enter particular data in a given 'field' on the form, which is subsequently saved in a known 'field' (and a known table) in the database.

The relational nature of the database adds efficiency, allowing the date and time of encounter to be stored in another table (thus only being entered once for all the data relating to that encounter) and demographic information about the patient in yet another. The table structure and their fields are called a (relational) schema and are unique to a particular vendor system and often, in large organisations, to a particular implementation. Most current systems use this approach to build an electronic health record, usually adding document management for externally generated information.

The problems of using a relational schema to provide the meaning of information are twofold:

1. The clinical concepts are not expressed in a manner with which clinicians can confer *meaning*, and as such the schematic representation is different in every system, even every implementation, and
2. these different schemata have to *evolve* as user requirements change, leading to ever more diverse representations of the health record data, as well as large development overheads for system developers.

These issues do not put great stress on healthcare record systems until patients and their advocates demand that key information be available wherever the patient presents. Further, this requirement for an enhanced or virtual unit record is matched by increasing demands for public health surveillance and organisational reporting, and demands for efficiency and patient safety. This approach cannot keep up with these demands.

The EHR is structured differently in different systems and settings, meeting different requirements and using different means of creating the 'paperless' experience for clinicians. It is worth standing back a little and considering the question, 'What is an electronic health record?'

What is an EHR?

Governments and providers want systems that meet modern requirements: they are prepared to pay money to achieve this, but the requirements themselves have proved difficult to state in a manner that is useful. This has led to a string of efforts to define the EHR. The Health Information Network for Australia (Commonwealth of Australia, 2000, p.xv) report in Australia proposed the following definition:

> ... an electronic, longitudinal collection of personal health information, usually based on the individual, entered or accepted by healthcare providers, which can be distributed over a number of sites or aggregated at a particular source. The information is organised primarily to support continuing, efficient and quality healthcare. The record is under the control of the consumer and is stored and transmitted securely.

Here the electronic health record is a personal record and designed to be available when and where the consumer seeks healthcare, and always under their control. This sort of definition concentrates on the record as a historical document, and as part of a system.

The International Standards Organisation (ISO) Draft Technical Report 20514 (2004, p.13) definition differs from this:

> ... a repository of information regarding the health status of a subject of care in computer processable form, stored and transmitted *securely*, and accessible by multiple authorised users. It has a standardised or commonly agreed logical information model which is independent of EHR systems. Its primary purpose is the support of continuing, efficient and quality integrated healthcare and it contains information which is retrospective, concurrent, and prospective.

Detailed requirements of an EHR architecture to address these requirements have been developed for ISO (2004), based on the Good Electronic Health Record (GEHR, 1995) and EHRA SupA projects in Europe (EHCR-SupA Consortium, 1998) and led by Dr Peter Schloeffel in Australia. This document is a definitive resource for those who are developing EHR services within their systems, and raises the possibility of a common (and standard) health record architecture such as *open*EHR. The advantages of such an approach are only just beginning to be measured in the Health*Connect* trials (Health*Connect*, 2004) in Australia.

In the existing health information environment, those offering EHRs in the marketplace claim that the way their systems are architected is proprietary. They argue that EHR systems need to be assessed on the basis of the functionality provided rather than the internal representation of information. In response, the United States government has funded HL7 (as a standards organisation) to develop a standard set of EHR functions called the EHR Functional Model – currently published as a draft standard for trial use (Dickenson et al., 2004). This avoids the difficulty of defining an EHR system, but enables profiles to be generated that express system functionality or requirements in a standard manner. The latest work in this arena is to add conformance criteria to each function, and agreed minimum functionality for EHR systems in a variety of settings. This 'demand-side' standardisation is a new development and is causing intense interest; the wording of the standard may mean that a system is recognised as conformant with major financial consequences.

It is worth considering the coarse grain functions as these reflect current attitudes. These functions are organised under three headings:

1. Direct care:
   - care management
   - clinical decision support
   - operations management and communication.
2. Supportive functions:
   - clinical support
   - measurement, analysis, research and reports
   - administrative and financial.
3. Infrastructure functions:
   - security
   - health record information and management
   - unique identity, registry, and directory services
   - health informatics and terminology standards
   - standards-based interoperability
   - business rules management
   - workflow management.

The name of the second group is somewhat euphemistic and reflects the interest of third parties in the EHR. These functions are largely meeting the needs of non-clinical interests and are supportive to organisations and populations.

A detailed list of one section of the Direct Care functions is given in Table 16.1. These functions have descriptions and a growing set of conformance criteria. Profiles, as described above, are the means used to describe specific systems (Ocean Informatics,

2004). So, for example, a profile for a medical office system in the community will not include DC.1.3.2, manage medication administration, but a hospital system is likely to require this.

Table 16.1: Example direct care functions from the HL7 EHR-S functional mode

DC.1	Care management
DC.1.1	Health information capture, management, and review
DC.1.1.1	Identify and maintain a patient record
DC.1.1.2	Manage patient demographics
DC.1.1.3	Manage summary lists
DC.1.1.3.1	Manage problem list
DC.1.1.3.2	Manage medication list
DC.1.1.3.3	Manage allergy and adverse reaction list
DC.1.1.4	Manage patient history
DC.1.1.5	Summarise health record
DC.1.1.6	Manage clinical documents and notes
DC.1.1.7	Capture external clinical documents
DC.1.1.8	Capture patient-originated data
DC.1.1.9	Capture patient and family preferences
DC.1.2	Care plans, guidelines, and protocols
DC.1.2.1	Present care plans, guidelines, and protocols
DC.1.2.2	Manage guidelines, protocols and patient-specific care plans.
DC.1.2.3	Generate and record patient-specific instructions
DC.1.3	Medication ordering and management
DC.1.3.1	Order medication
DC.1.3.2	Manage medication administration
DC.1.4	Orders, referrals, and results management
DC.1.4.1	Place patient care orders
DC.1.4.2	Order diagnostic tests
DC.1.4.3	Manage order sets
DC.1.4.4	Manage referrals
DC.1.4.5	Manage results
DC.1.4.6	Order blood products and other biologics
DC.1.5	Consents, authorisations and directives
DC.1.5.1	Manage consents and authorisations
DC.1.5.2	Manage patient advance directives

A range of other terms have been used to describe the EHR in various settings: the computerised patient record, the electronic medical record, the electronic patient record, and the continuity of care record to give a few examples. What is important is to understand the requirements, the setting and the communication patterns. No health information is an island, and none is precedent. It depends!

So ... the answer to 'What is an EHR?' has become, 'It depends'. It depends on if one understands an electronic health record to be an information-rich, patient-centric concept as defined above, or rather as a functionally delineated system. In the case of the latter, then it depends on what functionality you might expect from an EHR system in the setting in question. It also depends on the pattern of care and to what degree the record is shared or communicated.

Achieving the promise of the EHR

The advantages of paperless practice have been alluded to – fast and non-dependent retrieval of documents. If the EHR is considered to be a collection of documents then it is possible to add some information to each document that is machine-readable and begin to be able to find key information in the EHR. This overcomes some of the difficulties of this digital paper approach.

Facsimile interoperability

Achieving a basic level of communication is not straightforward. Web-browser access to web-enabled clinical applications remains the most popular approach, while forwarding of word processing documents (in, for example, rich text format or portable document format) and images is also popular. Immediately the communication technology must be mastered, even if it is only email. The HL7 Clinical Document Architecture (CDA) offers a standard way to communicate documents in Version 1, adding some Extensible Markup Language (XML) data to a semi-structured document so that it can be indexed within the clinical information system. This relatively straightforward approach has been adopted in a number of centres including the Mayo Clinic.

Terminology is required for accurate searches and, as a consequence, the LOINC document ontology (Regenstreif Institute, 2005) has been created. Unfortunately this has a strong cultural element reflecting the local (US) healthcare system – a problem with all terminologies. Nevertheless, a group called the Integrating the Healthcare Enterprise (IHE, 2005) has supported the communication of these semi-structured documents and proposes to coordinate a distributed document repository. One might call this level of sharing *facsimile interoperability* – people can read it – and like the paperless office, it is difficult to understand why it has taken so long to achieve.

Data and semantic interoperability

The demands for patient safety and automatic processing require that health information be represented in a way that enables the computer to determine the meaning. This deeper level of sharing information is called semantic interoperability. It is the search for this greater level of interoperability that has delayed the transmission of readable forms of the EHR; it has always seemed to be just around the corner.

There are two major efforts to achieve this end using somewhat different, but converging approaches: HL7 and openEHR/CEN[1]. Each of these will be discussed separately below.

The HL7 approach

The background to and discussion of Health Level 7 (HL7) has been presented in previous chapters and this will not be discussed in depth here. However, its use in the EHR will be discussed in some detail.

HL7 Version 2 is used widely throughout the world, but Version 3 has a multitude of outstanding issues. Version 3 differs little from Version 2 from a functional point of view, in that each defines numerous message models, one for each communication, based on requirements. Each model is used to generate a specification (or in Version 3 an XML schema) to describe the message.

Each message has a different model (and schema), and all rely heavily on terminology, as the models are usually quite simple and terminology-driven. Figure 16.1 depicts the HL7 approach. Although there is only one reference information model, the messages are based on refined models, so that each message has a unique schema. CDA aims to provide a single schema for all clinical documents.

Figure 16.1: The HL7 approach to messaging

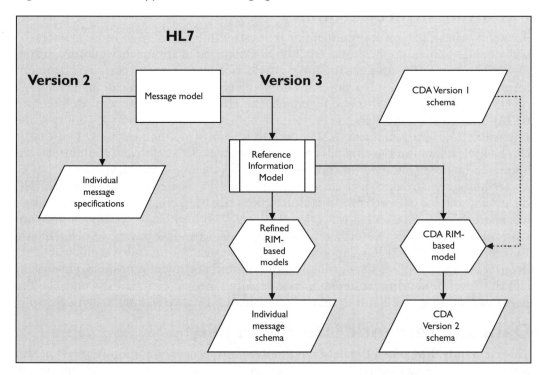

A great deal has been achieved using the simple Version 2 message – but the real successes have been when there are a very limited number of parties involved and the resources to generate the message definitions are available, such as the integration of different services (e.g. pathology, financial and radiology) within a hospital environment. The problems of maintenance and coordination grow when there are multiple senders and receivers of the same message. Getting a message moving in such a setting can take many years and may even be impossible!

Interest box

'Once you've seen one HL7 implementation, you've seen one HL7 implementation!'
(Wes Richel, Chair of HL7 1993–94).

Recent experience with the Australian HL7 pathology message has shown that the difference in implementation of a nationally standardised HL7 message specification by different vendors can be astounding – to the point that it is not recognisable as the same message.

Frustration with these difficulties led to the development of the CDA, which was strongly resisted by the HL7 power brokers in the first instance. It is now seen by some as their flagship and in release 2, the CDA adds the ability to describe some of the information in the document in a form that potentially allows semantic interoperability. The CDA has the advantage of providing a single schema, which has been aligned to some degree with the CEN and *open*EHR specifications. The approach is to provide a human readable document (as in Version 1 of CDA) while enabling machines to access any detailed information that accompanies it. The problem of representing detailed information covering a sufficient range of health information in a manner that can achieve machine interoperability is yet to be overcome.

*open*EHR and CEN

The *open*EHR Foundation is a non-profit organisation based in the United Kingdom that provides access to specifications, tools and clinical models to the health informatics community, encouraging collaborative development where this is appropriate. CEN has signed a memorandum of understanding with *open*EHR to bring this work to the new European EHR standard – a revision of Env-13606.

The *open*EHR specification differs from the HL7 approach in that it offers a logical health record architecture. The CEN definition of an EHR architecture offered in 1987 was refined during the development of ENV13606 in 1999 as:

> a set of principles governing the logical structure and behaviour of healthcare record systems to enable communication of the whole or part of a healthcare record.

The result is that a shared logical structure exists, to which all information that is communicated conforms. This provides another level of interoperability – data interoperability. One feature of the *open*EHR approach is that each system is guaranteed to be able to receive information and display it to the user because, as with CDA, there is a single schema (see Figure 16.2). The *open*EHR architecture provides folders for organisation of documents, which can also be shared in extracts, to make reading by the receiving clinician easier. A full versioning (change management) model is also part of the architecture to deal with all medico-legal requirements.

Figure 16.2: *open*EHR interoperability

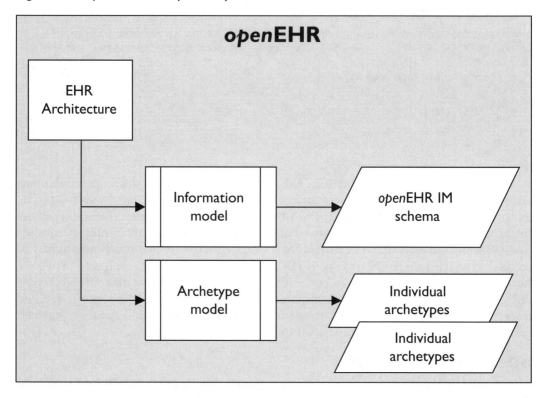

The innovation in the *open*EHR architecture is that the clinical meaning of the data, that is to say, the way the clinical concepts are represented in this shared schema, is defined in a separate artefact called an archetype. Archetypes can be shared, evolve, be specialised and deprecated all independent of the shared schema. They can dictate what terminology is used at which data points and ensure that only sensible values are allowed for all data types. These discreet clinical structures can then be reused in any EHR. One principle is that data conforming to the same archetype *always* has the same meaning.

The *open*EHR approach requires a greater level of agreement at the outset, and the ability to deal comprehensively with all health information requirements: this is a non-trivial task and has, from its roots in GEHR, been underway about as long as the HL7 Version 3 development, but with fewer participants. CEN has taken many of the *open*EHR design features and put them in the new 13606 standard. The archetype methodology is attractive to those in the messaging environment and is being considered for use within the HL7 context. The multilingual capability, the open specifications and source code of key tools, as well as simplified requirements for terminology, make *open*EHR attractive to countries that do not have the infrastructure required to deal with complex connectivity.

Archetypes

It is worth considering archetypes in a little more detail, as these are a way of representing clinical concepts formally within a known information model. An archetype is a formal expression of how a domain concept (in healthcare that is a clinical concept) is represented in an information model, including any necessary constraints that will apply at data entry, such as what values are allowable. The archetype editor is a new tool for clinicians to express clinical concepts in a manner that can be used in systems. The tool has been developed for *open*EHR to enable archetypes to be created consistently to ensure that they can be shared. The design of archetypes requires clinicians and other stakeholders to consider the direct care and the supportive functions that the data will support.

The benefit of the archetypes may not always be clear, but can be understood using some examples. First, all data that is stored in a health record is entered using an archetype to constrain it. Thus, a diagnosis is always entered using the archetype for diagnosis, part of which is shown in Figure 16.3.

Figure 16.3: HTML view of an archetype for diagnosis

Diagnosis as defined by the clinician: *EVALUATION*

Generated by the Ocean HTML generator: 22/06/2005   Comments to *Ocean Informatics*   Copyright *open*EHR Foundation © 2005

Concept description:	Identification:	Information structure:
A diagnosis defined by the clinician which is coded in an accepted terminology and may include the stage of the condition and the diagnostic criteria	*Id:* openEHR-EHR-EVALUATION.problem-diagnosis.v1 *Reference model:* EHR	Data ▢ Protocol ▩

Data: *TREE*

Concept *Ordered*	Description	Type	Cardinality	Values
T Diagnosis (*specialisation of:* Problem)	The index diagnosis	*Coded_text*	mandatory 1..1	*Terminology* Any term that 'is_a' diagnosis
T Status	The status of the diagnosis	*Coded_text*	optional 0..1	provisional working
Date of initial onset	The date that the problem began causing symptoms or signs	*Date_Time*	optional 0..1	Partial date yyyy-??-XX
Q Age at initial onset	The age of the at the onset of the problem	*Quantity*	optional 0..1	*Property* = TIME *Units:* yr, (0..200) wk, (0..52) mth, (0..36) day, (0..56)
Severity	The severity of the index problem	*Ordinal*	optional 0..1	1, Mild 4, Moderate 7, Severe
T Clinical description	Description of the clinical aspects of the problem	*Text*	optional 0..1	*Free or coded text*
Date clinically recognised	Date the problem was recognised by clinicians	*Date_Time*	optional 0..1	Partial date yyyy-??-XX

Location, Location of the problem in terms of body site.   *Cluster* (0..*, ordered) optional, repeating

Concept	Description	Type	Cardinality	Values
T Body site	The body site affected	*Coded_text*	optional 0..1	*Terminology* Any term that describes a body site
T Location description	A free text description of the location - may be in addition to a coded body site	*Text*	optional 0..1	*Free or coded text*

Aetiology, Agents or Factors known to have been of aetiological significance.   *Cluster* (0..1) optional

The full richness of the archetype for a diagnosis is more evident in the view from the archetype editor in Figure 16.4. It is immediately obvious that this has been constructed by clinicians and with some thought to detail. This sort of information is too complex to construct from terminology on the fly and will not be computable in such a form for the foreseeable future.

Figure 16.4: The diagnosis archetype from the *open*EHR Archetype Editor

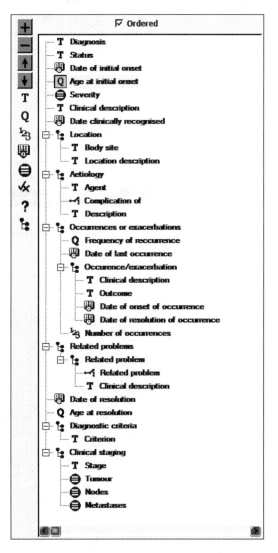

The archetype represents the clinicians' knowledge about what is required to record meaningful information about specific concepts, while the information model provides the containers and the other medico-legal and recording infrastructure for building a health record. Having recorded information using the archetype, it is always possible to retrieve it in the same manner, as all data is 'stamped' with the archetype used to create it.

Queries are generated using the archetype repository, built using the Ontology Language for the Web (OWL). As all data is archetyped, it is relatively straightforward to generate statements that can be interpreted and return the desired result.

Separation of knowledge and data

Archetypes represent knowledge and so can be dealt with inside a knowledge framework. The relationship between archetypes can be expressed in ontologies, and meaning anchored to reference knowledge bases of various sorts.

The innovation of separating knowledge and data formalisms in the *open*EHR architecture offers the hope of achieving comprehensive semantic interoperability in a sustainable manner. Terminology is still required to populate the archetypes when creating actual EHR entries, remembering that terminologies are capturing knowledge through the expression of ontological relationships. The next phase of EHR development will show us which of the approaches is the most successful:

- numerous rich schema, with meaning largely conveyed through terminology as identifiers and content, or
- one simple schema, plus archetypes and simplified terminology demands.

The problem for the rich schema and terminology approach is controlling the use in practice; the problem for the archetype approach is getting sufficient archetypes available to get communication started.

Conclusion

Electronic health records are here, and here to stay. At present they offer limited functionality and limited communication capacity. There are three levels of interoperability: facsimile or human readable, data level when information can be received but not necessarily processed, and machine readable or semantic interoperability.

Standardisation is proceeding from the payer side; this may do more for overcoming the barriers to achieving interoperability than at first imagined. As functionality in systems is rewarded, communication first, and semantic interoperability a close second, will be required. The EHR, as a safe and sharable resource for healthcare, is only achievable with agreed standards and cooperation.

Review questions

1. What is the difference between an electronic health record (EHR) and an electronic health record system (EHR-S)?
2. What levels of interoperability are useful in sharing health information? How do they differ?
3. What are some of the knowledge 'components' required for sharing electronic health records? How does their use vary in HL7 Version 3 and *open*EHR?

Exercises

- Describe three fundamental components required to achieve machine level interoperability. How are they related?
- Choose a function of an EHR System. Describe the data models and knowledge resources that would have to be shared in order that machines could provide this functionality in a distributed environment – using automatic processing.

Online reading

INFOTRAC® COLLEGE EDITION

For additional readings and review on electronic health records, explore **InfoTrac® College Edition**, your online library. Go to: **www.infotrac-college.com** and search for any of the InfoTrac key terms listed below:

➤ Electronic health Records
➤ EHR Records architecture
➤ OpenEHR
➤ Archetypes

INFOTRAC

References

Audit Commission (1995). *For your information: a study of information management and systems in the acute hospital*. HMSO, London.

CEN (n.d.). Revision of CEN 13606. Retrieved 23 May, 2005, from www.cenTC251.org.

Commonwealth of Australia (2000). A health information network for Australia. National Electronic Health Records Taskforce, Canberra.

Dickenson, G., Fischetti L., & Heard, S. eds. (2004). *Electronic health record system functional model and standard. Health Level 7*. Retrieved 12 June, 2005, from http://www.hl7.org/EHR/.

Dolan, B. et al., (2005). *Clinical Document Architecture. Health Level 7*, http://www.hl7.org.

EHCR-SupA Consortium (1998). *Electronic health care record: support action*. Retrieved 12 June, 2005, from http://www.chime.ucl.ac.uk/.

GEHR (1995). *The Good European Health Record Project. Advanced Informatics in Medicine*, DG XIII, European Commission, http://www.chime.ucl.ac.uk/.

Health*Connect* (2004). *A health information network for all Australians*. Retrieved 12 June, 2005, from http://www.healthconnect.gov.au/.

IHE (2005). *Integrating the healthcare enterprise, a vendor driven group coordinating the implementation of standards*. Retrieved 16 June, 2005, from http://www.ihe.net.

ISO (2004). *Technical Report 13808: Requirements for an Electronic Health Record Reference Architecture*. International Standards Organisation, Geneva.

Ocean Informatics (2004). *An EHR-S profiling tool based on the HL7*. Retrieved 10 June, 2005, from http://www.oceaninformatics.biz.

*open*EHR. (2005). *The openEHR Electronic Health Record Reference model*. Retrieved 12 June, 2005, from http://www.openehr.org/.

Regenstreif Institute (2005). *Logical Observation Identifiers Names and Codes (LOINC)*. Retrieved 12 June, 2005, from http://www.regenstrief.org/loinc/.

Weed, L. (1968). 'Medical records that guide and teach', *New England Journal of Medicine,* 278: 593–600.

Endnote

1   European Committee for Standardization, http://www.cenorm.be/cenorm/.

17

Clinical information systems

R.M. Ribbons

To many in the informatics community, clinical information systems represent the 'Holy Grail' of healthcare information systems. In many respects, the reason for this is related to the complexity of clinical data.

Outline

There is a plethora of challenges in dealing with clinical data, but once they are captured and identified they need to be stored in such a way as to allow efficient retrieval and their secure transmission to the appropriate clinician. This chapter discusses the development and implementation of clinical information systems (CIS) in the Australian healthcare environment.

The argument against paper-based clinical records

Traditionally, clinical records have been paper-based systems with varying degrees of contribution from electronic data sources such as laboratory results. Although paper based clinical records are easy to use, there is a number of obvious disadvantages in comparison with the hard copy record. One major disadvantage is that paper-based records can only be read by one person at a time and they must have physical possession of the document. It can only be organised in one format although multiple formats may be required to meet the clinician's information requirements. The traditional paper-based record only provides a third of the data that a clinician needs to provide adequate patient care (Anderson, 1999). This fact, combined with the difficulties in searching paper-based records, presents a major impediment to clinical research.

Paper records security is also a problem with almost any clinician (and others) able to access it regardless of their 'need to know' status. In addition to this, there is no method of tracking access. The ease of data entry is often offset by a lack of legibility, accuracy and clinical detail of the data entered. The poor quality of data increases the risk of clinical errors and, consequently, potential harm to the patient (Milholland Hunter, 2002).

Updating or simply adding a new page may require the same data to be written multiple times on multiple forms (a patient allergy for example). To make matters worse, different clinicians will use different terms to describe the same clinical phenomenon leading to a lack of compatibility with specific data standards and reducing the clinical usefulness of these data for both patient care and for clinical research (Hannan, 1996; Milholland Hunter, 2002). Over time, the clinical record becomes bulky requiring multiple volumes that, in turn, lead to the need for costly storage and archiving solutions. Poor indexing of the record may make it time consuming and expensive to retrieve.

It is frustrating, from the patient's perspective, to be continually repeating the same information to a number of different clinicians all asking the same or similar questions. Not only is this frustrating, it sends the worst possible message to the patient who is left wondering 'Why can't they get their act together and at least talk to each other?' In a paper-based system, the quality of the patient's history is often relative to their ability to recall important personal health related events. In the face of injury or illness, individuals are often unable to recall critical aspects of their health history. This, in turn, impacts on the clinician's ability to make accurate clinical diagnoses.

Because paper-based communication has historically been so slow, it has often been the case that information is not in the right place at the right time. This restricts the clinician's ability to provide a continuity of care across healthcare services. For example, a paper-based discharge summary that arrives two weeks after the patient is booked for GP review is useless. Often, slow communication leads to duplication of tests, clinical errors and inefficient administrative processes (Reinecke, 2005).

Case study

Mr Joe Lee is admitted to the Emergency Department unconscious following a single vehicle motor traffic accident. Paramedics stabilised his condition at the scene and diagnosed a closed head injury. The ED staff identify Mr Lee from his driver's licence. The admitting clerk searches the hospital Patient Administration System for previous admissions. The database reveals an episode of care three years ago for the repair of an inguinal hernia. No other data is available as Mr Lee's history has been sent to the hospital's off-site archiving service.

At 2.30 a.m. a request is placed to have the history retrieved from the archive 30kms away. A courier from the storage facility is paged and requested to retrieve the history. The courier arrives at the facility, accesses the archive area and locates the history, then drives the 30kms back to the hospital. This takes more than two hours. In the meantime, the ED staff are 'flying blind' totally unaware of the patient's past history, allergies or regular medications.

Imagine how much more effective and timely the emergency care of this patient could have been had the patient's health record been available electronically.

Purpose of CIS

The primary goal of any CIS is to make information and knowledge available to healthcare providers during care delivery (Geissbuhler & Scherrer, 2003). Velde and Degoulet (2003, p.271) define a CIS as a system 'that manages clinical data to support patient care and clinical decision making derived from various feeder systems such as laboratory and radiology'. It has only been since the early 1990s that the need for greater clinical and financial efficiencies heralded the development of CIS. These systems were designed to assist clinicians in the provision of patient care via clinical decision-support and by better managing medical resources.

CIS are purported to streamline clinical workflows and eliminate repetitive tasks that reduce productivity and lead to errors. Clinical decision-support inherent in many clinical systems acts to safeguard the patient and the clinician, enhancing safe practice. Automated clinical pathways and system alerts ensure that therapeutic measures are not overlooked. Collecting data at the bedside results in more accurate clinical data that should result in more accurate clinical decisions.

Initially, many health information/patient administration systems vendors simply added clinical modules to their applications. However, clinicians often found the resulting systems cumbersome to use and the need to make care delivery more cost effective meant that specialist clinical systems needed to be developed (Velde & Degoulet, 2003).

To achieve efficiencies, healthcare facilities must integrate health data from a number of different sources. Anderson (1999) suggests that the successful implementation of CIS will be heavily dependent on the integration of these data sources. Before discussing the complexities of CIS it is appropriate here to briefly describe the architecture that underpin them.

Clinical systems architecture

While it is not necessary for informaticians to possess an intimate technical knowledge of servers, *routers*, *bridges*, network *operating systems* and *protocols*, it is worthwhile to have some basic-level understanding of the underlying technical structure of clinical systems.

Prior to the widespread appearance of mass-produced microprocessor chips and the personal computer (PC), most hospital systems were based on *mainframe* technology. Mainframe computers were initially exceedingly large machines, often occupying an entire building or, at least, extensive amounts of floor space (McKeown, 2001). These character-based systems (they did not run a graphical user interface) featured '*dumb terminals*' linked to a centrally located computer. Figure 17.1 illustrates a typical dumb terminal, which consists of a screen and a keyboard with a connection directly to the mainframe.

Dumb terminals do not possess memory or processing chips and therefore are unable to perform processing functions unless they are connected to the mainframe; hence the term 'dumb'. Mainframes are very efficient at processing transactions and dealing with many users simultaneously. However, they require highly specialised programmers to maintain them, making them difficult and expensive to run. Clinical users often found these systems difficult, if not impossible to use (Velde & Degoulet,

2003) because often one needed to know the operating system language to issue the mainframe with processing commands.

Figure 17.1: A 'mock-up' of what a typical 'dumb terminal' character-based screen might look like.

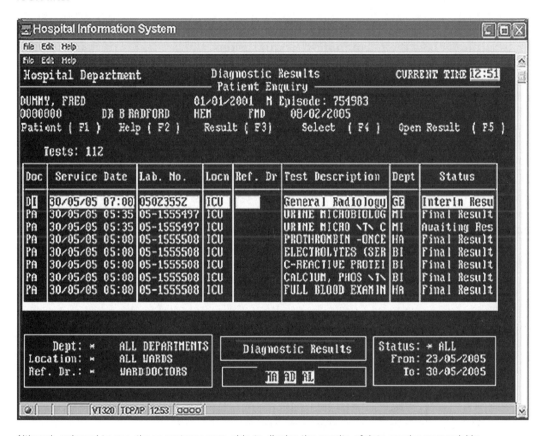

Although awkward to use, these systems were able to display the results of data queries very quickly.

The advent of the PC in the mid-1980s heralded a paradigm shift in the computer industry. Suddenly, departments within a healthcare facility could have their own computer. Using a local area network (LAN), stand-alone desktop PCs were linked creating a distributed computing environment. In many organisations, this resulted in the development of 'home grown' software solutions that essentially created 'information silos', in which information was only available to members of a particular department. Clearly, this creates problems when business critical information needs to be shared or when the department requires the processing power of a much larger computer.

To overcome these limitations client /server computing was developed. That means that information can be shared between multiple smaller computers or clients that are all connected via a network to a powerful host computer; the server (McKeown, 2001). Today's servers are significantly cheaper and easier to run and maintain than their monolithic mainframe counterparts. This has resulted in a move away from mainframes to these relatively compact network servers.

Velde and Degoulet (2003) suggest three reasons for this. Firstly, client computers with their graphical user interfaces (GUIs) provide consistency across applications and are therefore easy and safer to use. Secondly, this architecture enables the client to process data and finally, it is generally believed that the client/server architecture is more cost effective by offering better cost:performance ratios. Client/server architecture is now the norm in most organisations.

Perhaps the most widely used form of client /server architecture in contemporary CIS is known as three-tiered architecture (Velde & Degoulet, 2003). This architecture uses a client, an application server and a database server (Figure 17.2). In this environment, the user works on a client computer, a desktop PC for example. In many cases this architecture uses thin client software.

This software, usually a browser type application, shifts the data processing functions onto the server. The user sends a request for data to the application server that is actually running the application the user is accessing. The application server passes the query for this request to the database server, which processes the query and sends the results back to the application server. The application server processes the data into the form required by the client (McKeown, 2001).

This type of architecture allows patient data to be stored across departments and facilities in database servers that can be integrated in a patient-centric format by the application server. This provides clinicians with a comprehensive view of the patient's care, including progress notes, laboratory results, x-rays, health histories and care plans. The growing complexity of clinical data highlights the need to provide information at the point-of-care where it is needed most.

Figure 17.2: A typical three-tier client/server architecture. Most CIS now utilise this architecture.

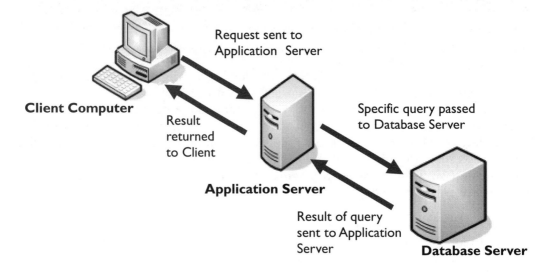

Request sent to Application Server

Client Computer

Result returned to Client

Specific query passed to Database Server

Application Server

Result of query sent to Application Server

Database Server

What are point-of-care clinical systems?

Point-of-care clinical systems are simply CIS located adjacent to where care takes place, in most circumstances at the bedside. These systems support clinical care by allowing easy input and retrieval of information. Examples of point-of-care systems include; *order entry*, *results reporting*, clinical documentation, *electronic decision-support*, *medication management*, online evidence retrieval and *telehealth* systems (Huges, 2000). These systems support the provision of safe, efficient and effective clinical care. Given the increasing demand for accurate, appropriate and timely clinical data, coupled with improvements in hybrid computer and information technology, point-of-care systems will form an integral component of future electronic health records.

The most common point-of-care clinical systems include electronic prescribing, electronic order entry, and results viewing systems (Westbrook & Gosling, 2002). Most of these systems are referred to as *e-ordering* systems, *physician order entry* (POE) or *computerised physician order entry* (CPOE). They enable the entry of clinical orders (investigations, medications, procedures, services) directly into the CIS. The ordering system then electronically transmits the order to the appropriate department. Once investigations are completed, the results are available online via the results viewing system.

A major benefit of these e-ordering systems is their ability to augment clinical judgement via integrated clinical decision-support software (Liaw, 1996). Decision-support systems (DSS) allow the process of ordering an investigation to go beyond the process of manually ordering the investigation by adding clinical value. Clinicians can access additional evidence-based information or may be automatically alerted to a range of clinical sequelae (a drug interaction or allergy alert for example) that may impact on patient care.

Huges (2000) indicates that the goals of any point-of-care system should be to:
- reduce the amount of time spent documenting patient care
- eliminate inaccuracies and data redundancy
- enhance the timeliness of data communication
- provide optimal access to information
- improve the quality of care by providing clinicians with the best possible information on which to base clinical decisions.

Capturing data at its source (from the patient) is critical in providing accurate, timely, cost effective, quality care. Contemporary CIS provide for point-of-care data entry, either manually or automatically via a medical device (for instance, IV pumps or haemodynamic monitor). This means that data are accurately transformed and available in a distributed fashion to other clinicians involved in the patient's care. Given their proximity to the source, point-of-care systems should ensure patient-centric care is delivered safely, effectively, efficiently, equitably and in a timely manner (Anderson, 1999; Sttig, et al., 2002).

Wireless clinical systems

There is the temptation to see point-of-care computing as simply moving computers closer to the patient, however this is really only a partial solution. In the absence of effective clinical systems, including clinical documentation, this approach lends little of the benefits expounded by proponents of point-of-care computing (Hughes, 2000). A truly integrated, mobile solution is required.

Integrating point-of-care clinical systems provides clinicians with a wide variety of clinical tools best suited to their specific work practices and this is crucial. Most hospital clinicians are highly mobile and, consequently, software applications must allow them to quickly review and interact with patient information while they are on the move. Mobile computing provides the right information, at the right time, for the right patient, in a user-friendly format. The development of wireless LANs over recent years has facilitated the move to mobile clinical computing solutions.

Internationally the use of wireless technology has become widespread in healthcare settings (Chen et al., 2004) but Australian hospitals appear to be lagging behind. This is unfortunate, as wireless technology provides clinicians with clinical decision-support tools constantly at their fingertips. Centrally located desktop computers (that is, those in the nurses' station) have proved inflexible in the clinical environment and access has been a problem. Mobile systems can reduce access time dramatically. Highly mobile clinicians such as resident medical officers and allied health professionals are able to manage patient lists, order investigations and receive referrals through handheld devices at any wireless-enabled location inside or outside the hospital.

Components of a CIS

Clinical documentation systems

Automated clinical documentation systems are designed to replace the paper-based systems. Their primary purpose is to support the documentation of care and provide a tool to manage the delivery of care. However, implementing a CIS is not simply replecating the paper-based model by scanning paper-based records into the system. It may overcome the physical limitations of the paper-based history, but they are unable to make an illegible entry legible.

Truly automated clinical documentation systems support the way that clinicians function, enhancing workflow. Allan and Englebright (2000) suggest that a well-constructed clinical documentation system can decrease documentation time, standardise documentation making clinical data more reliable, provide for multidisciplinary care coordination, and reduce the bulk of paper-based histories. Automation of clinical documentation can also improve clinician satisfaction. They can automatically calculate patient acuity, enabling nurse managers to make appropriate clinical and staffing decisions.

Clinical documentation systems should augment clinical practice by improving access to sophisticated information management tools. Internet databases such as Cochrane, decision-support tools and online policy and procedure manuals should ensure better informed, more evidence-based care is provided. The design of these systems should simplify the documentation process because many of the repetitious aspects of the traditional paper-based documentation process are eliminated.

Most hospitals require the completion of a large number of separate documents for each episode of care. A menu driven system is currently the most effective way to capture this volume of data. Menu driven forms are easy to use and guarantee high levels of data integrity because the user can only select specific highly structured data elements. Clinical documentation design should incorporate 'point and click' operations where possible.

Documentation using clinical pathways is becoming more prevalent in electronic CIS. These protocol-driven, evidence-based clinical documents are intended to provide improvements in the efficacy of patient care. Clinical pathways are constructed by critically reviewing research related to a particular diagnosis or diagnostic-related group (DRG) and analysing a significant number of patients with the same DRG. A series of protocols representing best practice are then built up to form the pathway. Essentially, these protocols create a grid used to define interventions and patient outcomes that should be achieved within predetermined time frames. Once established, pathways can be used for future patients with similar DRGs. If the patient deviates from the set care path in terms of required interventions or actual outcomes, a variance occurs.

Automated clinical pathways can alert clinicians when a variance occurs, thereby enabling appropriate adjustments to the patient's care and a timely correction of the variance. Clinicians can use variance analysis to evaluate patient care and determine why a variance occurred. Analysis can also predict when a variance might occur, enabling clinicians to readjust pathways accordingly (Donaldson & Conrick, 2004). CIS with preloaded pathway templates allow for rapid deployment of these systems and provide for local customisation of pathways.

Standardisation of concepts in clinical pathways is achieved through the integration of clinical dictionaries and clinical language systems such as the Systematized Nomenclature of Medicine (SNOMED), the International Classification of Diseases (ICD-10) and the North American Nursing Diagnosis Association (NANDA) (Andolina, 2000). Because pathways are multidisciplinary, they provide an opportunity for all clinicians to benefit from their automation. Implementing automated clinical pathways enables the provision of a more consistent, holistic and streamlined level of cost effective, quality patient care. They can also reduce a patients' length of stay (Davis & LaCour, 2002).

Order entry

Computerised physician order entry (CPOE), e-orders or simply order entry systems are an important aspect of CIS. Order entry systems may be an integral part of a much larger CIS, may be a separate component or module integrated with the clinical system. In either case, these systems allow clinicians to electronically prescribe medications, order laboratory or radiological investigations, or create referrals to allied health services.

When a clinician orders a particular investigation, the order entry system generates a request for direct transmission to the radiology or laboratory information system using standardised health data communication structures such as *Health Level 7* (HL7). During the ordering process, the system offers clinical decision-support in the form of duplicate order checking, additional information about the investigation being ordered or special requirements for the sample (for example, must be heparinised). The system can generate the appropriate labels and specimen forms at ward level and alert the clinician to the possibility of any duplicate order. Evidence suggests that these types of alerts can significantly improve patient care (Briggs, 2003; Bates et al. 2001). Figure 17.3 illustrates a typical browser-based GUI Order Entry system.

Figure 17.3: A browser-based order entry system (Soprano Workflow Orders™)

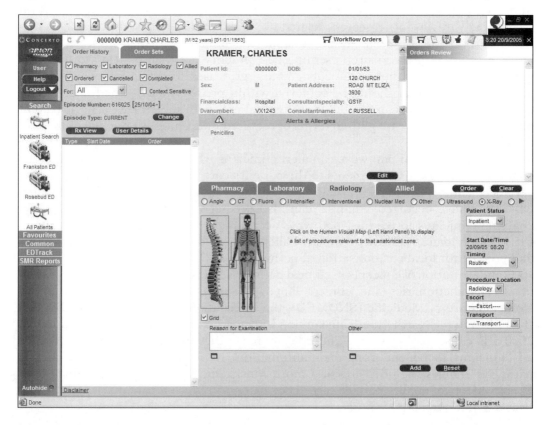

This system illustrates how pharmacy, laboratory, radiology and allied health services can be integrated into a simple, easy to use clinical interface. (Courtesy of ORION Systems International.)

On receipt of the order, the service provider system (such as the laboratory information system) sends an acknowledgement (using a HL7 message) back to the clinical system indicating the receipt of the order. The integration of ordering and provider systems using bi-directional HL7 messaging allows the ordering clinician to check the order status at any time.

Order entry systems can save significant time, as re-keying patients' details into the service provider system is unnecessary. This also reduces the possibility of data entry mistakes. Briggs (2003) suggests CPOE systems may, in the future, provide sophisticated research tools to facilitate data mining and improve long-term treatment outcomes.

e-prescribing is the process of ordering medications and creates a prescription using an order entry system. These systems should not be confused with medication management systems, which are discussed later in the chapter. Several researchers have found that e-prescribing systems improve the efficacy of the prescribing and ordering process and reduce the costs related to medication prescribing (Lehman et al., 2001; Briggs, 2003; Glemaud, 2000), while others assume that it provides safer, more accurate medication administration (Karow, 2002).

e-prescribing systems employ several forms of clinical decision-support systems targeted at increasing patient safety by decreasing the frequency of serious medication errors. Decision-support systems achieve this by performing error checks, providing relevant information quickly, and improving communication to other clinicians. The research reveals effective reductions in medication errors of between 55 and 81 per cent, and that computer-assisted prescriptions were more than three times less likely to contain errors than handwritten prescriptions (Briggs, 2003; Bates, Leape & Cullen, 1998; Bates et al., 1999; Oran, Shaffer, & Guglielmo, 2003). Despite this, the system seems undervalued and uptake limited, as only an estimated two to five per cent of all United States hospitals are installing electronic order entry systems (Briggs, 2003).

Medication management

Electronic prescribing systems can automate only a third of the medication management process. Medication management is a complex three-phased process involving medical staff, pharmacists and nursing staff. Due to the complexity of the process patients are at risk of adverse drug events at each stage of the process.

Automating the prescribing phase, but leaving the remaining two phases, brings with it a number of inherent difficulties. One obvious difficulty is that it deprives the pharmacists and nursing staff of clinical decision-support and is therefore only a partial solution to improving patient safety. Another difficulty is the necessity to reprint a paper-based administration chart every time a new medication is electronically prescribed and maintaining version control over these printed medication charts.

A medication management system that automates both the prescribing and administration process can overcome this, resulting in tangible improvements in patient safety and medications administration (Mekhjian et al., 2002). When coupled with barcode scanning technologies, medication management systems minimise the amount of manual documentation required of nurses and enhance patient safety by checking that the right patient receives the right medication.

Other systems

Systems that feed in to the CIS are discussed here in that capacity, and from a more detailed clinical orientation in Chapter 14.

Pharmacy

Pharmacy information systems are also concerned with three phases of medicating patients, with functions relating to both the e-prescribing and administration phases. Interfacing order entry or CIS to pharmacy systems provides drug file information allowing for medications not on imprest to be made quickly available to the ward. The order entry system maintains a history of the patients' medications while data in the clinical system, such as allergies, can be ported to the pharmacy system. Medications used during an inpatient episode can be easily scripted for discharge and the order sent to the pharmacy system for dispensing, saving both staff and patients' time, ensuring continuity of medications, and making the discharge process more efficient, increasing efficiency throughout.

Pathology

In Australia, all pathology providers use automated laboratory information systems. Many pathology providers maintain complex information and analysis technologies that support sophisticated messaging systems. This makes the task of integrating pathology and CIS relatively straightforward. If CIS and pharmacy systems are interfaced, the results are available to clinicians as soon as the analysis is completed.

Abnormal results can be flagged in the CIS by using pre-defined rules; some systems automatically page or text an alert to the responsible clinician. Some systems will automatically re-order an investigation if an abnormal result is returned. Figure 17.4 illustrates the cumulation and subsequent graphing of pathology results in a CIS.

Figure 17.4: Once downloaded from the pathology system, results are able to be cumulated and graphed (Soprano Results Viewer™).

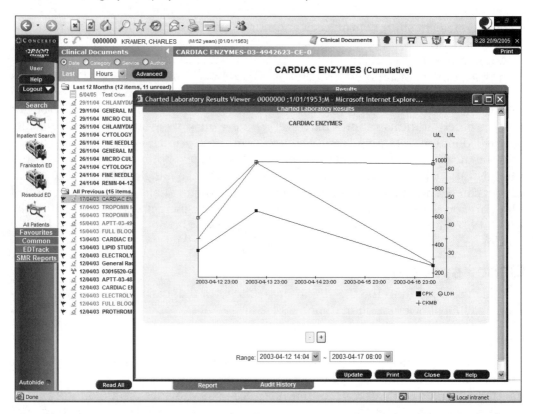

(Courtesy of ORION Systems International.)

Radiology

Radiology information systems have been available for more than a decade and provide improved management of medical images and enhance workflows in medical imaging departments. The introduction of more cost effective optical fibre network technology, together with high-density storage media, will accelerate the ability of hospitals to embrace digital imaging and to integrate the picture archiving and communication systems (PACS) that manages electronic communication of the images with CIS. This functionality will enable clinicians to view x-rays and other radiological investigations at the point-of-care via the CIS. It will significantly reduce the time clinicians spend looking for patients' films. The days of junior medical officers spending hours 'chasing' x-ray film bags are numbered!

Many health informaticians regard digital radiology as the future multimedia component of a patient's electronic health record. The integration of still images and digital video will enhance diagnostics, making the electronic health record far more data rich than traditional health records. Easy storage and retrieval of a patient's radiology record facilitates clinical review, reduces errors, and improves patient outcomes (Dodge and Reid, 2003).

Physiological monitoring systems

All medical devices, from ventilators to intravenous therapy (IV) pumps, have the ability to interface with database systems via what is known as RS-232 interface that allows these devices to download data to a CIS. They have been used for years to capture ventilatory parameters, heart rate, blood pressure, temperature, PaO_2 and numerous other physiological readings in critical care areas. Once in the database, these readings can be displayed in a graphical format that facilitates precise identification of abnormal trends. For example, IV pumps download data about the volume of fluids infused, and display these in tabular form or as a histogram in the CIS (see Figure 17.5 on the following page).

The ability to automatically capture physiological data significantly reduces the amount of manual documentation, freeing the clinician to spend more time in direct patient care. Physiological monitoring systems not only save time, but also ensure that accurate, timely data are available in a useable form. Wireless networks also have the potential of interfacing mobile patient monitoring devices such as Holter monitors with CIS.

Subsidiary systems

A number of subsidiary clinical systems can address specific needs of specialist departments within a healthcare organisation. One of these is the Emergency Department (ED) whiteboard system, which is an electronic version of the traditional physical whiteboard. This whiteboard automatically updates itself with the latest patient information at predetermined intervals. It provides staff with an on-screen, 'at-a-glance' list of the patients currently in the department, including their triage category, diagnosis, time in the department, admission details, location and attending clinician.

Figure 17.5: Physiologic data presented in Cerner's PowerChart®

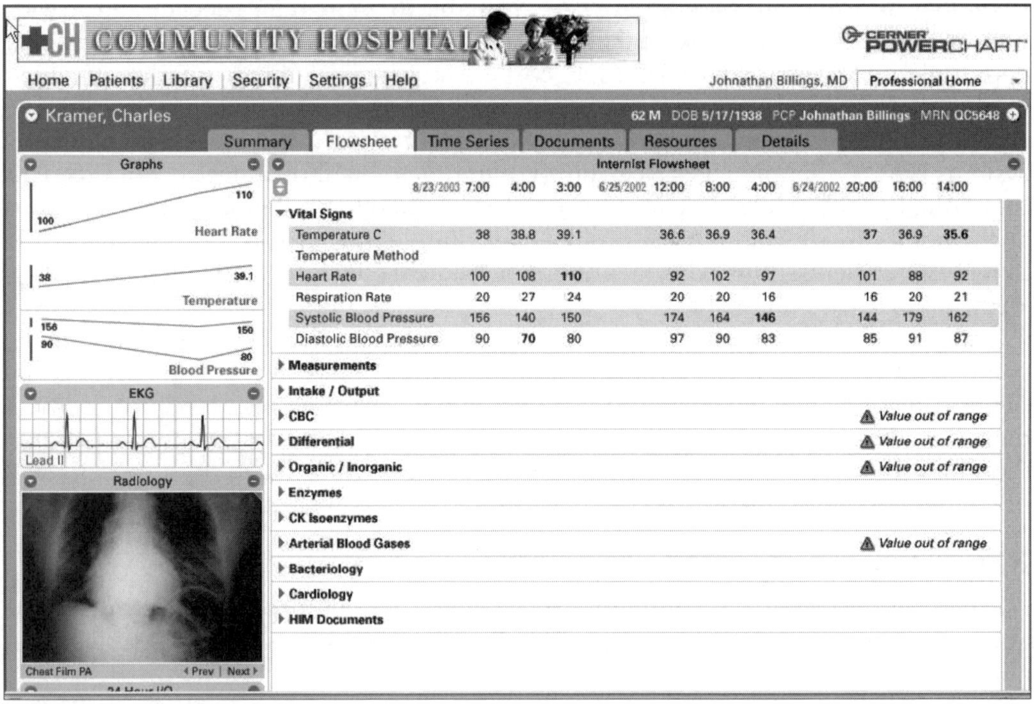

(Courtesy of Cerner Corporation)

Commonly, these electronic whiteboards are linked to other hospital CIS, so when new patient data becomes available, such as urgent lab results or x-ray reports, an automatic alert 'flag' appears on the screen. These systems provide clinicians with real-time, onscreen patient locator maps, for example the patient location in the ED or which department they have been sent to for further investigations. Similar software can be used throughout the hospital, providing ward staff with an on-screen ward map and an 'at-a-glance' view of their patients.

Over the past decade, in addition to the introduction of proprietary clinical systems, many hospital departments have developed their own databases. These in-house systems often work well, fulfilling the functions for which they were designed. However, they often lack robustness and rigour and frequently have inadequate backup capabilities and security to protect patient data (Geissbuhler & Scherrer 2003). It is critical that new CIS integrate these 'home-grown' databases to ensure the continuity of efficiencies these databases provide while reducing their inherent risks.

Conclusion

Increasing demands from state and federal departments of health, health professionals and the wider community for cost effective approaches to improving patient outcomes will drive the move towards more effective integrated CIS. Today's information silos will need to be replaced by clinical systems able to aggregate, synthesise, communicate and store patient information. It is only once these disparate, fragmented systems have been integrated that we will truly have the foundations of an electronic health record.

Review questions

1. What are some of the challenges facing acute healthcare facilities wishing to implement CIS?
2. How might standardised nomenclatures be integrated into a clinical documentation system and what form might they take?

Exercise

• The hospital you work for has decided to implement a CIS. You have been selected to be one of the clinicians on the project team. What specific application features, aimed at improving clinical workflows, would you be looking for as part of the system?

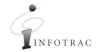

Online reading

INFOTRAC® COLLEGE EDITION
For additional readings and review on clinical information systems, explore **InfoTrac® College Edition**, your online library. Go to: **www.infotrac-college.com** and search for any of the InfoTrac key terms listed below:
➤ Clinical information systems
➤ Point-of-care
➤ Order entry systems

References

Allan, J. & Englebright, J. (2000). Patient-Centered documentation: an effective and efficient use of CIS, *Journal of Nursing Administration*, *30*(2), 90–5.

Anderson, J.D. (1999). Increasing the acceptance of CIS, *MD Computing. 16*(1). Retrieved 28 January, 2003, from: http://www.mdcomputing.com/issues/v16n1/ci_systems.html.

Andolina, K.M. (2000). The Automation of clinical pathways, in M.J. Ball, K.J. Hannah, S.K. Newbold and J.V. Douglas (eds). *Nursing Informatics: Where Caring and Technology Meet*, (3rd edn, pp.227–41). Springer-Verlag, New York.

Ball, M.J. (2000). Emerging trends in Nursing Informatics, in M.J. Ball, K.J. Hannah, S.K. Newbold and J.V. Douglas (eds). *Nursing Informatics: Where caring and technology meet*, 3rd edn, pp.301–4. Springer-Verlag, New York.

Bates, D.W., Leape, L.L. & Cullen, D. (1998). Effect of computerized physician order entry and a team intervention on prevention of serious medication errors, *Journal of the American Medical Association, 280*, 1311–16.

Bates, D.W., Teich, J.M., Lee, J., Seger, D., Kuperman, G.J., Ma'Luf, N., Boyle, D. & Leape, L. (1999). The impact of computerized physician order entry on medication error prevention, *Journal of the American Medical Informatics Association, 6*, 313–21.

Bates, D. (2000). Using information technology to reduce rates of medication errors in hospitals, *British Medical Journal, 320*, 788–91.

Bates, D.W., Cohen, M., Leape, L.L., Overhage, J.M., Shabot, M.M. & Sheridan, T. (2001). Reducing the frequency of errors in medicine using information technology, *Journal of the American Medical Informatics Association, 8*(4), 299–308.

Briggs, B. (2003). CPOE: Order from chaos, *Health Data Management, 11*(2), 44–8, 50, 52 passim.

Chen, E.S., Mendonca, E.A., McKnight, L.K., Stetson, P.D., Lei, J. & Cimino, J.J. (2004). PalmCIS: a wireless handheld application for satisfying clinical information needs, *Journal of the American Medical Informatics Association, 11*, (1), 19–28.

CHIK Services (2004). *Australian eHealth market: acute care 2003–2005*. CHIK Services, Gosford, New South Wales.

Commonwealth of Australia (2005). Health*Connect*. Retrieved 3 June, 2005, from http://www.healthconnect.gov.au/.

Davis, N. & LaCour, M. (2002). *Introduction to health information technology*. WB Saunders Co., Philadelphia.

Dodge, J. & Reid, B. (2003). Integrated PACS-RIS, in enterprise grabs RSNA spotlight, *Health-IT World Dec. 4*, Retrieved 25 May, 2005, from http://www.health-itworld.com/enewsarchive/e_article000207507.cfm.

Donaldson, P. & Conrick, M. (2004). *The effectiveness of using a patient dependency system to develop and audit clinical pathways*, paper presented at the HIC2004, Brisbane.

Dorenfest Integrated Healthcare Delivery System (IHDS +) Database (2003*). Healthcare information technology spending is growing rapidly*. Dorenfest & Associates, Chicago.

Economist (2005). Economist looks at the barriers to health IT, 5 May, p.45.

eHealth Implementation Group, Department of Health and Ageing (2005). *Lessons learnt from the MediConnect field test and HealthConnect trials*, Commonwealth of Australia, Canberra.

Geissbühler, A. & Scherrer, J.R. (2003). HCUG CIS, in R. Van de Velde & P. Degoulet (eds), *CIS: a component-based approach*, pp.243–52, Springer-Verlag, New York.

Glemaud, I. (2000). Use of a physician order entry system to identify opportunities for intravenous to oral levofloxacin conversion, *American Journal of Health Systems Pharmacists, 57*(suppl 3), S14-S16.

Harsanyi, B.E, Allan, K.C., Anderson, J., Valo, C.R., Fitzpatrick, J.M., Schofield, E.A., Benjamin, S. & Simundza, B.A. (2000). Healthcare Information Systems, in M.J. Ball, K.J. Hannah, S.K. Newbold and J.V. Douglas (eds.), *Nursing Informatics: Where Caring and Technology Meet*, 3rd edn, pp.264–83. Springer-Verlag, New York.

Hebda, T., Czar, P. & Mascara, C. (1998). *Handbook of informatics for nurses and healthcare professionals*, Addison Wesley Longman, Menlo Park California.

Hughes, S.J. (2000). Point-of-care information systems: state of the art, in M.J. Ball, K.J. Hannah, S.K. Newbold and J.V. Douglas (eds), *Computers in healthcare nursing informatics: where caring and technology meet*, 2nd edn, pp.144–54, Springer-Verlag, New York.

Karow, H.S. (2002). Creating a culture of medication administration safety: laying the foundation for computerized provider order entry, *Joint Commission Journal on Quality Improvement. 28*(7), 396–402.

Lehman, M.L., Brill, J.H., Skarulis, P.C., Keller, D. & Lee, C. (2001). Physician Order Entry impact on drug turn-around times, *Proceedings/AMIA Annual Symposium*, 359–63.

Liaw, T. (1996). Decision-support in clinical practice, in E. Hovenga, M. Kidd and B. Cesnik (eds.), *Health Informatics: An overview*, pp.161–72), Churchill Livingstone, South Melbourne.

McKeown, P.G. (2001). *Information technology and the networked economy*, Harcourt, Fort Worth, Texas.

Mekhjian, H.S., Kumar, R.R., Kuehn, L., Bentley, T.D., Teater, P., Thomas, A., Payne, B. & Ahmad, A. (2002). Immediate benefits realized following implementation of physician order entry at an academic medical center, *Journal of the American Medical Informatics Association, 9*(5), 529–39.

Milholland Hunter, K. (2002). Electronic Health Records, in S.P. Englebardt and R. Nelson (eds), *Healthcare Informatics: An interdisciplinary approach*, (pp.209–30), Mosby, St Louis.

Oren, E., Shaffer, B. & Guglielmo, J. (2003). Impact of emerging technologies on mediation errors and adverse drug events, *American Journal of Health Systems Pharmacists, 60*(14), 1447–58.

Reinecke, I. (2005, May). *Australia's e-Health agenda: what it means for older Australians*, paper presented to the NACIC 2005, National Aged Care Informatics Conference, Hobart, Tasmania.

Sttig, D.F., Hazlehurst, B.L., Palen, T., Hsu, J., Jimison, H. & Hornbrook, M.C. (2002). A CIS research landscape, *Permanente Journal, 6*(2), 62–8.

Westbrook, J.I. & Gosling, A.S. (2002). *The impact of point-of-care clinical systems on healthcare: A review of the evidence and a framework for evaluation*, Centre for Health Informatics, University of New South Wales, Sydney.

Van de Velde, R. & Degoulet, P. (2003). *CIS: a component based approach*, Springer-Verlag, New York.

18

Decision support systems

Jim Warren and Jan Stanek

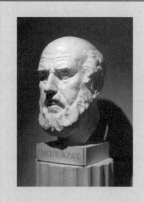

'Life is short, and Art long; the crisis fleeting; experience perilous, and decision difficult.'
(Hippocrates – Aphorisms. 400 BC)

Has the situation changed?

Outline

Decisions lie at the very core of medicine and healthcare. Attempts to make decisions easier are as old as the profession itself – rules of thumb were once included into verses so they would be easier to memorise. In the modern era, we strive to organise the best available clinical evidence into guideline documents and, increasingly, to produce automated models for decision support. This chapter examines the use of clinical decision support systems (CDSS) as a means of achieving this.

Introduction

A decision support system (DSS) can be thought of as any computer-based system that supports decision-making. However, the term DSS now carries some more precise connotations that usefully separates the concept of a DSS from other computer applications. A DSS has at least two distinct architectural components: (a) models, using knowledge and/or data about the world to support inference; and (b) a query interface, by which a decision-maker asks questions of the model (typically getting results in graphical and/or tabular form). As such, DSS generally support unstructured or semi-structured decision-making, which excludes a system where the user is simply given an answer by the computer and has no discretion in terms of interpretation of options.

A narrow conception of the role of a DSS is as an executive information system (EIS) – a workstation through which an executive weighs up the pros and cons of strategic decision options. Health, like any industry, makes use of DSS as EIS in strategic planning. For instance, a health industry executive may use a DSS to decide on the most effective location for a new hospital or how to market a new health insurance policy.

Where DSS for health become special, however, is in support for clinical decision-making. By 'clinical' we do not mean only medical decisions; clinical decision-making includes the assessment and care decisions made by nurses, pharmacists and allied health workers, and (taking the definition to its broadest extent) reasoning about health choices as made by consumers. A clinical decision support system (CDSS) provides patient-specific healthcare advice.

How and when decision support systems are used

A system is not innately a DSS – it becomes a DSS because of how it is used. DSS can be partitioned into several categories of use:

Research/exploratory – in this use the process is highly directed by the user. The system is queried to retrieve support for one or more courses of action under consideration or to simply describe a situation for users to make their own judgement. The process may be highly iterative, with query results suggesting further questions to the user.

Diagnostic/classification – in this case the interaction is more directed. The system attempts to classify the case into a pre-existent category (diagnostic entity) given the information supplied by user. Information gathering is driven mainly by the system – depending on what is needed to infer the diagnosis. Final outcome is typically accompanied by some measure of confidence and, ideally, with an explanation.

Constructive – these systems attempt to construct a solution from pre-existing components given specific constraints (e.g. recommended an antibiotic treatment given individual patient characteristics, type and location of infection, and given other concomitant diseases). Typically these systems are mixed initiative – exploiting strengths of computers (in quick calculations, searches, visualisation) and humans (in 'intuition' and formulating reasonable solutions from experience).

Critiquing – in this case the user does not interact directly with the DSS until the DSS detects a pattern that it evaluates as unacceptable or questionable. At this point the system provides an alert to the possible problem, including an explanation and possibly a recommendation of what its model indicates as a superior course of action.

The diagnostic use of CDSS is well known, especially for those familiar with the history of Artificial Intelligence. In the 1970s, the technology of expert systems (ES) was being developed based on inference from machine-encoded rules (see *symbolic reasoning systems* below). The most famous early medical ES, MYCIN, was designed at Stanford to diagnose infectious diseases and recommend antibiotic treatment.

While MYCIN was technologically pioneering, and in fact outperformed Stanford medical staff in evaluation, it was never used in practice. The chief barrier to use was a medico-legal one – it was unacceptable for a machine to be 'the expert' in a clinical setting. MYCIN-like technology has since found useful deployment, but it is important that a CDSS be seen as a tool to support human decision-making, not as an authoritative source of decisions.

A further important use of DSS is as an education tool. This is particularly powerful when the DSS is combined with illustrative case data to quiz the user or critique student decisions. One might say that when a DSS is used this way it is no longer a DSS, but is acting as an Intelligent Tutoring System (ITS). However, many historically important DSS, such as MYCIN and Iliad, have proven to be successful educational tools.

The technology of decision support systems

Decision support systems are dependent on their models – abstract representations of clinical knowledge – to provide users with help in decision-making. There is a great diversity in the types of models, and a resultant diversity in the forms and implementations of DSS.

Forms of DSS

Given a wide definition of computer-based DSS, we can classify decision support approaches into the following major categories:
- data presentation/visualisation tools
- problem-solving by search
- case bases reasoning
- symbolic reasoning systems
- artificial neural networks
- simulation modelling tools
- statistics/data-mining.

Data presentation/visualisation tools

Data presentation or visualisation tools support the decision-maker by rearranging existing data (facts, observations) such that the data is easier and much quicker to grasp. Typically, some precision is lost, but this is often acceptable.

What time is it?
A digital clock shows precise information: 15:58:34. A glance at an analogue watch allows us to say that it is 'almost 4 p.m.' How often do we really need more precision? How much time do we spend calculating that 15:58:34 is in fact very close to 4 p.m?

A medical example of data visualisation is a star diagram with colour coding for presentation of the biochemical profile of a patient. The decision-maker learns to recognise shapes and colour patterns characteristic of certain disorders.

Strengths: Visualisation is usually straightforward and tools are broadly available (for example, a spreadsheet package). Visual presentation of information fits well into the humans' decision-making process, using the broadest information channel (vision).

Traps: Ill-designed visualisation (or misused visualisation, for example, for advertising purposes) can obfuscate certain relationships and lead to incorrect decisions.

Problem-solving by search

Searching for a solution in a database is another approach. The basic idea is that the solution does already exist, is stored in a data structure, and can be retrieved given an initial set of parameters as a search query such as an alert system for drug interactions, for example:

> 'Given drug A and drug B, search an interaction table and return all entries involving both A and B.'

Strengths: Typically very quick, so can be used in real-time (this depends on the size and efficiency of the underlying data structure).

Traps: 'Knowledge' in the system is rather static and needs to be regularly updated. It usually has rather low flexibility.

Case-based reasoning (CBR)

Case-based reasoning simulates reasoning by experience. The system's knowledge is embodied in a library of past cases typically containing a statement of the problem (for example, symptoms and signs), the solution (such as diagnosis or treatment), and the outcome (for example, success of the proposed treatment). Finding a solution amounts to being able to match the underlying case to the cases already successfully solved.

All case-based reasoning (CBR) methods have the following process in common. They:

- retrieve the most similar cases by comparing the case to the library of past cases
- re-use the retrieved cases as a basis for solving the current problem
- revise and adapt the proposed solution if necessary
- retain the final solution as part of a new case (eventually including the outcome of the solution).

Strengths: It is relatively easy to set up the database of cases; evolution is also relatively simple – new cases are added into the database. Sets of solved cases are sometimes more available than models or rules, allowing use of CBR even when the problem is not very well understood.

Traps: A fairly large database of cases has to be built before the system starts to be useful. A major problem is *designing* a measure of similarity, that is, to decide what the important parameters are and how *similar* cases can be identified and ordered according to their similarity for the problem under consideration. Proposed solutions require interpretation as the system does not provide any explicit hints on 'correctness' of the solution.

Symbolic reasoning systems

Human experts are distinguished by knowledge and their ability to reason. This idea led to systems using formalised knowledge to produce a solution. A repository of knowledge (knowledge base) and a set of programs using that knowledge for reasoning (inference engine) are at the core of such systems (see Figure 18.1). A typical system consists of a knowledge base (KB), inference engine, and a database storing data about the patient case being processed.

Figure 18.1: General structure of a symbolic reasoning system

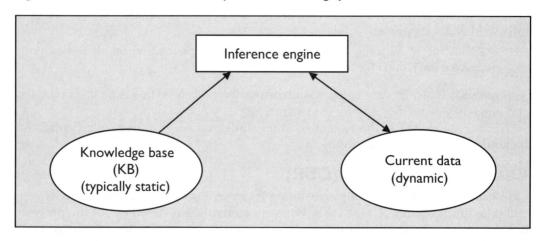

Before a piece of knowledge can be included into a KB, it has to be formalised. Knowledge representation methods to achieve this formalisation have become a separate field of study: knowledge engineering. The simplest knowledge representation is a rule (variously called a *production rule*, *condition-action rule*, or *if-then rule*); for example:

if [fasting plasma glucose > 7.0 mmol/l] then [infer the Dx: Diabetes mellitus]

A simple inference engine evaluates left-hand (if) parts of the rules, and whenever there is one evaluated to True, the right-hand (*then*) part is executed and a value is written into the case database. This is repeated in cycle until a stopping condition is reached, or there are no more rules with true-evaluated left-hand side. In large rule bases, the inference engine may work from a desired or likely right-hand (then) part to then seek values (for example, by querying the user) for the left-hand (if) part. This process is known as *backward chaining*. For more complex problems, a *frame* representation is useful to manage the complexity: a frame has a set of slots containing descriptions, rules for value assignment (to the frame), rules for messages, rules for setting goals, etc.

Strengths: Explicit knowledge representation allows generation of explanation on why and how the results were inferred – this can be important when the system proposes a surprising solution, and the decision-maker wants to scrutinise or challenge this proposal.

Traps: Building knowledge bases is difficult and expensive and will not be able to represent all tacit knowledge from experts. Large knowledge bases are difficult to maintain. There is no reliable automated procedure to test for completeness, implicit contradictions or even correctness of a large KB.

Coping with uncertainty: Inherently, in reasoning we face uncertainty issues – imprecise or incomplete rules, imprecise or incomplete observations or measurements and so on. There are many possible ways to deal with this issue; some examples are:

- *Qualitative reasoning* – in situations where no exact information is known, it is still possible to work with qualitative information (symptoms are present/absent), or with semi-quantitative data (taking into account a notion of magnitude – low/normal/high, or trend increasing, stable, decreasing)
- *Endorsements* – using crisp rules to express steps of confidence in an inference; possible, suspected, definitive
- *Scoring systems* – a broad range of relatively simple to highly sophisticated methods to calculate an overall score to express the confidence in the proposed decision
- *Bayesian reasoning* is using conditional probabilities to reason under uncertainty – see 'Information box'
- *Fuzzy sets* – fuzzy logic is an extension of Boolean logic that allows a continuum of values between True and False. Fuzzy sets can contain members that are less than completely in the set as defined by a membership function giving a value from 0 to 1.

Artificial neural networks (ANNs)

Artificial neural networks (or simply 'neural networks') are designed to be analogous to the neurological functions of the brain. Neural networks use a data set (with known outcomes – a 'training set') to build a structure capable of making predictions or classifications (decisions) on data sets describing the problem to be decided. Alternatively, neural networks can be used to reveal natural clusters in data where no specific 'right answer' is given (unsupervised learning).

Strengths: ANNs can be trained on a set of cases decided by an expert – thus eliciting eventually also some of the tacit knowledge of the expert. This is discussed further in Chapter 6. This process has to be carefully designed, but is much easier than knowledge engineering a knowledge base in a rule-based system. Like the human brain, neural networks are composed from many units – as a result they can extensively exploit parallel processing in computer hardware that supports this.

Traps: Selecting the training set is crucial – with a wrong or insufficient set of cases a neural network can produce misleading conclusions that are difficult to check (no explanation can be given). Also the number of possible training methods is rather high; selecting a good one can be a challenge.

Simulation modelling tools

Frean in Chapter 4 discusses the use of models to create simplified representation of the real world for analysing information structures, predicting outcome or explaining the observed behaviour. It also examines their ability to take into account structure, functionality, behaviour and causal relations between the components of a real world system. Chapter 4 also discusses the necessity for the model to be close enough to its real world counterpart to be able to provide usable solutions. In this chapter, modelling is applied to decision-making and its use in developing dosage models for drugs with narrow therapeutical range (as in cytostatics, some antibiotics, digoxin) to adjust dosage to patient body size and renal function, and to take into account previous plasma concentrations of the drug.

Strengths: Closeness of the model to the real world provides significant advantage in interpretation and explanation of the real world itself. Solutions can be obtained for rare situations never experienced before (and not expected). Completeness of the model can ensure that exceptions do not exist, and that the solutions provided are reliable. 'What if?' questions can provide answers on how the real world system might behave in certain situations.

Traps: Building models is difficult, lengthy and expensive. Until it is fully built, utility of the model is very low. Once *built*, the model is relatively rigid and difficult to change. Extensive testing is often required to make sure that the model behaves correctly in extreme cases.

Statistics/data mining

Statistical methods and data mining summarise information about the population (and specific subpopulations) of interest (typically used in public health – such as morbidity statistics, mortality statistics) and show associations between various parameters like morbidity and types of industry. While statistical methods are typically used to assess assumed/expected associations (or relationships), data mining can help to discover such associations.

Strengths: When applied correctly, it provides strong support for/against a proposed solution, and using some of the learning algorithms it can help to find associations in the dataset. Data mining, especially when combined with data visualisation, can provide good results in looking for new knowledge ('knowledge discovery').

Traps: Reliability of DATA can be a challenge – data can be biased, noisy, etc and data cleaning can be highly challenging. Rules discovered by data mining can be trivial (such as pregnancy occurs in females), difficult to interpret, or possibly spurious random associations that will not generalise (the result of what statisticians call 'data dredging').

Information box

Bayes' Rule

A key concept in CDSS technology is that of Bayes' Rule (or more formally, Bayes' Theorem), which is commonly written as:

$$P(H \mid e) = \frac{P(e \mid H)P(H)}{P(e)}$$

Bayes' Rule gives us a very specific, rational and evidence-based way of dealing with uncertainty.

Underlying Bayes' Rule is the idea of *probability*. Probability is simply the chance of some hypothesized outcome, denoted P(H). One can denote the probability of rain tomorrow as P(rain) = 0.2, which would be read as 'the probability of rain equals 0.2' or, just as accurately as 'there is a 20% chance of rain'. Taking the example of rain, we can see that a specific assertion, P(rain) = 0.2, is a statement of local, contextual knowledge; at its best, this assertion may represent fundamental knowledge of meteorology, combined with knowledge of current and regional conditions, as well as perhaps historical knowledge specific to the area to which the predication applies. And, for all of this, it is of course just a type of educated guess. For some scenarios the estimate of probability may be quite accurate without consideration of a great deal of external variables. A theoretical 'fair coin' will come up heads 50% of the time, and a real coin, if it isn't bent or asymmetrically layered, is likely to behave in very close accordance with this model over the long term.

The situation becomes more interesting when we think in terms of *conditional probability*, P(H | e), the probability of some hypothesis, H, given some evidence, e (read the vertical bar as 'given'). We know that the probability of rain is higher in the presence of falling barometric pressure than it would be 'on average' for any particular region and season. Thus we may estimate that the probability of rain prior to hearing about the barometric pressure is P(rain) = 0.2, but after hearing about the barometric pressure we decide the more relevant estimate is P(rain | falling barometer) = 0.6; these estimates are known as *prior* and *posterior* probability, respectively.

Bayes' Rule gives us a computational way to relate prior and posterior probabilities. Let's say that we know that 10% of our patients are smokers [take this as P(e)], 5% have lung cancer [P(H)] and 50% of the patients with lung cancer are smokers [P(e | H)]. We could then compute, by Bayes' Rule, that the probability a patient has lung cancer given that they are a smoker [P(H | e] is P(smoker | lung cancer)P(lung cancer) / P(smoker) = (0.5)(0.05) / (0.1) = 0.25 or 25%.

The application of Bayes' Rule can be extended to consider multiple influencing factors, and to relate a number of factors into a sequential chain of inference. The resultant structures are known as Bayesian Networks (or sometimes Belief Networks or Influence Diagrams). Reasoning on these networks, inferring specific probability estimates from evidence can be computationally complex. Neapolitan (2003) provides a comprehensive, but reasonably approachable, source for further reading in this area.

Instances of clinical DSS (CDSS)

Most of the popular DSS in existence today have had a long history of development (see 'Interest box – *CDSS implementations*'). Some of these well-known CDSS represent widely available off-the-shelf solutions or nationwide implementations, but there also exists a multitude of local and custom-built CDSS implementations working with minimal fanfare in healthcare centres throughout the world. Many of these are relatively simple DSS as compared to systems like DxPlain or QMR – the model may be a locally trained ANN, a set of algorithms implemented into a spreadsheet, or a query interface to a local data warehouse.

Other systems, while local, may be quite advanced and well proven. For instance, Evans et al. (1998) reported on an anti-infectives management DSS deployed to a twelve-bed intensive care unit, observing significant reductions in excessive drug dosages and other adverse events, along with reductions in costs and length of hospital stay. This system – part of a decade-long DSS development program – was integrated with the hospital's computerised patient record, greatly reducing redundancy in data entry. The *Electronic Decision support for Australia's Health Sector* report (National Electronic Decision support Taskforce, 2002) provides Australian and international perspectives on CDSS implementations and evaluations.

Interest box

CDSS implementations

DxPlain uses a set of clinical findings to produce a ranked list of diagnoses, which might explain (or be associated with) the clinical manifestations. DXplain provides justification for considering each of these diseases, suggests what further clinical information to collect, and lists clinical manifestations, if any, which would be unusual or atypical for each of the specific diseases.

GIDEON is used for diagnosis and reference in tropical and infectious diseases, epidemiology, microbiology and antimicrobial chemotherapy. It was designed to diagnose all infectious diseases, based on symptoms, signs, laboratory testing and dermatological profile. The database incorporates 327 diseases, 205 countries, 806 bacterial taxa and 185 antibacterial agents. GIDEON's major modules address diagnosis, epidemiology (disease status by country), therapy and microbiology (such as expected test results).

Iliad uses Bayesian reasoning to calculate the posterior probabilities of various diagnoses under consideration, given the findings present in a case. Iliad covers about 1500 diagnoses in this domain, based on several thousand findings. Iliad is primarily used as an education tool for medical students, but can also be used in diagnostic and research modes.

PRODIGY (Prescribing RatiOnally with Decision Support In General Practice studY) is a major initiative in the United Kingdom to develop and evaluate a computerised prescribing decision support system for the United Kingdom General Practice. PRODIGY is based at the Sowerby Centre for Health Informatics at Newcastle (SCHIN) and is funded by the NHS Executive.

QMR (Quick Medical Reference) is a diagnostic decision support system with a knowledge base of diseases, diagnoses, findings, disease associations and lab information. With information from the primary medical literature on almost 700 diseases and more than 5000 symptoms, signs, and labs, QMR can suggest relevant diagnoses, give advice regarding cost-effective workup strategies, and explain relationships of findings to diseases.

(Berner, 1999; National Electronic Decision Support Taskforce, 2002; OpenClinical, 2005; Sittig, 2003).

Implementing and deploying decision support systems

Kawamoto et al. (2005), found four factors that significantly contribute to DSSs' improving clinical practice:

1. providing decision support automatically as part of clinician workflow
2. delivering decision support at the time and location of decision-making
3. providing actionable recommendations (not just assessments)
4. enabling computer-based generation of the decision support.

In particular, the provision of automatic decision support in clinical workflow is the most critical factor for DSS success. How can this be achieved?

Organisational challenges

The first challenge in addressing a promising area is to overcome the 'knowledge acquisition bottleneck'. Authoritative experts in the domain of interest must be involved, and must engage with technology experts who can produce executable models (can 'knowledge engineer') based on what is in the domain experts' heads. After the model has been programmed, further involvement of domain experts (the same ones or, better still, different ones) is needed to test that the resultant DSS program provides an adequately accurate reflection of expert judgement. There is some possibility of avoiding the knowledge acquisition bottleneck by using machine learning techniques such as Artificial Neural Networks, assuming large amounts of training data are available; but the practical applications where an automated decision is useful on its own, lacking the human touch in either explanation or evaluation, are extremely limited.

Once a working DSS for the application domain is programmed, or sourced from elsewhere, the next barriers are in organisational and professional resistance, intentional or otherwise. The barriers for introducing a computer-based DSS are not fundamentally different from those for introducing any change of policy or procedures. Here experiences from the implementation of paper-based clinical practice guidelines are particularly relevant. A successful guideline implementation requires the support of local clinical expert(s) to 'champion' the change and lead customisation to the local context, advertising the availability of the guideline and a method of measuring its effectiveness (Waitman & Miller, 2004). In this sense, a DSS implementation is a guideline implementation, and if the above requirements are ignored is likely to fail in its integration with the organisation and run foul of the attitudes of the local professional community.

A further requirement to successful DSS implementation is integration with workflow. What this means is that the intended user (for instance, the clinician) must find it natural (or at least reasonable) to combine the use of the DSS with their normal, core work duties. Rousseau et al. (2003), examining factors influencing the adoption of a CDSS for chronic disease management in General Practice, found that major areas of concern centred on timing of advice (or advice inappropriate to the particular consultation), ease of use of the system, and perceived usefulness of the advice. Regarding ease of use, a key problem is related to the users not being able to access all necessary clinical information without exiting the system – integration of the DSS to the electronic health record (EHR) is a technical issue (see below), but one that must be achieved for a truly smooth integration of the DSS into the organisation.

A further ease-of-use issue observed by Rousseau et al. (2003) is that user training appeared ineffective for allowing the users to exploit the system's capability. Insufficient (or absent) training is a common problem in all health information systems deployments and DSS deployment is no exception. Finally, the perceived usefulness of the advice relates back to the knowledge-acquisition bottleneck (engineering a sufficiently deep and current model to be a real help to the clinicians). Rousseau et al. observed clinician complaints about the lack of actionable advice specific to the patient – a DSS does not fit the organisational workflow unless its advice is relevant and provides some specific basis for action by the user at the time that the advice is given.

A final organisational issue to consider relates to the medico-legal context and allowing clinicians to feel free to exercise judgement and have appropriate flexibility in light of the automated recommendations from a CDSS. A DSS does not have as complete a model of the patient as a healthcare provider will have; there are always boundaries to the DSS's viewpoint on the world as reflected in the set of factors it considers. However, the presence of a DSS can create an intimidating situation for a clinician who believes it appropriate to deviate from the DSS recommendation.

The clinician may well fear the professional and legal implications of non-adherence, especially if the patient's ultimate outcome is unsatisfactory. Such a situation is unacceptable – humans, not machines, should drive decisions and care. To avoid this intimidation however, DSS deployment must proceed with a culture of understanding that the DSS's model is useful (especially for its consistency), but is more limited than human understanding and will legitimately be over-ridden on a fairly regular basis. The best system feature to accommodate DSS over-rides is the facility for a clinician to provide an explanation in any case of variation from recommendations, accompanied by an ongoing organisational process of reviewing reasons for variation and progressive update of the DSS where possible to improve the relevance of its recommendations.

Technical challenges

A young medical student approaches a patient who has been rushed to the ER in a distressed state. The student dutifully asks questions and types details into his CDSS. Finally, he reads off a prominent suggestion from the system: 'Pain in the back between the shoulder blades, sweating, chills – could be a gallstone attack! Perhaps an ultrasound will show them up.' At this point, the patient loses patience and turns around to indicate the arrow jutting prominently from his back.

CDSS, especially when used in diagnostic mode, are notorious for not 'knowing' their limitations. It can be said that the DSS, while rich in knowledge, is lacking *meta-knowledge*. It is up to the human operator to know the appropriate scope of application for DSS tools, and elements of this can be conveyed in training. However, from a technical perspective there is also scope to ensure that the menuing systems by which a healthcare professional accesses the DSS provide appropriate explanations of both systems and their uses and, as much as possible, that CDSS are deployed only where they are appropriate to the scope of clinical work generally undertaken at the site of deployment.

Developers of new CDSS should always consider the opportunity to embed in the system user interface statements about appropriate scope or even meta-knowledge whereby the system prompts the user to consider whether the problem is outside the scope of the CDSS. In the case of embedded DSS functionality (such as a critiquing CDSS inside a computer-based order entry system), the system's integrator should have the critiquing criteria only applied to those parts of the host system that match the CDSS knowledge base.

Appropriate accessibility of a CDSS is essential to its successful use. Terminals must be located conveniently (for instance, the bedside is ideal, and 'down the corridor' is generally useless). Displays must be appropriate to show all relevant information without excessive scrolling or paging. Processing and network delays (latency) can make system use frustrating, if not simply unacceptable. In an interactive session, a delay of more than one second will cause a user's mind to wander; variable-length delays will create anxiety. All of this is required to achieve integration with clinical workflow.

Integration with clinical workflow will be limited unless the CDSS is integrated with the relevant healthcare data in electronic format. Failing such integration, the decision-maker must enter decision variables interactively. In addition to the time this requires if the data are already held elsewhere, the user is likely to resent the 'duplication' involved in what seems an unnecessary data entry task. Deployment of an electronic health record is a huge enabler of CDSS. However, there is often still a huge technical data integration task to query the data elements from the EHR into the CDSS decision variables, including assurance that they are in the appropriate format (and units) for the CDSS.

A number of efforts have been made to formalise the representation of clinical guideline knowledge for CDSS. Tu, Johnson and Musen (2001) divide electronic guideline models into flowcharts, disease-state maps, plans and workflow specifications and provide examples of each of these four guideline types. Among these guideline models, Arden Syntax, which encodes clinical algorithms in medical logic modules (MLMs), has been incorporated into the Health Level 7 (HL7) family of standards. The HL7 Arden Syntax for Medical Logic Systems has achieved approval as an American National Standard, making it the most accepted standard for electronic guideline representation. The standardisation of medical logic representation brings with it the potential for both models of clinical knowledge and the inferencing systems that process these models to become more of an open, commodity market.

In whatever format knowledge may be implemented into a computer-based system, there is no escaping the need for comprehensive and ongoing maintenance and quality assurance. The complexity of the models is such that formal verification is intractable – there will be errors in full-scale CDSS implementations. Procedures must be in place for the reporting and fixing of errors. Even with a perfect implementation, the software cannot remain static while 'best practice' moves on. For these reasons, CDSS must incorporate processes and methods for routine update of the fielded systems. Moreover, the complexity of medical logic is such that any change in a function of the system has the possibility of creating unintended side effects on other functions of the system (this is known as 'coupling' in the jargon of software engineering). Strong modularisation (the second 'M' in Arden Syntax MLMs) is a technique to reduce side effects, but comprehensive testing after revisions is always necessary.

Who monitors the medical literature to identify relevant changes in best practice? Who undertakes the required updates and error fixes? Who does the testing? Presumably these tasks fall to the CDSS software vendors. Then who sets their standards? Given that clinicians differ in their interpretation of medical evidence, who decides what knowledge should be put in a given CDSS module and in what way? How do we balance the fact that CDSS will contain defects, with their proven ability to reduce error and cost when successfully deployed? These issues form a concept known as clinical governance, which is still in its infancy. As the use of CDSS further matures, the roles of governments and professional bodies in setting quality and maintenance standards will become more formalised.

Conclusion

DSS are computerised systems that apply knowledge-based models to help users make better decisions. Clinical DSS provide support for patient-specific healthcare decision-making. A wide variety of DSS forms have been implemented across a range of healthcare settings. Successful CDSS implementation requires a careful plan of integration with the clinical context, and will require ongoing maintenance.

Review questions

1. What is the purpose of a Decision Support System (DSS)?
2. Discuss why it has been found unacceptable for Clinical DSS (CDSS) to make decisions *for* health professionals.
3. What are some key barriers to integration of CDSS with clinical workflow?

Exercises

- Describe how uncertainty can be taken into account in CDSS. Contrast two methods of handling uncertainty from the perspective of a healthcare professional trying to make use of the CDSS recommendations in a patient care setting.

- Identify several CDSS products (such as the ones described in the CDSS 'Interest box'. Say you are trying to identify a solution to be used by a local health service provider. Can you identify how the CDSS products would be licensed? Develop an Evaluation Table comparing at least four CDSS on what you believe are key selection criteria.

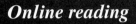

INFOTRAC® COLLEGE EDITION

For additional readings and review on decision support systems, explore **InfoTrac® College Edition**, your online library. Go to: **www.infotrac-college.com** and search for any of the InfoTrac key terms listed below:

➤ Decision support
➤ Clinical decision support
➤ Probability
➤ Bayes' rule

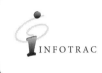

References

Berner, E. (ed) (1999). *Clinical decision support systems: theory and practice*, Spring-Verlag, New York.

Kawamoto, K., Houlihan, C., Balas, E. & Lobach, D. (2005). Improving clinical practice using clinical decision support systems: a systematic review of trials to identify features critical to success, *BMJ* 330(7494): 765.

National Electronic Decision support Taskforce (2002). *Electronic decision support for Australia's health sector*. Retrieved 14 January, 2005, from http://www.ahic.org.au/.

Neopolitan, R. (2003). *Learning Bayesian Networks*, Prentice-Hall, Upper Saddle River.

OpenClinical (2005). AI systems in clinical practice. Retrieved 20 March, 2005, from http://www.openclinical.org/.

Rousseau, N., McColl, E., Newton, J., Grimshaw, J. & Eccles, M. (2003). Practice-based, longitudinal, qualitative interview study of computerised evidence based guidelines in primary care, *BMJ* 326: 314–18.

Scott Evans, R., Pestonik, S., Classen, D., Clemmer, T., Weaver, L., Orme, J., Lloyd, J. & Burke, J. (1998). A computer-assisted management program for antibiotics and other antiinfective agents, *NEJM* 338(4): 232–8.

Sittig, D. (2003). Clinical decision support systems, The Informatics Review. Retrieved 15 March, 2005, from http://www.informatics-review.com/.

Tu, S., Johnson, P. & Musen, M. (2001). A typology for modelling processes in clinical guidelines and protocols in, *Proc. AMIA Annual Symposium*, Hanley & Belfus, Philadelphia.

Waitman, L. & Miller, R. (2004). Pragmatics of implementing guidelines on the front lines. *J Am Med Inform Assoc* 11: 436–8.

19

Telehealth and communication

Sisira Edirippuligé and Richard Wootton

'Transmission of documents via telephone wires is possible in principle, but the apparatus required is so expensive that it will never become a practical proposition.'

(Dennis Gabor, British physicist and author of *Inventing the Future*, 1962)

Outline

The use of telecommunications technologies to deliver health services is not a new concept. In fact the telephone has become so ubiquitous in healthcare that it is taken for granted. This chapter discusses telehealth and its implications for the health system. It provides the history of telehealth and introduces the participants served by this tool, the methods and technologies used, and the areas in which technology can be applied for enhanced communications.

Introduction

The prefix 'tele', which derives from the Greek, means 'at a distance'. Telehealth has been defined as the use of telecommunications to provide health information and services, that is, a health-related activity carried out at a distance. Some see telehealth as all forms of electronic healthcare delivery over the Internet, ranging from educational products to direct services offered by professionals, non-professionals and even consumers themselves (Maheu, Whitten & Allen, 2001). Another definition with more business emphasis states that 'e-Health is the use of computers and the Internet to increase practice efficiencies and knowledge bases, to exploit market inefficiencies in heath and medicine-related commerce, and to disseminate information to consumers and providers' (Grigsby & Brown, 1999). In fact, a number of similar terms, such as telemedicine, telecare and e-health have been coined and are often used interchangeably.

Telehealth therefore encompasses many aspects of healthcare practice, including the provision of health information, health administration and education, as well as diagnosis and management. It is important to emphasise that telehealth is not just about technology, but the use of it to improve healthcare delivery, particularly to communities who are disadvantaged in terms of their access to healthcare. Consider this factual case study.

Case study

A baby born late on Saturday night in a regional hospital shows symptoms of heart problems. Its condition is deteriorating and the doctor is unsure of what to do. It is the middle of winter and transport is difficult. The choices are to manage the baby conservatively in the regional hospital, or to activate emergency arrangements, which will result in a retrieval team being sent to the hospital, by air, to take the baby to the nearest tertiary hospital, some 1000kms away. If conservative management is not appropriate, the baby may die. Of course, if the retrieval team arrives and finds the baby too ill to move, then an expensive trip will have been wasted.

Luckily the hospital has a telehealth link and a telephone call to the telepaediatric service initiates a video consultation with a paediatric cardiologist at the tertiary centre. The cardiologist examines the baby over the video link. The real-time echocardiography examination shows that the baby is too ill to move, but treatment to stabilise the baby's condition can be started, with a view to making an elective transfer for cardiac surgery after a few days. The baby is later treated successfully for a major heart defect.

This is telehealth, or at least this is one aspect of a wide field: putting a doctor in touch with a specialist in order to obtain an expert opinion.

History of telehealth

The exchange of health information and the delivery of healthcare at distance have a long history. Table 19.1 summarises some of the most important developments in telehealth over the years.

Telehealth covers a very wide range of healthcare interactions for many different purposes. It is useful to classify these interactions by:
- participant: doctor-to-doctor, doctor-to-patient
- type: real-time, non-real-time
- information transmitted: audio, video.

Table 19.1: Timeline of telehealth (adapted from Wootton & Craig, 1999)

Period	Technical development	Telehealth application
1835	Telegraph	Used in the American Civil War to deliver casualty lists and order supplies. Later used to transmit x-ray images.
1876	Telephone	Initially used for voice communication. About 30 years later, used to transmit ECGs and EEGs.
1895	Radio	Used to supply medical advice to seafarers. In 1920 the Seaman's Church Institute of New York provided medical care using radio. The CIRM in Rome has been using radio to provide medical advice to shipping since 1935.
Late 1960s	Video/television	A two-way closed circuit television link was set up between the Nebraska Psychiatric Institute in Omaha and the state mental hospital in Norfolk for educational purposes.
1990s	Videoconferencing	Videoconferencing for health purposes became more common.
Mid-1990s	Internet	Use of the Internet for health purposes.

Participants in the telehealth interaction

Telehealth can involve a wide range of participants and the exchange of information may take place locally within a hospital or internationally between hospitals or practitioners. The nature of the communication in health can be:

- patient with practitioner
- practitioner with practitioner
- patient with patient (that is, mutual support)
- practitioner or patient accessing educational material (that is, sources of health information).

Patient with practitioner

Telepsychiatry is a common telehealth application. It is usually performed by videoconferencing, since this provides audiovisual communication. The telephone can also be used for some purposes (Simon et al., 2004; Evans et al., 2004). An evaluation of telepsychiatry services in Alberta, Canada, showed that it was acceptable to users and there were significant cost savings from avoided travel by psychiatrists and patients (Simpson et al., 2001). There have been recommendations to integrate telepsychiatry into existing mental healthcare (Stamm, 1998).

Practitioner to practitioner

Teleradiology is one of the most widespread of telehealth applications. It involves the transmission of digital radiographs between institutions using a telecommunications network. The technology required is well understood and there are agreed standards for performing teleradiology (see the American College of Radiology http://www.acr.org). It can be highly cost-effective to transmit radiographs using a telecommunication network rather than hiring a radiologist for every small hospital (Hayward & Mitchell, 2000). Teleradiology consultations may also take place internationally, which can be particularly effective for out-of-hours reporting (Kalyanpur et al., 2003).

Patient with patient

The use of health support groups has become popular, because they allow communication between people who have similar conditions, enabling them to share experiences. There is a large number of Internet-based support groups facilitating this interaction within a wide range of problems, from mental health to obesity to parenting. Communication in support groups can be in real-time where patients meet online or via telephone, or it may be asynchronous, for example by email. A study of the use of audio conferencing by breast cancer patients in rural Newfoundland showed that it provided valuable mutual support, despite the distances (Solbers, Church & Curran, 2003).

Types of telehealth interaction

The interaction in telehealth can be classified as either real-time or store and forward.

Real-time: The closest alternative to a conventional, face-to-face consultation is a real-time telehealth consultation, otherwise called synchronous or interactive, and is where parties communicate simultaneously via a telecommunication network. During a videoconference, both sound and vision are transmitted. The primary advantage of real-time telehealth is that there is no time delay between the information being transmitted and received, that is, the parties can interact as though they were present in the same room.

Real-time telehealth has proven to be effective for providing specialist consultations to rural health workers and for educational purposes (Callas, Ricci & Caputo, 2000). Videoconferencing has also been used for home nursing (Tran, Buckley & Prandoni 2002) and there is evidence that videoconferencing in fields such as dermatology, geriatrics, speech therapy and psychiatry can be effective (Hakan et al., 2003).

It is commonly assumed that real-time telehealth consultation is expensive, and certainly high quality videoconferencing equipment can be costly. However, videoconferencing is also possible with low cost equipment. For example, low cost videophones used over the public telephone network can enable community nurses to provide care and support to patients at home (Chambers et al., 2002).

Store and forward: Store and forward telehealth involves the non-interactive transmission of information from one site to another (Loane & Wootton, 2001). It is sometimes referred to as asynchronous or pre-recorded and involves information being captured and then transmitted to the other party for advice, opinion or specialist consultation. The main advantage of this method of working is that those involved can work independently from one another, that is, they do not have to be present at a pre-arranged time. Those who send the information can do so at their convenience and those who view and use the information can do the same.

In addition, store and forward telehealth is usually relatively inexpensive in comparison with real-time telehealth, which requires sophisticated and expensive equipment. Examples of store and forward telehealth include the transmission of ECGs using a simple fax machine (Srikanthan et al., 1997) or a second opinion using email (Vassaleo et al., 2001). Obviously not all consultations can be done by store and forward telehealth. However it is ideal where specialists rely on image interpretation, such as in radiology, dermatology and pathology.

In these cases, digital images of microscopy specimens, radiographs, wound and skin lesions, can be stored on a computer and then transmitted via email to a specialist. A number of studies prove the feasibility of this approach (Swinfen et al., 2003). Acquisition of information stored in websites on the Internet can also be considered as asynchronous telehealth and there are increasing numbers of websites with health-related information (Ball, 2001).

The major disadvantage of store and forward telehealth is that the specialist is entirely dependent on the information that the referrer sends, so if a poor quality picture of a dermatology lesion is sent it may be impossible to make a diagnosis.

Technology for telehealth

Whether the telehealth interaction is in real-time, or store and forward, the technology required for the telehealth system comprises three main components:
1. equipment to capture the information at each site
2. communication equipment to transmit this information between the sites
3. equipment to display the information at the relevant sites.

It is important to understand that videoconferencing is not the only mode of communication in telehealth or even necessarily the best. The suitability of a system depends on the needs, which will vary from one application to another.

There are four types of information transfer common in telehealth:
1. *Audio:* The most common form of audio is the transmission of speech. It is also possible to transmit heart or breathing sounds using an electronic stethoscope.
2. *Text:* Messages can be transmitted by use of a fax machine for instance. However, better quality transmission can be achieved if the documents are transmitted in digital form. If the information already exists as a computer file this is easy. Alternatively, printed documents can be digitised using a flatbed scanner or a digital camera and then transmitted as still images.
3. *Still images:* These may be transmitted for various health purposes such as diagnosis, management and education. Low-cost digital cameras are capable of capturing good quality images that can be transmitted to specialists for consultation. A flatbed scanner can be used to produce digital images of charts such as ECG traces. X-ray films can also be digitised this way, although when high quality diagnostic images are required, the equipment involved can be costly (see Figure 19.1).

Figure 19.1: X-ray digitiser

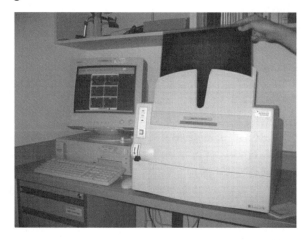

4. *Video:* Commercial videoconferencing equipment enables high quality online meetings. A specialist can see and communicate with the patient almost naturally. Setting up a sophisticated videoconferencing studio (see Figure 19.2) can be expensive although equipment costs are reducing.

Figure 19.2: High-quality videoconferencing studio

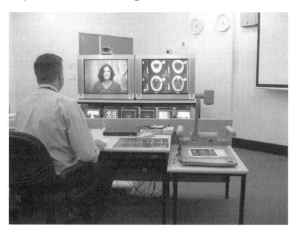

Audio and visual transmission does not allow a consultant to access aspects like touch, smell and physical feeling. However, a consultant can see the patient's wounds and skin lesions from different angles, and obtain close ups. This seems to be sufficient for many consultations.

The reliability of the technology is a critical factor in a successful telehealth implementation. Analogue telephone transmission is not appropriate for many telehealth purposes, since signals may be degraded because of noise on the lines and low bandwidth. Digital signal transmission is preferable, since the data can be transmitted over networks for long distances without degradation and bandwidths are usually much higher.

Information box

Issues of bandwidth

Bandwidth is the data-carrying capacity of the transmission medium, measured in bits per second (bit/s). It ranges from 1200 bit/s in some mobile phones to more than 1000 Mbit/s through a fibre-optic cable. Some successful telehealth applications have used 9600 bit/s modems and ordinary telephone connections, while others require the capacity of fibre-optic cable networks. The type of clinical information to be transmitted dictates the minimum network bandwidth. In practice, the main question is what telecommunications are available between the sites. Rural areas where patients are most in need of telehealth services are often those where network communications are limited. Providing high bandwidth connections to such sites can be extremely expensive.

Telecommunications

There is a wide choice of telecommunications options for telehealth. All have their positives and negatives.

Standard telephony

The conventional telephone system is the PSTN (public switched telephone network) that provides analogue telephone lines almost anywhere in the world. This is the most widely used communication medium in health, although paradoxically no longer considered as novel due to its ubiquity. The bandwidth available to users is limited to 56 kbit/s. In practice it is often considerably less. As a result, use of standard telephony in telehealth is limited.

The Internet

The Internet is a very popular communications medium generally and its use in health communication is growing. The advantages of the Internet are that it is ubiquitous and the cost is low, for example, when access is via the ordinary telephone network. The disadvantages are that the Internet is an open system and it is not secure. It is also difficult to guarantee the quality of services it delivers because normally it provides only a low bandwidth transmission. Therefore, the Internet it is not very suitable for transferring large quantities of data, particularly internationally. However, there have been some studies of the feasibility of Internet-based telehealth applications (Jacko, Sears & Sorensen, 2001; Monnier, Laken & Cindy, 2002).

Mobile phones

In some circumstances, data networks based on digital mobile phones can be used for health purposes. Mobile phones can be used to access the Internet and transmit live video images. The mobile phone system is most suitable for applications where real time transfer is needed and access to a standard modem is not possible. Trials have been carried out where mobile phones were used to take pictures of injuries and send them to consultants for immediate specialist advice (Lam, Preketes & Gates, 2004). Mobile phones have also been used to assist people with disabilities in communication (Lauruska & Kubilinskas, 2002).

ISDN

ISDN is a fully digital service, which provides a digital connection from end to end. Compared to the conventional telephone network, the ISDN provides higher bandwidth. There are two data rates available to ISDN users – a basic rate service, which provides two user channels each carrying 64 kbit/s, or the primary rate service providing 30 user channels each carrying 64 kbit/s. Basic rate ISDN can transmit low quality video, which is sufficient for many telehealth purposes. Primary rate ISDN gives improved transmission, but is more expensive.

Satellite

Satellite communication provides global coverage and therefore has great potential for telehealth. Since the mid-1990s, a number of activities have been initiated in Europe by national and international organisations to demonstrate the use of satellite communication for telehealth (Lamminen, 1999). The main disadvantage is the high cost, but it is expected that future cost reductions will stimulate the use of satellite communications in healthcare. Recently the Indian space agency announced plans to launch a communications satellite to provide specialist medical consultations to remote and rural areas (Indian Space Research Institute, 2005).

Current telehealth practice

The 2001 report of the Association of Telemedicine Service Providers (ASTP) documented an overall growth in telehealth practice and an increase in network sizes in the United States of America. The survey of telehealth in the United States identified nearly 130 programs and estimated that 40 000 teleconsultations were performed annually. However, these consultations constituted only 0.004 per cent of all US consultations (Health United States, 2004).

The ATSP survey showed that over thirty-five specialities were using telehealth and that there was a wide acceptance of store and forward techniques. Interactive videoconferencing also showed a steady growth in usage (TRC Report on US Telemedicine Activity, 2004). There has also been growth in telehealth in other industrialised countries, particularly Japan, Australia, United Kingdom and Scandinavian countries (Takahashi, 2001; Bend, 2004).

The introduction of electronic health records will create information networks linking hospitals, physicians, pharmacists and other healthcare professionals, allowing the sharing of health information. These will form an important foundation for telehealth.

Health education

Telehealth offers great gains in health education particularly for geographically isolated health care workers (Chang, 2001). Systematic and regular updating of skills and knowledge are essential elements in effective healthcare provision and the Internet supports this development (Zimitat, 2001). Research has demonstrated that health education delivered through new technology is effective and viable (Harris, 2001) and online education has been used successfully for various specialities (Kingsnorth, Vranch & Campbell, 2000).

Health information and the Internet

The Internet has revolutionised access to healthcare information for both healthcare professionals and consumers. The Internet has also become an important source of health information for healthcare providers (Gregg & Wozar, 2003) and is used for health-related commercial activity.

Advantages of telehealth

Telehealth offers a number of advantages. In particular it has the potential to make specialist care accessible to underserved rural and remote communities. The lack of specialist care in rural areas is widespread. In Australian specialist psychiatric care for example, there are 5.8 physicians per 1000 population in major cities and 2.7 in very remote areas (AIHW, 2005). Reduced travel time, expenses, and inconvenience for patients and their families are also significant advantages offered by telehealth.

Several programs in correctional facilities, particularly in the United States, have demonstrated the efficiency of telehealth in providing healthcare to prisoners and avoiding transporting them for consultations (Ellis et al., 2001).

Telehealth can be advantageous for health professionals and has helped dispel professional isolation, particularly for those in geographically isolated areas. It enables isolated practitioners to update their skills and knowledge, communicate with specialists, reduce transportation costs and inconvenience, and avoid interruptions to their practice. There is evidence that healthcare professionals accept telehealth as an essential part of the healthcare sector (Demiris, Edison & Schopp, 2004).

Patient empowerment is another advantage of telehealth. Patients are no longer dependent on the limited information provided by the doctors and they can take greater control over their health conditions. The changing nature of the doctor/patient relationship is an important advantage of telehealth (Ball & Lillis, 2001) and research has shown high levels of patient satisfaction with it (Gustke et al., 2000).

Barriers to telehealth

Despite obvious advantages under appropriate circumstances, telehealth has not entered the mainstream of healthcare as there is a number of barriers to its widespread introduction. Human and organisational factors represent the major barrier (Wootton, 1997). A lack of financial support has often been a serious obstacle to research and development in telehealth (Myers, 2003). Sometimes a lack of trust, commitment and dedication by healthcare personnel reflect a lack of readiness for telehealth (Hibbert et al., 2004). It is also noteworthy that there is a lack of appropriate training and educational facilities (Edirippulige, 2005).

One frequently cited barrier is the lack of information about the cost-effectiveness of telehealth, but there has been little research into this (Bynum et al., 2003). However, if it is to become integrated into mainstream healthcare, convincing evidence for its cost-effectiveness is required. Depending on the perspective, the financial benefits of telehealth applications may vary. Cost shifting is a common situation in telehealth. For example, patients can save (such as in travel), while the costs accrue to the hospitals in terms of payment for telehealth equipment and communications.

Many potential telehealth projects, especially in rural areas and in the developing world, have been hampered by the lack of an adequate telecommunication infrastructure. Other barriers in telehealth are the legal and ethical issues (Terry, 2000). These include licensing, privacy and confidentiality (Stanberry, 1998). Reimbursement, or the lack of it, is also an obstacle for potential telehealth practitioners (Edlin, 2003).

Conclusion

Telehealth has significant potential to address a range of healthcare problems, especially in underserved areas. However, it is erroneous to think that telehealth is a panacea, which will entirely replace conventional methods of healthcare delivery. Instead, if used properly it can complement the traditional healthcare system to provide service to a wider population. The benefits and advantages of telehealth are well recorded. But there is a number of barriers to overcome before widespread adoption occurs.

Review questions

1. Why is telehealth the natural result of the evolution of healthcare in the digital age?
2. What factors should be considered when selecting a telehealth system?
3. What are the advantages and disadvantages of telehealth where you live?

Exercises

*   Discuss the criteria you would use for evaluating the success or failure of a telehealth application.
*   Discuss the advantages, disadvantages and major barriers to the adoption of telehealth into mainstream healthcare delivery where you live.

Online reading

INFOTRAC® COLLEGE EDITION
For additional readings and review on telehealth or ehealth, explore **InfoTrac® College Edition**, your online library. Go to: **www.infotrac-college.com** and search for any of the InfoTrac key terms listed below:
➤ Telehealth
➤ Telecommunications
➤ Communications

References

Australian Institute of Health and Welfare (AIHW) (2005). Mental health services in Australia 2002–03, *AIHW*, Canberra, Cat No. HSE-35.

Ball, M.J. (2001). Welcome to e-Health, *Healthcare Informatics*, October, 45–9.

Ball, M.J. & Lillis, J. (2001). e-health: transforming the physician/patient relationship, *International Journal of Medical Informatics*, 61, 1–10.

Bend, J. (2004). *Public value and e-Health*, Institute for Public Policy Research, UK. Retrieved 22 March, 2005, from http://www.ippr.org/research.

Bynum, A.B., Irwin, C.A., Cranford, C.O. & Denny, G.S. (2003). The impact of telemedicine on patients' cost savings: some preliminary findings, *Telemedicine Journal and e-Health*, 9(4), 361–7.

Callas, P.W., Ricci, M.A. & Caputo, M.P. (2000). Improved rural provider access to continuing medical education through interactive videoconferencing, *Telemedicine Journal*, 6, 393–9.

Chambers, M., Connor, S., Diver, M. & McGonigle, M. (2002). Usability of multimedia technology to help caregivers prepare for a crisis, *Telemedicine Journal and e-Health*, 8(3), 343–7.

Chang, B.L. (2001). Can telehealth technology be used for the education of health professionals?, *Western Journal of Nursing Research*, 23(1), 107–14.

Demiris, G., Edison, K. & Schopp, L.H. (2004). Shaping the future: needs and expectation of telehealth professionals, *Telemedicine Journal and e-Health*, 10, Suppl. 2, 60–3.

Edirippulige, S. (2005). Perception of Australian nurses on e-Health, *Journal of Telemedicine and Telecare*, 11, 266–8.

Edlin, M. (2003). Electronic medicine: pilot programs define uses and payment for online consultations, *Managed Healthcare Executive*, 13(3), 26–9.

Ellis, D.G., Mayrse, J., Jehle, D.V., Moscati, R.M. & Pierluisi, G.J. (2001). A telemedicine model for emergency care in a short-term correctional facility, *Telemedicine Journal and E Health*, 7(2), 87–92.

Evans, M., Kessler, K., Lewis G., Peters, T.J. & Sharp, D. (2004). Assessing mental health in primary care research using standardised scales: can it be carried out over the telephone?, *Psychological Medicine*, 34, 157–62.

Gregg, A.L. & Wozar, J.A. (2003). Delivering Internet health resources to an underserved health care profession: school nurses, *Journal of the Medical Library Association*, 91(4), 398–403.

Grigsby, B. & Brown, N. (1999). *ATSP report on US telemedicine activity*, Association of Telehealth Service Providers, Portland.

Gustke, S.S., Balch, D.C., West, V.L. & Rogers, L.O. (2000). Patient satisfaction with telemedicine, *Telemedicine Journal*, 6(1), 5–13.

Hakan, G., Thoden, C.J., Carlson, C. & Harno, K. (2003). Realtime teleconsultations versus face to face consultations in dermatology: immediate and six month outcome, *Journal of Telemedicine and Telecare*, 9(4), 204.

Harris, J.M. (2001). The Internet and the globalisation of medical education, *BMJ*, 323, p.1106.

Hauber, R.P., Vesmarovich, S. & Dufour, L. (2002). The use of computers and the Internet as source of health information for people with disabilities, *Rehabilitation Nursing*, 27(4), 142–5.

Hayward, T. & Mitchell, J. (2000). The cost-effectiveness of teleradiology at the women's and children's hospital in Adelaide, *Journal of Telemedicine and Telecare*, 6, Suppl. 1, 23–5.

Health United States, Centers for Disease Control and Prevention, National Center for Health Statistics, National Ambulatory Medical Care Survey and National Hospital Ambulatory Medical Care Survey (2004). Retrieved 8 April. 2005, from http://www.cdc.gov/.

Hibbert, D., Mair, F.S., May, C.R., Boland, A., O'Connor, J., Capewell, S. & Angus, R.M. (2004). Health professionals' response to the introduction of a home telehealth service, *Journal of Telemedicine and Telecare*, 10(4), 226–30.

Indian Space Research Institute. Retrieved 11 April, 2005, from http://www.isro.org/.

Jacko, J.A., Sears, A. & Sorensen, S.J. (2001). Framework for usability, *Healthcare professionals and the Internet*, 44(11), 989–1007.

Kalyanpur, A., Weinberg, J., Neklesa, V., Brink, J.A. & Forman, H.P. (2003). Emergency radiology coverage: technical and clinical feasibility of an international teleradiology model. *Emergency Radiology*, 10(3), 115–8.

Kingsnorth, A., Vranch, A. & Campbell, J. (2000). Training for surgeons using digital satellite television and videoconferencing. *Journal of Telemedicine and Telecare*, 6, Suppl.1, 29–31.

Lam, K.T., Preketes, A. Gates, R. (2004). Mobile phone photo messaging assisted communication in the assessment of hand trauma, *ANZ Journal of Emergency*, 74(7), 598–602.

Lamminen, H. (1999). Mobile satellite systems, *Journal of Telemedicine and Telecare*, 5(2), 71–83.

Lauruska, V. & Kubilinskas, E. (2002). A system for teleconsulting communication and distance learning for people with disabilities, *Journal of Telemedicine and Telecare*, 8, Suppl. 2, 49–50.

Loane, M. & Wootton, R. (2001). A review of telehealth, *Medical Principles and Practice*. 10(3), 163–70.

Maheu, M., Whitten, P. & Allen, A. (2001). *e-Health, Telehealth and Telemedicine: A Guide to start up and success*. Jossey-Bass, San Francisco, p.2.

Monnier, J., Laken, M. & Cindy, L. (2002). Patient and caregiver interest in Internet based cancer services, *Cancer Practice*, 10(6), 305–10.

Myers, M.B. (2003). Telemedicine: An emerging health care technology, *Health Care Manager*, 22(3), p.221.

Simon, E.G., Evette, J.L., Tutty S., Operskalski, B. & Korff, M.V. (2004). Telephone psychotherapy and telephone care management for primary care patients starting antidepressant treatment, *JAMA*, 292(8), 935–42.

Simpson, J., Doze, S., Urness, D., Hailey, D. & Jacobs, P. (2001). Evaluation of telepsychiatry service, *Journal of Telemedicine and Telecare*, 7(2), 90–8.

Solbers, S., Church, J. & Curran, V. (2003). Experiences of rural women with breast cancer receiving social support via audioconferencing, *Journal of Telemedicine and Telecare*, 9(5), 282–7.

Srikanthan, V.S., Pell, A.C., Prasad, N., Tait, G.W., Rae, A.P., Hogg, K.J. & Dunn, F.G. (1997). Use of fax facility improves decision making regarding thrombolysis in acute myocardial infarction, *Heart*, 78(2), 198–200.

Stamm, B.H. (1998). Clinical applications of telehealth in mental health care, *Professional Psychology: Research and Practice*, 29(6), 536–42.

Stanberry, B.A. (1998). *The legal and ethical aspects of telemedicine*, Royal Society of Medicine Press, UK.

Swinfen, P., Swinfen, R., Youngberry, K. & Wootton, R. (2003). A review of the first year's experience with an automatic message-routine system for low-cost telemedicine, *Journal of Telemedicine and Telecare*, 9 Suppl. 2, 63–5.

Takahashi, T. (2001). The present and future of telemedicine in Japan, *International Journal of Medical Informatics*, 61, 131–7.

Terry, N.P. (2000). Structural and legal implications of e-health, *Journal of Health Law*, 33(4), 605–14.

Tran, B.O., Buckley, K.M. & Prandoni, C.M. (2002). Selection and use of telehealth technology in support of homebound caregivers of stroke patients, *Caring*, 21(3), 16–21.

Grigsby, W. (2004). *TRC report on US telemedicine activity*, Civic Research Institute, Kingston, USA.

Vassaleo, D.J., Hoque, F., Patterson, V., Roberts, M.F., Swinfen, P. & Swinfen, R. (2001). An evaluation of the first year's experience with a low-cost telemedicine line Bangladesh, *Journal of Telemedicine and Telecare*, 7(3), 125–38.

Wootton, R. & Craig, J. (1999). *Introduction to telemedicine*, Royal Society of Medicine Press, UK, p.6.

Wootton, R. (1997). Telemedicine: the current state of the art, *Minimally Invasive Therapy and Allied Technologies*, 5(6), p.400.

Zimitat, C. (2001). Designing effective online continuing medical education, *Medical Teacher*, 23(2), 117–22.

20

Information across the health system

Moya Conrick

> When news of the telephone reached England, the chief engineer of the post office was asked whether this new Yankee invention would be of any practical value. He gave the forthright reply: 'No, sir. The Americans have need of the telephone – but we do not. We have plenty of messenger boys.'
>
> (Sir William Preece)

Outline

Emerging information and communications technologies, such as electronic health records (EHR) systems, offer new ways of accessing health information and assisting clinicians and consumers in decision-making that improves the quality and safety of care delivery (Commonwealth of Australia, 2003c). These technologies create an awareness of the holistic needs of patients because information is readily available from multiple sources, across geographical boundaries and within flattening information silos. Using scenarios, this chapter draws together the discussion in previous chapters to illustrate information flows and to contrast the papers and automated record systems.

Introduction

Healthcare consumers have multiple entry and exit points in a complex system that support an increasingly transient community. There is a diverse array of providers from traditional disciplines and the alternative therapies in a variety of practice areas and geographical settings. Providing healthcare services is an ongoing struggle, particularly in rural and remote Australia, where healthcare workers are often isolated from other practitioners. They are often asked to make decisions about patients with sketchy information or no information at all.

Reports of problems with paper health records are numerous with issues of illegibility and access well documented. Electronic health records (EHR) systems are thought to negate most of these problems and lead to more efficient, safe and cost-effective healthcare. Earlier chapters have shown that in the current system, information is often locked away in silos inside organisational or professional boundaries leading to gaps in information flow across the health sector. The patient record is the only place that an episode of care and its outcomes can be documented, but it is widely acknowledged that the quality of documentation in the paper record is poor. The following scenarios will follow Vera through her episodes of care to illustrate the flow of information across the health system.

Information flows across care

Vera is a 72-year-old woman living alone. She felt unwell and visited her General Practitioner (GP) who drew blood for testing. She was given a script for angina medication and antibiotics, to be taken after meals but before her arthritis tabs. She is to return in two days for a check up and results of her tests.

If current system	*If automated system*
A form is written and wrapped around the blood vials and secured with a rubber band. They are left on the bench (just washed, and still wet) awaiting the courier.	An electronic order is sent to the pathology lab. The plastic coated, bar coded vials are left on the bench (just washed, and still wet) awaiting the courier.

Vera goes home. She has heard of an acupuncturist who is also a herbalist and works 'magic' with arthritis. Her arthritis is really bothering her so she makes an appointment for the next day.

Vera arrives for her session. Relates her history – what she can remember of it – and tells the acupuncturist about her symptoms, which he notes in a new paper chart.	The acupuncturist has Vera's EHR and full history, notes that she visited her GP yesterday and has had blood tests. Vera views her record and notes a mistake that is corrected by the acupuncturist in a new notation.

Vera has her treatment and her joints feel much improved, although she is still 'off colour'

The acupuncturist dispenses a herbal remedy after Vera recited her current medications. None were contra-indicated. The paper chart is filed. Whoops … she forgot the little blue pill!	The acupuncturist does not prescribe herbal medications because, according to the current medications list, the herbs are contra-indicated. The acupuncturist treatment is noted on the shared EHR.

The next day Vera goes to the chemist to have her scripts filled

(No hurry, she has plenty of old tablets in her cupboard [she just knew she would need them one day!] and she also has the new herbal remedy.) A locum pharmacist dispensed her oestrogen as per his reading of the handwritten script from the GP.	An electronic prescription has been sent to Vera's local pharmacist. A locum pharmacist checks her current medications list for contra-indications or alerts. The erythromycin was individually packaged and dispensed and she is handed a printout of instructions.

Next day Vera returns to the GP	
(The receptionist knows she has filed Vera's record... She is sure it started with V.) After reading the 1946 *Readers Digest*, Vera sees her GP. No results yet, the fax is 'playing up'. Phone call to the pathologist: 'V-e-r-a ... no, not Dora... Vera!' The results are read over the telephone. The GP jots them down on a note pad.	After watching a health promotion video in the waiting room, Vera sees her GP. Her EHR is open on the desktop. The visit to the alternative therapist is noted. The test results are in the in-box and the current medications list shows that the correct medications have been dispensed.

Vera is to be admitted to hospital immediately	
The GP writes a quick note: Dear Dr... please admit this lovely woman ... who has been off colour for a week.	Vera's GP sends a summary record to Health*Connect* repository and provides her with printed information about diabetes from the practice computer's knowledge database.

The receptionist phones an ambulance. On the way to hospital Vera has 'a turn'.	
The ambulance officers are unsure of the cause, her diagnosis is sketchy and she is not able to give them any information. They give her oxygen, monitor her and hope the traffic isn't too heavy.	Vera's chart is downloaded to the ambulance's mobile videoconferencing equipment and consultation begun between the emergency department (ED) specialist and ambulance. Real-time physiological monitoring data is available to the specialist. The ED is prepared for her arrival.

Information technology (IT) has permanently transformed the way in which we communicate; however one of the constraints in the Australian eHealth agenda is the inadequacy of the mainly copper wire communications network. Sending large amounts of data through the existing network is painfully slow and largely ineffective (Conrick, in press).

In 2004, the Commonwealth Government committed $35 million over three years to provide broadband Internet access to GPs across Australia to ensure that all general practices and Aboriginal Community Controlled Health Services have access to high quality, secure broadband services. Secure e-mail communication between GPs and other healthcare providers, and rapid online delivery of referrals, requests, hospital discharge summaries and test results such as pathology, x-ray and ultrasound images will be facilitated (Australian Health Information Council, 2004). The broadband rollout will also support the national electronic health record – Health*Connect*.

IT also has the capacity to rein in the unacceptable levels of errors and adverse events resulting from illegible handwriting and mistakes in the prescribing and administration of medications. Medications management is an ongoing concern in most countries with errors responsible for considerable morbidity. Tamblyn (Institute of Medicine, 2001) reveals that drug-related adverse events are reported as the sixth leading cause of death and contributes substantially to morbidity in Canada. Inappropriate prescribing is identified as a preventable cause of at least 20 per cent of drug-related adverse events with elderly patients at greatest risk of receiving such prescriptions. Because GPs write approximately 80 per cent of all their prescriptions for people 65 years of age and older, Tamblyn argues that effective interventions to optimise prescribing are a priority.

The United States Institute of Medicine (2001) report that over 98 000 deaths each year in America were related to medical error, 40 per cent of outpatient prescriptions were unnecessary, and patients receive only 55 per cent of recommended care. It noted that, on average, consumers visit six different healthcare providers each year (range 2–14) and because the multiple records do not interoperate, health providers have incomplete knowledge of their patients. Patient data was unavailable in 81 per cent of cases in one clinic and an average of four missing items per case was reported. It was estimated that 8 per cent of medical errors were due to inadequate availability of patient information.

In Australia, misuse, under-use, overuse and reactions to therapeutic drugs result in 140 000 hospital admissions every year and cost approximately $380 million each year in the public hospital system alone (AIHW, 2002). In this scenario, the use of sophisticated medication management and comprehensive online databases to enhance prescribing safety is apparent. A database that supports discharge summaries, procedure summaries, laboratory data and investigation reports is also critical to ongoing care. The ability to catch errant orders with decision-support alerts and prompts for the clinician can mean the difference in the outcomes and cost of care.

The Medi*Connect* trials demonstrated the benefits of improved provider and consumer access to medicines information and the usefulness of using technology to link patients, doctors, pharmacists and hospitals (Commonwealth of Australia, 2003b). Access to more complete consumers' medicines information improves quality and safety in prescribing, dispensing and managing medicines. This will help to reduce the incidence of duplicate prescriptions, and allergic or adverse reaction – both major problems and cost in the Australian health system.

Delivering data and information to participants where and when it is needed relies on proven technologies such as the Internet, leveraging emerging technologies such as Extensible Markup Language (XML) and web services (Commonwealth of Australia, 2003a). According to the Australian Government, electronic records must be 'future-proofed' by explicitly allowing for changing definitions or new technologies. The technical models used for sharing information across healthcare must be robust and reliable. For example, Health*Connect* is expected to include a storage system that consists of three layers:

- a coordination layer representing the infrastructure, metadata and services needed to integrate Health*Connect* into a common national network of records
- a federated record system layer, which comprises multiple nodes (potentially with a range of system owners), each of which has an independent records system servicing a defined user population
- the user layer comprised of the consumers' and providers' local information systems used to access Health*Connect* (Commonwealth of Australia, 2003a).

Adaptable mobile computers and scalable, point-of-care devices that are easily integrated with a variety of wireless medical devices and healthcare sensors are available. They enable the rapid collection and transmission of vital patient data from the scene from the emergency response team. Digital images and vital sign measurements are quickly captured and transmitted to the appropriate clinician, wherever that person might be situated. This technology enables an accurate patient assessment before the patient is moved from the site or arrives at the receiving hospital. Continuous vital signs monitoring coupled with high-speed digital network connections and interactive videoconferencing capabilities, enable the consultant and emergency personnel to discuss and monitor patient care en route. All care and interventions are accurately recorded and stored automatically in the patient's EHR using voice recognition software.

Vera arrives at the Emergency Department

If current system

Vera's chart is ordered from Medical Records Department storage. She is resuscitated and sent to Intensive Care. A paper progress note is used to admit her and to document progress. It will be placed in her chart when it arrives.

Vera is admitted into a high dependency unit; her details are recorded (again). A medical student does a thorough admission as does the resident and the registrar repeats the dose. All ask about current medications and each documents a full past and present health history. Vera's vague status is noted and yesterday's tests are repeated (the former results are in the GP's silo). A nursing assessment is also carried out and documented.

Vera is prescribed medications and the nursing staff makes sure that these are given at the right time, in the right dose. She is asked about allergies before being given the first dose of ampicillin. Vera is unsure, but after ingesting the medication remembers having 'a funny turn' some years ago after taking penicillin.

If automated system

The current EHR is displayed on the point-of-care device and as Vera has been stabilised en route a routine admission follows. All clinicians have access to all information. Vera is transferred to the ward.

The EHR is available in the ward and had been automatically updated. It includes Vera's past and present health history and a list of current medications and dispensing dates. Yesterday's and all previous test results are also in the EHR.

Vera is due for her medications. She has a bar coded armband with all information – demographics, allergies etc. The bar code reader crosschecks this with her chart and an allergy alert is received. The antibiotic is changed.

Next day Vera is sent for a chest x-ray

A paper referral is sent to the x-ray department. Vera is x-rayed and waits for the quality to be checked. She returns to the ward. The film will be read, the results typed and a paper copy sent later. Some time later it is received but not glued into her chart, as it cannot be located. The result slip is placed in the filing box.

The x-ray appointment is made electronically. A digital x-ray is taken, and uploaded into her EHR. The radiologist comments on the x-ray using voice recognition to populate the EHR. This is immediately available to all concerned in Vera's care long before she returns to the ward.

The physio has received a referral slip sent yesterday. He has visited the ward twice to see Vera while she was still in the x-ray department.

The physio referral was sent electronically and treatment began yesterday. He goes online and notes that Vera has returned to the ward. Treatment is completed and documented although three other clinicians are simultaneously using the record.

The Open Architecture Clinical Information System (OACIS) project in South Australia has demonstrated that improvements in information flow are possible in EHRs and that the provision of timely provider access to results makes duplicate pathology and radiology tests unnecessary (Commonwealth of Australia, 2003a). The majority of providers seem to support OACIS because they see efficiency gains through improved access to information. Benefits reported by the Toronto Electronic Child Health Network were also impressive and include reduced human and financial costs for repeat testing; better coordination of care; and the ability to inform clinical care by trending results over time (Commonwealth of Australia, 2003b).

The Walsall study of EHRs (Orion Health, 2004), report a reduced number of appointments to effectively treat patients and that reviewing the record prior to consultations reduced the number of referrals to chiropody, physiotherapy and other areas. Owens and Foord (2002) also report a reduction in time spent by clinicians chasing information for complex cases, with critical results being at hand much faster than previously possible.

Other benefits of EHR have been demonstrated, although it is premature to quantify these in most instances. The fledgling Gloucester ERDIP project for example, points to major reductions in the average length of stay as well as significant savings on chemistry, haematology, transfusion and microbiology tests (Owens & Foord, 2002). The national summary EHR (Health*Connect*) should achieve similar results in Australia because it enables real-time downloading of current patient information at the point-of-care. It focuses on automating the capture, exchange, transmission and collection of health data (Commonwealth of Australia, 2003b).

IT enables the sharing and storage of data not before possible with paper-based records and other current means of communication. In the United States of America for instance, 30 billion healthcare transactions are conducted electronically via mail, fax, or phone every year (Institute of Medicine, 2001).

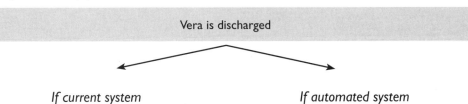

Vera is discharged

If current system	*If automated system*
A discharge summary is written for the community nurse and given to Vera. It contains current medications and diagnosis. The resident forwards a letter to the GP with a brief reintroduction to Vera and her care. It should arrive in the next few days/ weeks. One-month's supply of medications is dispensed.	A clinical discharge summary is automatically uploaded into Health*Connect* via a fast broadband connection. Her health team has immediate access to this. All are aware of Vera's medications and a sufficient supply has been pre packed and dispensed. Her GP will review her next week.
Vera returns home and rings the Community Health Nurses for assistance, but she requires a referral. Her GP does not do this via telephone and it will have to wait until she see can see him. The first available appointment is next week. The community nurse makes an appointment to see Vera after that. Eventually …	An automatic referral is sent to the community nurse who makes an appointment with Vera the day after she returns home.

Vera is seen by the community nurse

The community nurse arrives a little late, as she was lost. She quizzes Vera about her past history and hospital stay and asks about her treatment and outcomes (unfortunately the discharge summary is still in the taxi). Vera does not seem to remember much. The nurse asks about medications. Vera produces an apple box containing medicines from 1956 to the latest supply from the hospital, oh … and her herbs. She seems confused about which of the little red pills she should take.	The community nurse arrives on time thanks to the GPS built into her Tablet PC. She has immediate access via a wireless network to Vera's full history, current medications and care plan. Vera has surfed the net and has printouts about her condition that she wishes to discuss with the nurse. In future they will meet via a telehealth home link.

To take informed health action, individuals, families and communities must have access to meaningful accurate information delivered in a culturally effective and timely manner. The last decade has seen advances in telehealth that have put it at the forefront of the digital revolution in healthcare and home-based care. This clearly demonstrates the capabilities of the technology discussed by Wootton and Edirippuligé in the previous chapter.

Interest box

The Royal District Nursing Service (RDNS) in Victoria first trialled mobile computing in 1994. It demonstrated the ability to improve data integrity, and reduced documentation and duplication. It enabled nurses to begin their shift from home because of their access to up-to-date client information and the day's schedule. Following another trial in 1997–98 computers were rolled out to all field staff. In 2003, the service became fully mobile with over 800 Tablet PCs selected for field use. These offer a wide range of usability and incorporate wireless networking, GPRS, modem functionality, pen-based computing, handwriting and voice-recognition data entry.

(RDNS, 2005)

Mobile computing enables the collection and sharing of quality data to reduce errors, improve patient safety, and enhance service provision. However, community healthcare providers also offer a range of services that have very specific obligatory reporting requirements. In such a diverse environment, data collection is potentially confusing and extremely complex. To overcome this, the Royal District Nursing Service introduced a data-mapping matrix that supports the use of quality data and information while enabling the organisation to respond and comply with the many health-related minimum data sets (RDNS, 2005).

Telehealth in home healthcare is available in many forms and is transmitted in three basic forms – text data, audio, and images. However, home-based telehealth tools require the provider to exhibit cognitive and observational skills to assess patient status – from a distance (Lisetti & LeRouge, 2004). Although physiological measurement and so forth can be effectively communicated using current telehealth systems, the often crucial affective state assessment provides a greater challenge. A system currently under development builds a model of user's emotions (MOUE), while monitoring the patient using multi-sensory devices (Lisetti & LeRouge, 2004). These types of innovations will be a timely addition to the data and information available on a remotely monitored patient.

However, with the increasing transience of the population, the triangular model of health services between general practitioner, community nurse and hospital is dated and probably does not reflect healthcare of the future. Roggiero (Chapter 28) demonstrates the use of information technology in an isolated Aboriginal Community Health Centre and the necessity for a rethink about the way people engage with the health system.

Conclusion

Changes around funding, resource allocation and models of healthcare have increased the demand for sharing quality data and information across the health system. Fragmented patient records and inadequate methods of communication are no longer acceptable and indeed, the general population expects better. Patients and healthcare providers require timely, relevant information at the point-of-care, to improve decision-making, and provide quality, cost-effective services when and where they are needed. Patients expect their health information to be shared between providers and are bemused to find that this does not automatically happen.

IT has the potential to support healthcare by providing timely, quality data and to largely negate the tyranny of distance through high speed broadband and satellite access. It has the capacity to take clinicians into the future as informed, aware knowledge workers. Digitalisation of health services has the capacity to change healthcare as never before and, in time, the health system as we know it will no longer exist.

Review questions

1. What are the most efficient methods of data transfer across healthcare?
2. What infrastructure is necessary for this to occur?
3. What benefits are derived by the interoperability of systems?

Exercise

There are many factors necessary in the transfer of data across healthcare. Create a flow chart that depicts this information flow.

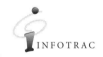

Online reading

INFOTRAC® COLLEGE EDITION
For additional readings and review on electronic data exchange, explore **InfoTrac® College Edition**, your online library. Go to: **www.infotrac-college.com** and search for any of the InfoTrac key terms listed below:
- Communication
- Information technology
- Information interchange

References

AIHW (2002). *Australian hospital statistics 1999–00*. Retrieved 4 January, 2005, from http://www.aihw.gov.au/publications/.

Australian Health Information Council (2004). *Health workforce health informatics capacity building: national statement 2004*. Department of Health and Ageing, Canberra.

Commonwealth of Australia (2003a). *HealthConnect interim research report: overview and findings Vol.1*, Department of Health and Ageing, Canberra.

Commonwealth of Australia (2003b). *HealthConnect: interim research report Vol.1*, Department of Health and Ageing, Canberra.

Commonwealth of Australia (2003c). *HealthConnect: interim research report overview and findings*, Department of Health and Ageing, Canberra.

Conrick, M. (in press). Using informatics to expand awareness, in J. Daly, S. Speedy and D. Jackson (eds.), *Contexts of nursing: an introduction*. Sydney. Churchill Livingstone.

Institute of Medicine (2001). *The use of computers in healthcare can reduce errors, improve patient safety, and enhance the quality of service*. Quality Chasm Report, Bethesda.

Lisetti, C. & LeRouge, C. (2004). *Affective computing in Tele-home health*, paper presented at the 37th Hawaii International Conference on System Sciences, Hawaii.

Orion Health (2004). *Walsall Health Partnerships – case study*. Retrieved 23 March, 2005, from http://www.orionhealth.com/.

Owens, N. & Foord, R. (2002). *ERDIP N2 Core national evaluation report – Section 1–3*. NHS Information Authority, Gloucester.

Royal District Nursing Service (2005) (RDNS). *Information services/ IT*. Retrieved 23 March, 2005, from http://www.rdns.com.au.

Part 5

The human issues in health informatics implementations

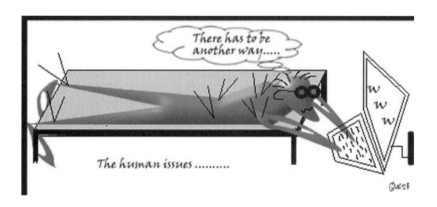

21

Informatics professional roles and governance

Moya Conrick

'If computers get too powerful, we can organize them into a committee – that will do them in.'

Anonymous

Outline

Information has always been fundamental to healthcare. The pace and scale of developments in IT have meant that many roles have been developed and people seconded or appointed to positions that have previously not existed. In this climate strong governance structures are imperative because of the significant business and organisational risk, lengthy development times, and substantial costs involved. This chapter discusses the roles that have emerged in the sector and the issues of governance that manage it.

Introduction

Over the last decade there has been an increased push from some governments, including the Australian Government, for the uptake of technologies in healthcare as a way to reduce the cost of an increasingly unaffordable health system and, at the same time, to deliver improved healthcare outcomes. The United States government has been vocal in recommending the adoption of technology to reduce medical errors. The British government has set aside $3.5 billion for the 2003–08 period to provide the healthcare professions with easy access to essential data in order to improve the delivery of health services (National Health Service (NHS), 2004).

In Australia, the Health*Connect* project has been a major driver for the use of information technology in healthcare and is being supported by all states in partnership with the Commonwealth Government. The 2004–08 budget for Health*Connect* is $128 million (Commonwealth of Australia, 2004).

The push for greater automation at all levels of healthcare has increased the need for skilled professionals who understand both the healthcare and information technology environments, and good governance for it to be successful. However, healthcare is different from other sectors in its requirements and complexity and this requires specialists in health informatics rather than specialists in technology or health alone.

What makes health informatics different?

The definition of health informatics (HI) discussed in Chapter 1 reveals that HI professionals work in two domains, health and information technology, whereas in most other industries information technology (IT) implementations can be undertaken with purely IT knowledge. However, it is only in the last few decades that health and IT have come together for the good of healthcare.

Health demands are unique because there is a need to respond to market forces, while providing for consumers, who are different from payers (Tuttle, 1999). The workforce is diverse and includes multiple provider groups, administrators and managers, IT specialists, academics, scientists, business specialists, statisticians, and librarians. The sector also has a very mobile, increasingly casual workforce that works around the clock, seven days a week. Staff turnover is high in most areas, but it is even more so in major teaching organisations where clinical rotations and rapid staff turnover are commonplace. The adoption of IT has taken a somewhat torturous path with health lagging behind other industries. This can be directly related to the extremely complex nature of health, the fiscal investment required, and end user resistance. Only in healthcare can resistance endanger the lives of consumers.

Clinicians generally embrace systems that support their practice and improve patient outcomes. Resistance to the introduction of some technology has resulted in part from 'burned fingers' when poor system design and minimal change management processes resulted in technology implementations that were inappropriate. The lack of involvement or poor integration of the input of healthcare professionals in the planning stages and during implementation has also resulted in resistance, as has the lack of appropriate education. At the same time, some members of the health workforce perceive a diffusion of power in their professional groups and react negatively.

The differences between IT and health informatics can also be found in the environment in which HI takes place as health requirements are more challenging in a number of areas (Tuttle, 1999). For example, the implications for violations of privacy and confidentiality are much greater in healthcare than in other industries and, unlike other sectors, support for personal values is essential. The complexity of the health knowledge base and multiple terminologies required across so many professional and administrative groups is not seen elsewhere. The responsibility for public health planning and the management of populations is also unique to health.

Perceptions of high risk in the implementation of health IT persist, but at the same time there is substantial pressure to make rapid critical decisions about deployment. Adding to the challenges is the difficulty in providing evidence for the adoption of IT because the outcomes in health are poorly defined and not easily quantifiable (PricewaterhouseCoopers LLP, 2005).

The health informatics workforce

Health informatics is a broad field encompassing the 'whole of health' and all technological implementations that relate to health information management in the sector. Health informaticians are involved in all facets of the development and deployment of health information systems and technologies that are capable of pushing the boundaries of health knowledge. They find new ways of making health services safer and more efficient by maximising outputs for clinicians and managers while supporting and educating users. The scope for people with different interests, skills and qualifications is enormous and the entry requirements for the health informaticians vary. Depending on the role, it may be possible to enter a career in HI without formal qualifications, but other roles may require specific professional qualifications.

Health informaticians also come from diverse backgrounds. They might be clinicians who, because of an interest in technology, are seconded and later move into full-time HI roles. Informaticians may be IT specialists who bring their expertise to health or, more recently, university educated health informatics professionals. The diversity in health informatics enables informaticians to operate in more dynamic roles than those usually found in the healthcare sector alone.

Roles in HI

The roles in health informatics are as diverse as healthcare itself and as governments and others sectors adopt IT, there are many opportunities for health informaticians into the foreseeable future. Many roles are well described and have been for some time, but there may be roles undertaken in the future that do not exist yet.

Informaticians can move between health settings and work closely with a variety of health professionals and teams. They take integral roles in the development and implementation of systems and networks across healthcare organisations at all levels of management and the workforce more generally. The implementation of systems such as electronic health records has ramped up the demand for HI professionals to analyse the information in these systems, in the form that health workers require it (Tuttle, 1999) and to make it available when and where it is needed. Support is also necessary for clinical decision support and point of care systems. Because of the nature of IT implementations, health informaticians are often change agents and so must possess the knowledge and skills to effectively manage change.

Tuttle (1999) describes the roles that are frequently advertised in international health information management and information systems trade journals. The following outline is based on this work and includes the:

- *Clinical System Analyst* who is involved in coordinating, analysing, implementing and monitoring system integrity for health information management or clinical systems.
- *Database Administrator* who coordinates the projects structure between users, vendors or programmers and assist in planning, training, testing, installation and support of databases.

- *Database Reporting Analyst* who assists in analysis, planning, creation and maintenance of simple to moderately complex database projects, develops reports and analyses data.
- *Clinical Systems Trainer* who has primary responsiblility for end-user education.
- *Security Officer* who is responsible for managing the security of all electronically maintained information, including the promulgation of security requirements, policies and privilege systems, and the audit of performance.
- *Health Information Manager,* a high-level position requiring an in-depth knowledge of information systems, who works with information executives and users. This position is responsible for advancing systems, data quality, data usability and information security.
- *Data Quality (DQ) Manager* who monitors data integrity throughout the organisation and is responsible for the quality of and access to information, in addition to the presentation of information and how information is indexed on a site.
- *Data Resource Administrator* who provides the long-term integrity of and access to information and uses media such as electronic health records, data repositories and electronic warehousing to meet current and future care needs across the continuum of care.
- *Research and Decision Support Analyst* who uses a variety of analytical tools and databases to support senior management with information for decision-making and strategy development. They work with product and policy organisations on high-level analysis projects such as clinical trials and outcomes research..

There is also a variety of areas that employ health information specialists. The major players and their roles are:

- *Private practioners' practices* that require IT support for in-house systems, their connectivity and integration and the skills of data management
- *Consulting companies* that advise and assist governments and healthcare organisations in the development and implementation of information systems. They also provide knowledge management solutions.
- *Software companies* that hire people with strong programming skills and good knowledge of the healthcare sector.
- *Public health agencies* that requires workers who can design and implement surveillance and disease reporting systems for the collection and analysis of information on populations and communities.
- *Government and non-governmental agencies* that require staff with a diverse range of skills, including data collection, storage retrieval and analyses for health planning at various levels of government.
- *Insurance companies* that hire staff capable of analysing health insurance claims and health records.
- *Academia* that requires candidates to have an advanced degree in HI and teaching.

The current phase of development and implementation of IT in Australia is creating opportunities across all health informatics areas. However, all of these must be supported by efficient governance processes and frameworks.

Informatics governance

Many nations, organisations, institutions and individuals grapple with how best they can guide the implementation of IT and this depends a great deal on the governance frameworks used. The practice of 'good governance' is increasingly seen as critical for the good management of organisations, both public and private. It has a legal and ethical responsibility to ensure that decisions are taken in the interests of stakeholders, and that the organisation behaves like 'a good corporate citizen' (Weill & Ross, 2004).

IT governance is seen as 'the structure of relationships and processes to develop, direct and control IS/IT resources in order to achieve the enterprise's goals' (Korac-Kakabadse & Kakabadse, 2001, p.9). It is about people, culture, relationships, and leadership and, according to the Organisation for Economic Cooperation and Development (2004), provides structures for determining organisational objectives and monitoring performance to ensure that objectives are attained. However, it is only effective when participants have the will to make it work.

Governance should be an active and focused process that has its outcomes recorded and endorsed and, according to Exiner (2004), it requires an individual approach in each organisation. Protocols must be developed for areas such as decision-making, liaison, access to information, roles, and so on. Recording these embeds them in the organisation and also serves as a reminder and prompt for participants. Written protocols can also serve to strengthen accountability and transparency of both processes and the organisation (Exiner, 2004).

Structures and approaches are also usually unique to an organisation and these have to be achieved by agreement and followed voluntarily; they are protocols and conventions, rather than rules. There are some frameworks in use such as the Governance Design Framework (Weill & Ross, 2004) and The Control Objectives for Information and Related Technology (COBIT) framework 'which is being used increasingly by a diverse range of organisations throughout the world' (Pathak, 2003, p.33). These frameworks assist organisations to ensure alignment between IT and their business goals and are fundamental to efficient and effective IT governance.

The necessity for good governance is obvious because large organisations reportedly spend over 50 per cent of their capital investment on IT (Koch, 2002). In fact, governance has been recognised as a critical factor in achieving corporate success (Ridley, Young & Carroll, 2004). However, it is complex and depends on cooperation, communication and respect from all involved. An understanding of roles and role differentiation is critical, but must be sophisticated and flexible. Good relationships must be nurtured and consideration given to how groups work together, communicate and respect each other. Players must be mindful of and understand the issues and pressures that exist, all of which requires a significant investment in time, attention and effort. Good relationships mean good communication and a willingness to address and solve issues and problems.

Governance concepts are dynamic and should be revisited regularly to ensure their ongoing relevance and applicability. Organisations should have systems and processes in place for evaluating governance structures and this should be a regular part of a governance evaluation cycle (Exiner, 2004). In health informatics governance has two distinct areas, the first is that related to the adoption and implementation of IT and the second is governance of the professional bodies.

Governance in a digital environment

A report by PricewaterhouseCoopers LLP (2005) stresses the role of effective governance in the digitalisation of health saying that effective leadership and management by boards are imperative because of the significant business and organisational risk, lengthy development times, and the substantial cost involved. They also agree that a clear vision of the project's purpose and goals is essential to ensure that all stakeholders share a common view of the organisation's direction because, often, major organisational transformation is necessary (PricewaterhouseCoopers LLP, 2005; Exiner, 2004; Weill & Ross, 2004). The impact of this is a significant factor in determining the success of failure of any project.

According to Saunders (2005, p.28) process and technology are interdependent, 'it's a hand-in-glove thing … technology can only be as good as the process'. Process design, technology acquisition and implementation must be interwoven and is not as simple as buy-and-install. Implementing a digital hospital, for example, requires the deployment and integration of a complex, connected series of technologies to create a smoothly running system that fully exploits the technology and empowers the health workforce to more effectively fulfil their responsibilities. This is impossible if effective governance processes are lacking (PricewaterhouseCoopers LLP, 2005).

The digitalisation of hospitals entails major organisational transformations and substantial business risks that need to be managed. These risks include cost overages, failure to gain expected returns on the investment made, and even user refusal. Again healthcare is a rarity, as few other industries spend tens of millions of dollars on IT while facing the risk that when the project goes live a significant proportion of staff will refuse to use it (PricewaterhouseCoopers LLP, 2005).

Transforming healthcare process through technology can have a powerful impact on an organisation, and the board or governance group must provide both direction and explicit support for projects. However, unless they have an adequate understanding of the issues entailed in the project, this might not be possible and educational activities are crucial. Miller (in PricewaterhouseCoopers LLP, 2005 p.29) considers that 'The educational component for the board is as important as getting them aside for a couple of days and having them go through this in excruciating detail. Let them ask the questions, because it's (often) new to them, too'.

The impact of organisational transformation is a significant factor in determining whether a project is ultimately judged as a success or a failure. Effective governance protocols and practice are essential in this transformation.

Government governance structures: Health*Connect*

Health*Connect* came into existence in 2001. Since moving from its initial research and development phase to implementation and, following the Boston Consulting Group report into the project in 2004, the project has taken new directions with the establishment of the National eHealth Transition Authority (NeHTA), that is discussed below, and a trim Health*Connect* project office. As governance arrangements are still being developed, discussion is somewhat curtailed. However, the original Health*Connect* governance structure consisted of a board and its advisory groups that included a stakeholder reference group.

The Board was established in 2001 to oversee the research and development stages of Health*Connect* and provide guidance on strategic directions, including the establishment of trial sites and exploratory projects (Commonwealth of Australia, 2005). It involves representatives from State and Territory Governments' Departments of Health, a health consumer representative, a health provider representative and a health informatics expert. The Health Insurance Commission, the New Zealand Ministry of Health and the AMA have observer status on the Board. Nursing was invited as an observer for two meetings prior to its recess and allied health are not represented. In the restructure, the Stakeholder Reference Group was disbanded and a decision on the continuation of the board is pending.

In the interim, the Commonwealth Government (2005, p.18) have affirmed the following governance structures:

- a cross-jurisdictional national Health*Connect* Implementation Steering Committee will report to the National Health Information Group (NHIG) and take responsibility for the successful implementation of the Health*Connect* Strategy across Australia
- the Implementation Steering Committee will manage the policies and business issues of Health*Connect* and will have accountability for achieving agreed outcomes using available resources
- an Implementation Advisory Group will be set up to advise the Implementation Steering Committee on stakeholder issues. Working parties may be formed to focus on specific issues. Roles and membership of the Implementation Advisory Group and its working parties will be determined in the wider context of other health information advisory committees, such as the Australian Health Information Council (AHIC).

NeHTA

NeHTA's (2005) work program is focused on e-health informatics standards and includes developing standards for the exchange of clinical information. It also focuses on integrating infrastructure and considering the issues of the unique identification of patients, providers, products and services, providing shared information resources. It is looking to increase sectoral efficiency by facilitating reform, including the adoption of specifications for a national shared electronic health record (NeHTA, 2005).

NeHTA reports directly to the Australian Health Ministers Advisory Councils' Information and Information and Communications Technology working group. It is supported by an advisory committee that has specialist advisors from 'clinical', legal policy and technical areas – nursing, allied health and alternative practitioners are not included in this.

Professional governance in health informatics

The organisation and governance of HI as a professional group began in 1967 (see Chapter 1) with the establishment of the International Medical Informatics Association (IMIA) that has since become the most visible of the international informatics groups. Generally, membership of IMIA is limited to organisations, societies and corporations and it aims to:

> bring together, from a global perspective, scientists, researchers, vendors, consultants and suppliers in an environment of cooperation and sharing. The international membership network of National Member Societies, IMIA Regions, Corporate and Academic Institutional Members, and our Working and Special Interest Groups that constitute the 'IMIA family' is uniquely positioned to achieve these goals.
>
> (IMIA, n.d.)

IMIA is governed by a General Assembly that meets annually. It consists of one representative of each member country, Honorary Fellows, Chairs of IMIA's Working Groups and a representative from IFIP, the World Health Organisation, and each of IMIA's Regions. Only National Members have full voting rights (IMIA, n.d). Closer to Australia, APAMI is Asia's official representative body to IMIA and includes fourteen countries in the Pacific Rim from Japan to New Zealand.

Although there is a number of informatics organisations in Australia, the Health Informatics Society of Australia (HISA) is regarded as the major umbrella group and is the member of IMIA. Nursing informaticians were the driving force behind the formation of HISA, which is now an incorporated company. The membership comes from across the informatics spectrum, that is, from students to corporate affiliates. HISA has a number of branches (Queensland, New South Wales and Western Australia) as well as special interest groups such as nursing (NIA), pathology, aged and community care, industry and medical imaging.

The HISA board has ten members, one representative from each member group and two general positions drawn from members at large. The members have a two-year term in office, with half of those holding office the longest since the last Board election retiring each year.

Conclusion

Recent developments in technology have unlocked the power of information and knowledge and have provided a potent means for harnessing data and using it for the good of healthcare.

In this climate, governance must be strong, flexible and inclusive, because the degree of commitment of senior management and ownership by staff are the greatest success factors in IT implementations. Health is a dynamic industry and for organisations to remain strategic and relevant requires governance structures that are agile because change in traditional structures is cumbersome, slow and costly.

The restructure of programs such as Health*Connect* demonstrates the changing nature of IT implementations. It also demonstrates the refinement and streamlining that is essential in aligning IT and business processes. In the future, IT will integrate with health becoming an embedded process rather than a separate program with distinct governance structures.

Review questions

1. Why are IT professionals at a disadvantage if they have never worked in the health sector and do not have an understanding of the health industry?
2. Name four roles in which informatics specialists might be employed?
3. 'Governance is not something that is of interest to clinicians.' Discuss this statement.

Exercises

*   Go online and find three advertisements for health informaticians. Discuss the position and criteria for the position.

*   You are a manager preparing to interview aspiring informaticians applying to work as clinical systems specialists. What five questions would you ask to gauge their suitability?

Online reading

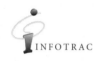
INFOTRAC

INFOTRAC® COLLEGE EDITION
For additional readings and review on governance, explore **InfoTrac® College Edition**, your online library. Go to: **www.infotrac-college.com** and search for any of the InfoTrac key terms listed below:
➤ **Informatics roles**
➤ **Governance**
➤ **IMIA**
➤ **HISA**

References

Commonwealth of Australia (2005). Health*Connect*. Retrieved 3 June, 2005, from http://www.healthconnect.gov.au/.

Commonwealth of Australia (2005). Health*Connect* implementation strategy. Retrieved 23 June, 2005, from http://www.healthconnect.gov.au/.

Commonwealth of Australia (2004). Budget Papers. Retrieved 20 October, 2004, from http://www.health.gov.au/.

Exiner, R. (2004). *Good governance guide*. Good governance advisory group, Melbourne.

Health Informatics Association of Australia (HISA) (2004). *Health Informatics Society of Australia (HISA) Plan (2004–2005)*, Melbourne. Retrieved 10 March, 2005, from http://hisa.org.au/.

International Medical Informatics Association (IMIA) (n.d.). *About IMIA*. Retrieved 4 February, 2005, from http://www.imia.org/.

International Medical Informatics Association (IMIA) (n.d). Retrieved 3 March, 2005, from http://www.imia.org/membership.html.

Koch, C. (2002). The powers that should be: IT decisions have to reflect the goals of the business and engage the attention of the business, often without the participation or even the interest of the business, *CIO, 15*(23), 48–54.

Korac-Kakabadse, N & Kakabadse, A (2001). IS/IT governance: need for an integrated model, *Corporate Governance, 1*(4), 9–11.

National Health Service (NHS) (2004). *Knowledge management*. Retrieved 22 February, 2005, from http://www.nelh.nhs.uk/knowledge_management.

NeHTA (2005). *About NeHTA*. Retrieved 23 June, 2005, from http://www.nehta.gov.au/.

Organisation for Economic Cooperation and Development (2004). *Governance culture and development: a different perspective on corporate governance*. Retrieved 22 February, 2005, from http://www.oecd.org/.

Pathak, J. (2003). Internal audit and E-Commerce controls, *Internal Auditing, 18*(2), 30–4.

PricewaterhouseCoopers LLP (2005). *Reactive to adaptive: transforming hospitals with digital technology*, PricewaterhouseCoopers, Delaware.

Ridley, G., Young, J. & Carroll, P. (2004). *COBIT and its utilization: a framework from the literature*. Paper presented at the 37th Hawaii International Conference on System Sciences, Hawaii.

Saunders, N. (2005). *Reactive to adaptive: transfroming hospitals with digital technology*. in PricewaterhouseCoopers LLP, Delaware.

Tuttle, M. (1999). Information technology outside health care: What does it matter to us?, *J Am Med Inform Assoc, 6*(5), 354–60.

Weill, P. & Ross, J. (2004). *IT governance*, Harvard Business School Press, Boston.

22

Workforce capacity building

Moya Conrick

> 'A health worker was asked to send a copy of a floppy disk to the IT department. He took a photocopy and posted it internal mail.'
>
> Anonymous

Outline

Healthcare workers are often asked to use information systems that are foreign to them and often have limited appreciation of the power and potential of IT to support their practice. It is crucial in a modern health system for the workforce to use technology efficiently and effectively and this has led to an urgent need for systematic health informatics education. This chapter explores the most crucial issues of building capacity in the health sector.

Introduction

Progress in information and communication technology (ICT) and information processing has changed society and its expectations of the health system. Society expects the latest technology to be available for those who need it and that clinicians be knowledgeable about technology and abreast of the latest research evidence. However, health knowledge has become available at such an extraordinary rate, it is difficult to for health workers to remain current, much less be able to store, organise and retrieve it in a timely fashion.

At the same time poor processes, systems and individual performance plague the healthcare system and are the main factors in adverse events according to a New South Wales Health report (2004). This report sees patient safety, quality improvements and reducing the cost of healthcare as the principal drivers in the adoption of information technology (IT), while escalating costs and decreasing confidence in the healthcare system are the catalysts for changes in the health sector.

Improvements in information management have the potential to address many of these problems and to produce significant health gains for the community and across the health sector in general. The New South Wales Health report (2004) calls for all clinicians, managers, patients and their carers to engage if this is to occur. However, 'engaging' is not simple or something that will happen without an informatics prepared workforce and a systematic and sustained approach to health informatics education across Australia.

IT is ubiquitous in health; some adoptions are as large as a hospital information system, others as discrete as the chip in a thermometer. No matter the setting, the importance of informatics to health cannot be overestimated because it is used across all health domains – clinical, administrative, education, research and planning. It involves all healthcare workers and is the most pervasive tool that has ever been introduced into the sector. Complex and changing environments, different models of care (with an increasing emphasis on non-institutional care), increased patient and client expectations and economic pressures have prompted significant changes in health service delivery over the last decade.

The Australian Health Workforce Officials Committee has developed several reports on workforce requirements and acknowledge that the types of healthcare workers will change and that these changes will be deeply impacted by technology (Australian Health Ministers' Conference, April 2004). They also noted the need for 'continually improving health workforce data collections; putting in place a common language, minimum data sets, and consistent collection and processing arrangements' (p.18). Regrettably, the importance of health informatics (HI) for the future health workforce and the need to develop skills in this area is not addressed in this report. Yet, to support healthcare, in this environment it is crucial to increase the range of people, organisations and communities who are able to address problems.

The Australian Health Information Council (2004) have realised the importance of raising the profile of HI and suggested that provision be made for capacity building in HI in any future workforce planning activities. Hawke, King, Noort, Jordens and Lloyd (2000, p.4) define capacity building as:

> the process of integrating vision, leadership, resources and support into the existing health system structure. The development of skills and resources and also problem solving capabilities at five levels: individual, within health care teams, within the health organization, across the organization and within the community

These authors acknowledge that this requires the development of sustainable skills, education structures, resources and a commitment to improvements in health to prolong and multiply health gains many times over.

The sheer size and disparate backgrounds of the health workforce make the provision of education challenging, but as ICT is the contemporary tool of practice, HI skills are fundamental to a modern health workforce. The very large amount of spending by government and the private sector on health IT infrastructure across the world stems from the realisation that information technology will improve patient care and deliver quality health outcomes. Although it is difficult to assess improvements in the quality of healthcare, interim reports suggest that it is enhanced by the systematic application of information processing and ICT (Commonwealth of Australia, 2003).

Automation has much to offer healthcare workers and, indeed, the last few years have seen the beginnings of a transformation triggered by a rapid rise in the use of information technology across healthcare and the rapid increase in the sophistication of information systems (Conrick et al., 2004). However, no matter the quality of systems or money spent, the projected improvement in clinical care and health outcomes will not eventuate unless all members of the health workforce have the skills in HI. There are already reports of systems failure related to user apathy or ignorance.

The skills gap in health informatics

Assumptions are made that many health workers, particularly those who have undertaken professional training in the past five years, and those who have undertaken specific systems training in individual workplaces, have some HI expertise (AHIC, 2004). Yet, a recent comprehensive study of 2020 nurses across a wide range of specialties and care environments in the United Kingdom places doubt on this (NHS Information Authority, 2003). The findings of this study are similar to anecdotal reports from Australian nurses and reveal that insufficient or inappropriate IT training was one of the issues raised most frequently by the respondents.

Training ranged from none at all (60 per cent), and being expected to just 'get on with it', to being trained, but having either no system or a different system in their practice area. Training was also rigid and unmatched to individual learning needs. Release from the clinical area was problematic and often there was no provision to 'back fill' the ward, necessitating some participants to undertake training in their own time. One participant noted that 'IT is not seen as essential when staff numbers are low' (NHS Information Authority, 2003, p.23).

In Australia the lack of computer knowledge of health workers is seen as impeding the realisation of the full potential of health information technology in advancing practice (Conrick et al., 2004; General Practice Computing Group, 1999). The lack of well-trained clinical informaticians is also acknowledged in Public Health (National Library of Medicine, 2001) and indeed across all health sectors.

As the deployment of technology in healthcare accelerates around the world, so does the demand for health informaticians. In Australia, this demand cannot be supported across both private and public health institutions from the available pool of HI specialists. This pattern is repeated around the world. Granger, the National Programme for IT at the NHS (NpfIT, 2003, p 24) makes this assessment: 'There are real difficulties getting high-quality, properly leveraged teams to deliver complex programmes'.

Although this shortage is acute in health, it is widespread across the IT sector and according to Collins (2005), recruitment of skilled IT professionals will be difficult over the next year as demand for staff rises. Exacerbating this is the disappearance of jobs from the IT industry itself; over the last five years this has been estimated at between 100 000 and 250 000 jobs in the United Kingdom alone. This causes the traditional succession from analyst to team leader, junior project manager and inter-program director, to 'fall apart' causing enormous problems (Granger, 2005).

Project managers and IT staff with business, industry sector knowledge and integration skills may also be in particularly short supply. According to a Quarterly Survey of Appointments Data and Trends there was a 20 per cent jump in the number of advertised job vacancies from the end of the 2003 to the third quarter of 2004. This is a doubling of jobs advertised at the end of 2003 (Collins, 2005).

These gaps in HI skills are set to continue because the entry requirements and qualifications for health informaticians are so varied, there is no clear career pathway for graduates as yet. Those involved in informatics range from the co-opted clinician to the experienced IT professionals.

Closing the informatics gap

Many factors influence the likelihood of individuals having adequate skills in HI, including the availability of subjects/courses in undergraduate programs, the length of time since finishing professional education, the rate of technological change and the rapid turnover of the workforce. These factors, coupled with difficulties accessing the necessary education and training, mean that skill gaps in HI capacity will be present for some time.

Changes to policy making, governance structures and research funding are required as is a fundamental change to education so that the health sector can remain abreast of ICT developments. This will necessitate change to undergraduate curricula, program design and course content. Unless these issues are addressed at all levels, the approach to informatics will continue to be fragmented, duplication of effort will continue, and the workforce capacity in informatics will remain very low.

What skills are required?

One of the key determinants of the IT skills required for the health workforce is the type, or model of care, that is being delivered. The AHIC for instance, recognises that the requirements for an aged care nurse will be different from an emergency nurse and that General Practitioners in rural and remote Australia may not require the same skills as those working in metropolitan areas. Other professional groups will also have different requirements and these will change between private and public practice (AHIC, 2004, p.18). There are commonalities and differences in the IT skills required for professional health groups just as they are in their practice (see Figure 22.1).

Figure 22.1: Relationship between health professionals (Conrick et al., 2004)

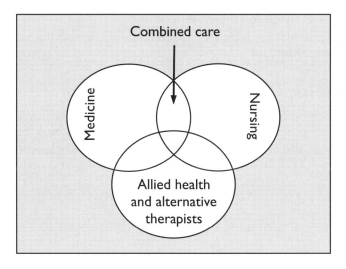

The health setting will also dictate the skills required, for instance, administrative staff and clinicians in private practice will have overlapping HI 'skill requirements surrounding the management of hardware and software, privacy and security, quality and safety, incident reporting, infection control, performance monitoring and management of knowledge resources' (AHIC, 2004, p.18). AHIC acknowledge the enormity of the task, saying that:

> Health service managers (clinical and administrative) need to make decisions about software purchases, while staff involved in implementations, need to be conversant with the whole health industry, as well as information systems, technologies and workflow processes, to ensure that appropriate decisions are made.

The emergence of the discipline of HI is beginning to blur traditional professional boundaries in the workplace and is generating completely new positions and work descriptions.

Many clinicians have found their way into informatics by simply showing an interest and aptitude for computers in their workplace, but as HI matures so do the requirements for employment. Skills such as those required to analyse large amounts of health data and information, and to communicate this across healthcare as knowledge will never change. Health workers require HI basic computer and information technology skills, to specialist clinical information management and health informatics expertise.

Although little work has been carried out in Australia, the International Medical Informatics Association (IMIA) provides an internationally endorsed approach to matching skills and competencies in ICT with the various roles and responsibilities of healthcare providers (IMIA, 2000). These include:

- an understanding of the healthcare industry
- communication skills
- management and leadership
- strategic planning
- information technology skills
- information analysis and organisation
- knowledge of system infrastructure design and networking
- programming skills.

Competencies

Defining competencies in health informatics has been slow and, while some professions have begun this work, competencies have yet to be widely adopted. Most employers set the levels of competence expected of their workforce, for example the NHS (2005, p.3) sets the following generic skills level for members of various staff groups:

	Level	Expectations
0	None	No skills or knowledge are required in a particular Health Informatics topic.
1	Basic	A fundamental knowledge only, with few basic skills at most, is required in a particular Health Informatics topic.
2	Intermediate	Moderate skills and knowledge are required in a particular Health Informatics topic.
3	Advanced	Indicates that specialist skills and knowledge are required in a particular Health Informatics topic. This means members of the staff group need to understand and/or have the ability to use a particular Health Informatics topic in order to fully carry out their job role without specialist support or supervision.
4	Expert	Needs to *completely* understand and/or have the ability to use *all* aspects of the particular topic.

Internationally, nursing and public health have been quite rigorous in developing competency levels for their constituents. A Delphi study carried out by Staggers et al. (2002, p.385) in America has resulted in four areas of competence being validated by nurses. Because of their universal nature they are presented here.

Beginning nurses (Level 1) have fundamental information management and computer technology skills and use existing information systems and available information to manage their practice.

Experienced nurses (Level 2) have proficiency in their domain of interest (e.g., public health, education, administration). These nurses are highly skilled in using information management and computer technology skills to support their major area of practice. They see relationships among data elements, and make judgements based on trends and patterns within these data. Experienced nurses use current information systems but collaborate with the informatics nurse specialist to suggest system improvements.

Informatics specialists (Level 3) are registered nurses prepared at least at the baccalaureate level who possess additional knowledge and skills specific to information management and computer technology. They focus on information needs for the practice of nursing, which includes education, administration, research and clinical practice. Informatics specialists' practices are built on the integration and application of information science, computer science and nursing science. In their practice, informatics specialists use the tools of critical thinking, process skills, data management skills (includes identifying, acquiring, preserving, retrieving, aggregating, analysing, and transmitting data), systems development life cycle, and computer skills.

Informatics innovators (Level 4) are educationally prepared to conduct informatics research and to generate informatics theory. These nurses lead the advancement of informatics practice and research because they have a vision of what is possible, and a keen sense of timing to make things happen. Innovators function with an ongoing healthy skepticism of existing data management practices and are creative in developing solutions. Innovators possess a sophisticated level of understanding and skills in information management and computer technology. They understand the interdependence of systems, disciplines and outcomes, and can finesse situations to maximise outcomes.

Public Health has developed nine core competencies, demonstrating that health informatics is extremely diverse and multifaceted, as are the responsibilities and role descriptions. The IMIA working group for education is considering developing credentialing criteria in the near future to serve as a guide for teachers wishing to participate in health and medical informatics education (IMIA, 2000).

HI education

The pressure for a skilled global health workforce makes it imperative that beginning practitioners have some competence in informatics because they are at the beginning of the workforce supply chain. The lack of informatics education at this level perpetuates the capacity problem and, without informatics knowledge and skills integrated into undergraduate curricula, providers are abrogating their responsibility to prepare graduates for the demands of a modern health system.

Workers engaged in clinical activity must understand the importance of IT as a tool of practice. They must also understand data and information management in clinical information systems and use this to produce clinical knowledge. This is an ongoing process that provides for the further development of informatics knowledge and skills that must be integrated into the continued development of practice.

However, there is little visibility of HI in undergraduate programs and little integration of HI skills in general postgraduate courses. The majority of clinical informatics programs that exist are at postgraduate level, in the form of Graduate Diplomas or Master level qualifications. There is a limited number of these programs so graduate numbers remain relatively small. Some certificate programs are offered, but there are no large-scale professional training programs in Australia at present.

Even if all postgraduate education providers integrate informatics into their programs a sizeable percentage of clinicians have little intention of undertaking postgraduate education programs in HI or any other area. Therefore, the needs of those already practicing must also be met. However, there is little incentive for health workers to gain HI skills post-graduation as there is scant recognition of HI expertise in most employment awards. In several health departments, for instance, HI qualifications are not recognised as postgraduate qualification for nurses, and no allowance is forthcoming.

Some organisations are developing activities to identify the requirements of their members and to provide training. For example, continuing professional development programs in informatics exist (and are largely funded) in the medical colleges, but these are the exception, rather than the rule. Other professions are not funded and, in the main, education efforts are piecemeal and uncoordinated, often resulting in gaps and duplication of effort. There needs to be a systematic and concerted effort to address this problem.

AHIC (2004, p.6) has released a (draft) report on capacity building that addresses some of these issues and provides a nationally agreed vision, a set of priorities for action, and recommends a number of initiatives including that:

- Funding is provided to develop a nationally agreed set of basic health informatics competencies that all health professionals need to acquire. These are to be incorporated in all undergraduate curricula and be used as the basis for staff development programs.
- The delivery of HI education and training should be available though a number of different mechanisms, such as through universities and the TAFE system, professional associations and private sector trainers.
- Incentives for offering HI training should be provided to organisations with the capacity to do so.
- Funding is provided to medical colleges and/or professional associations to assist members/fellows in undertaking appropriate and relevant educational activities to advance their core competencies in HI and, ideally, to recognise such activities as a form of continuing professional development.
- A scholarship program is developed to enable study in health informatics. Scholarships could be awarded each year to a general field of applicants and have identified places for indigenous health workers and aged care health workers. The scholarship program should be available to clinical workers, health service clerical and administrative staff and health managers.

A set of basic clinical informatics competencies would ensure a level of competence for all health professionals and could also form the basis for staff development programs. This may take the form of a certification or some other tangible award. Postgraduate programs could also help to increase the informatics capacity by embedding of informatics skills as a core competency.

A set of core competencies agreed to by the professions and industry seems sensible, but incentives (both stick and carrot) may be required to initiate this. Funding of professional bodies might also be necessary to assist members undertake appropriate and relevant educational activities and, ideally, this activity should be recognised as a form of continuing professional development (AHIC, 2004). A scholarship program would further ensure the development of the discipline and this should be open to general candidates and have places set aside for disadvantaged health groups.

Conclusion

A huge amount of financial and human resources will be wasted and the health sector will not receive the potential benefits of automation if capacity issues are not urgently addressed. This means that education and support must be provided to the appropriate people, in a timely fashion.

Funding, administration and delivery of health services in Australia is a complex partnership among many levels of government (national, state and local), and between the public and private sectors. All of these players have a stake in a well-educated workforce competent in HI and able to engage with and use embedded technologies when they enter the workforce. Educational providers must respond to the problems of informatics illiteracy in the health workforce in a more positive manner, as they have a responsibility to fully prepare students for their professional lives. In the modern health system informatics is an essential tool 'of the trade'.

In the recent past, informatics was seen as the computerisation of healthcare and the domain of a few enthusiasts. Today, computers are a part of routine daily life; they are ubiquitous in healthcare and permeate the everyday work of healthcare professionals. IT enhances communication, the sharing of knowledge across geographic boundaries, supports decision-making and the complex social and functional needs of healthcare organisations and services. Although there is some scepticism and debate about the effectiveness of IT in health, one thing is certain: without commitment to an informatics-educated health workforce, clinicians and managers will continue to 'drown' in paper and decisions will continue to be made on fragmented and questionable data.

Review questions

1. Why is human capacity building important in healthcare?
2. Whose responsibility is it?
3. What are the commonalities and differences in IT requirements for health workers? Take into account the differences in clinical, management and administrative areas.

Exercise

* Discuss this statement: 'Workers engaged in clinical activity must understand the importance of IT as a tool of practice'.

* Develop a matrix and map the HI skills required by at least four groups in the health workforce.

Online reading

INFOTRAC

INFOTRAC® COLLEGE EDITION
For additional readings and review on workforce capacity building, explore **InfoTrac® College Edition**, your online library. Go to: **www.infotrac-college.com** and search for any of the InfoTrac key terms listed below:
➤ Health informatics
➤ Education
➤ Skills gaps
➤ Human capacity building

References

Australian Health Information Council (2004). *Health workforce health informatics capacity building: national statement 2004*, Department of Health and Ageing, Canberra.
Australian Health Ministers' Conference (April 2004). *National health workforce strategic framework*, Sydney.

Collins, T. (2005). *Head of NHS IT acknowledges severe shortages of skilled staff*. Retrieved 1 April, 2005, from http://www.computerweekly.com.

Commonwealth of Australia (2003). *HealthConnect: Interim Research Report, Vol 1*, Department of Health and Ageing, Canberra.

Conrick, M., Hovenga, E., Cook, R., Laracuente, T. & Morgan, T. (2004). *A framework for nursing informatics in Australia: a strategic paper*, Department of Health and Ageing, Melbourne.

General Practice Computing Group (1999). *Survey of information technology activities in the Australian Divisions of General Practice*, Australian Medical Association, Barton.

Granger, R. (2005). *An update of progress on England's National Programme for NHS IT*. Paper presented at the HC2005, Harrogate.

Hawke, P., King, L., Noort, M., Jordens, C. & Lloyd, B. (2000). *Indicators to help with capacity building in health promotion*, NSW Health Department, Sydney.

International Medical Informatics Association (IMIA) (2000). *Recommendations of the International Medical Informatics Association (IMIA) on education in Health and Medical Informatics*. Retrieved 10 April, 2005, from http://www.imia.org/wg1/rec. htm.

National Health Service (2005). *Health informatics competency profiles for the National Health Service*. Retrieved 22 February, 2005, from http://www.nelh.nhs.uk/.

New South Wales Health (2004). *The NSW Patient Safety and Clinical Quality Program – Technical Paper*, New South Wales Health, Sydney.

NHS Information Authority (2003). *ERDIP: Lessons learned, benefits topic, final version*. Retrieved 2 February, 2004, from http://www.nhsia.nhs.uk/.

Staggers, N., Gassert, C. & Curran, C. (2002). A Delphi study to determine informatics competencies for nurses at four levels of practice, *Nursing Research, 51*(6), 383–90.

23

Human technology interfaces and ergonomics

Karen Guest and Moya Conrick

> 'Software development for different cultures requires attention to technical detail that goes beyond translation.'
>
> (Badre, 2002, p.213)

Outline

Technology is seen as one way to deliver healthcare across the continuum of care in a bid to rein-in expenses and to encourage consumers to become more autonomous and responsible for their healthcare decisions. Interface and ergonomic design that are essential for healthcare are those that are error-free, safe, effective and appropriate for clinicians and consumers to relate to technology. This chapter highlights some of the basic principles of interface design and ergonomics and will hopefully act as a trigger for the enthusiast to explore these issues further.

Introduction

Achieving a balance between useability and effectiveness of a software application is an important consideration for the human technology interface. Related to this is ergonomics and how physical design issues can be overcome to enable accessibility by the majority of stakeholders. Systems have become smaller and faster compared to the technology of a decade ago and this has ramifications for both interface design and ergonomics. The challenges of designing software applications and achieving high rates of use in a culturally diverse and ageing population of consumers and practitioners may be overwhelming unless appropriate and accessible human technology interfaces are developed.

The future of healthcare is currently focused on electronic healthcare records that are accessible by clinicians and patients. Governments are working collaboratively to enable this to occur, because it is a crucial issue when 78 per cent of the Australian population have complex chronic health conditions and co-morbidities (Australian

Bureau of Statistics, 2001) and this figure is set to rise. In this climate, access to information technology (IT) is essential and the human interface and ergonomic design are essential enablers of this.

The drivers for development

The human technology interface can be understood as the composition of the human population, the issues of technology and how the human population interacts with technology. Therefore, interface design must be compatible with both population demographics and the development of solutions for healthcare that increasingly include computers, the Internet and point-of-care devices. As public and private healthcare providers move towards a model of care that will see consumers having greater access to their health information and clinicians working in digital environments, the attention to interface design and need for some standardisation is now crucial.

The drive for ergonomically sound solutions also comes from the introduction of information technology as a tool of practice and its enhanced role in supporting consumers. Education will largely determine the success or failure of these developments and the provision of access to consumers will be especially challenging. Relative to this are issues of English proficiency in the general population.

It would seem that without government intervention healthcare is at the crossroads of developing a community of the 'haves or have nots' particularly as the Internet is becoming the tool of choice for exchanging data outside of institutions. Berners-Lee (inventor of the World Wide Web), had a noble vision of universal access to the web, but in Australia the proportion of households with access to a computer in 2003 was 66 per cent and access to the Internet 53 per cent (Australian Bureau of Statistics [ABS], 2003).

Outside of households it is hard to judge the true figures as communities have access to computers in libraries and some schools. Nonetheless, access to electronic health information is becoming an equity issue. While physical access is an issue, it is the secure, efficient and effective use of technology that is central to this discussion and design and ergonomics are fundamental in achieving this.

Ergonomics

Derived from the Greek *ergon* (work) and *nomos* (laws) to denote the science of work, ergonomics is a systems-oriented discipline that extends across all aspects of human activity. It considers physical, cognitive, social, organisational, environmental and other relevant factors (International Ergonomics Association [IEA], 2001). Ergonomists work across three main domains, the physical, cognitive and socio-technical systems all of which are relevant to digitalised health environments.

The physical domain is concerned with human anatomical, anthropometric, physiological and biomechanical characteristics as they relate to physical activity. Included in this area are issues such as working postures, materials handling, repetitive movements, work-related musculoskeletal disorders, workplace layout, safety and health (IEA, 2001).

Cognitive ergonomics is concerned with mental processes, such as perception, memory, reasoning and motor response, as they affect interactions among humans and other elements of a system. Relevant issues here are mental workload, human–computer interaction, decision-making, skilled performance, work stress and training as they may relate to human-system design.

The optimisation of socio-technical systems is the third domain of organisational ergonomics and includes organisational structures, policies and processes. Here, issues of communication, work design, teamwork, participatory design, new work paradigms, virtual organisations and telework are paramount. All three domains of ergonomic environments must be considered along with the basic principles of design when interfaces are being built for the health sector. Elements of both should be seamlessly incorporated into interface design and this chapter takes that route.

Design principles and issues

The first design principle in health should be that interfaces are designed in a way that makes it impossible for practitioners to make mistakes. Incorporating user-friendly elements such as menu selection as opposed to form fill-in, no alphabetic characters where numbers are expected, check before proceeding with major actions (for example, save before exit prompting), and feedback on errors including simple, specific instructions for recovery all assist with this (IEA, 2001). There are other strategies that also reduce error such as:

* making them detectable by providing feedback on effects of action
* reducing the potential for slips by simplifying and indicating input modes
* reducing the potential for mistakes
* reducing the consequences of error or make actions undo-able in areas such as navigation.

There are many standards available in interface and ergonomic design and in terms of website development. The best known and most widely used are those made available by the World Wide Web Consortium (W3C). This extensive resource is freely available for designers and other interested people.

Researching the end user

In recent years, user centered design has become of significant interest to academic researchers around the world. However, solutions are ultimately judged by how successful the requirements are for the user and the organisation (Cooper & Reimann, 2003). In healthcare, the reason for access and outcomes expected from the encounter are important if consistent use is to be encouraged. For example, a clinician accessing an electronic health record has a totally different need from a consumer surfing the web for health information.

The complexity of exploring the human technology interface in terms of large and diverse audiences should be taken into consideration when developing software applications for the health sector. In Australia, for example, the total population and therefore potential health consumer base in 2002 was over 19 million, with 63 per cent between 15–59 years; projections have this increasing to 22.7 million in 2020, and 26.5 million in 2050 (ABS, 2005). Australia is also a culturally diverse country with many minority groups. In the 1996 census, 13 million people were born in Australia and almost four million in other countries (ABS, 1996). Sensitivity to cultural issues in interface design is also essential.

User-centred design is described as a philosophy and an interactive design method that places the user at the centre of the design process. In websites it focuses on useability (Dey, 2002). The cultural diversity and accessibility issues for the Australian population discussed earlier, coupled with the diversity and complexity of the health sector, provides a challenging environment for interface designers. It also makes the development of a 'one-size fits all' interface strategy undesirable as providers' needs are quite different from that of consumers.

However, the design of common health provider interfaces that fit with work practices is essential as non-standard interfaces may lead to errors and increase the workload. The transience of staff also makes the standardising of interfaces crucial because in one week providers may not work twice in the same institution, unit or practice.

Different devices have different design issues that need consideration, for example, a computer, website or hand-held point-of-care device will all have fundamentally different requirements. Consider for a moment the issues of transferability of an interface developed for use on a large plasma screen to a personal digital assistant (PDA).

One of the basic principles in designing an interface is to understand the end user's mental construction of various elements and idioms. Cultural differences can be quite significant, for example, for light switches in Australia down is on; in America down is off. In Australia the colour red generally means danger, but this is not universally the case. How users make sense of what they see is important because often the user has a mental model of an image that is presented to them, and how they determine what that image represents depends greatly on their real life experiences. 'Users tend to form mental models that are simpler than reality which leads a user to a better understanding of what is being represented' (Cooper & Reimann, 2003, p.23). For example, a user may believe that email arrives as it is sent – as an entire message; they do not necessarily envisage that it is broken down and reassembled during transmission.

How users interact with the Internet gives important insights into how interfaces and ergonomic design can support their activities. A survey of online reading habits found that health professionals preferred to access documents using online databases, many health professionals also preferred either to read the entire full-text journal online or print it to read later (de Groote & Dorsch, 2003). Rho and Gedeon (2000) surveyed university researchers and research students, reporting that 96 per cent of their participants located articles using the web. The majority skimmed part of the journal articles online and then printed it for reading; only three per cent reported reading an entire article online.

Torre et al. (2003) found that among physicians the two main barriers to reading electronic publications were the inability to read them anywhere and a preference for print. Shaikh (2004) and De Groote and Dorsch's (2003) research agree with this and reports the following online behaviour:

- The *size of documents counts*, short documents (1–5 pages) were read online while long documents were printed.
- The *purpose* of the document was important. Research presentations or documents supporting a point were printed; entertainment material was read online.
- *Ease of navigation* was a major factor in determining whether or not to read online. Users more frequently printed a document with difficult navigating or if navigation back to it was challenging.
- *Convenience* was a major factor in determining to read online. Locating online documents was considered more time efficient than a trip to the library or bookstore, as was the ability to read them anytime.
- If the *quality of the document* was poor a printed version was sought because of the better quality of graphics, the ability to highlight the article, retention of original formatting, and tables were more legible.
- Respondents preferred to read *complex documents* or those needed for later reference on paper. The ability to highlight and make comments on the paper was also a positive.
- *Portability* of printed material was seen as a benefit.

Community sensitivity

There are already culturally sensitive developments that provide alternative health information to minority groups and many government organisations also provide interpreter services. The design of appropriate interfaces and use of ergonomically sound practices is essential for universal access to electronic sources and must be considered as new health models are embraced. We must accommodate a multicultural society that is complex and diverse, that has an increasingly ageing population, minority groups, groups for whom English is a second language, and non-English speaking people.

Interest box

The Health*Connect* program development team in the Northern Territory produced two CD ROMs that target the Aboriginal and Torres Strait Islander communities. These are written in keeping with traditional 'story telling' methods of education used in those communities. It used a frill-necked lizard in CD1 and a 'wise' kangaroo in CD2 to attract attention and reinforce the message.

Basic design principles

The first basic design principle is that of KIS (Keep It Simple) with a focus on navigation, layout, and colour. Appropriate language, the use of fonts, font sizes and an understanding of the user's understanding and construction of various interface elements are also crucial for an ergonomically safe and error-free interface.

Navigation

Hornbæk and Frøkjær (2003) report that if navigation is difficult, users turn to the tangibility of paper documents. To avoid this, the use of elements such as meaningful mnemonics, icons, and abbreviations can be used with good effect. Consistency and predictability are essential in interface design and particularly in health, because inconsistent provider interfaces can cause catastrophic incidents.

Cooper and Reimann (2003) also see the use of words, language, graphics, icons, commands and actions that always have the same effect in equivalent situations as simplifying navigation and making use consistent and predictable. This issue is of paramount importance because, if improperly designed, navigation can actually become an obstacle to useability and increases the potential for user error. Also important are the navigation design requirements for different devices because of screen size and resolution issues (Cooper & Reimann, 2003).

Error reduction

The use of simple, user-friendly language and presentation of relevant information is important in reducing errors and giving users a sense of control, as is the provision of online, context-driven and accessible help. Across the system consistent syntax is required for consistent input and readability. Legibility is also an issue and although Bernard et al. (2003) found no significant differences in reading efficiency between font types at any size, they did find significant differences in reading time.

Interest box

Generally, Times and Arial are read faster than Courier, Schoolbook, and Georgia. Fonts at the 12-point size are read faster than fonts at the 10-point size and Arial, Courier, and Georgia are perceived as the most legible. Overall, Verdana is the most preferred font, while Times is the least preferred. Text is also more difficult to read when it is in UPPERCASE, and when it blinks or moves.

(Bernard et al., 2003, p.82)

The use of symbols for navigation is also important because they enable quick access and enhance useability. Incorrect symbols may be thought offensive or be misunderstood.

Information box

All users worldwide have an accurate understanding of some symbols. For example, ♿ is the international sign for disability. However, a red cross can refer to the Red Cross organisation, first aid or a financial calculation tool. This symbol without any textual information may be confusing.

Shortcuts that provide more experienced users with quicker ways to negotiate devices deserve consideration to reduce frustration levels; these could include auto completion of commands, function keys and skipping instructions. Integrating ways to keep users informed by providing useful feedback also reduces frustration and encourages effective and efficient use; this might include sound, highlighting, animation and any combination of these (Chaparro, Shaikh & Baker, 2005). The hourglass is a good example here, but waiting as the hourglass fills makes one wonder if something is about to happen or has the device hung-up? Therefore, feedback should be prompt and as specific as possible, but not irritating and overdone by using intrusive, harsh tones and pop-ups, or constantly blinking or spinning text.

Because of concerns over confidentiality and privacy of health information, login processes are a challenge. They should be user-friendly to avoid the sharing of passwords and other unsatisfactory processes, but at the same time secure. Just as essential are clearly identified completions and exits to encourage healthcare workers to log off before moving away from the machine. The user should have easy way out wherever possible and should not find the logout process confusing.

Layout

In terms of layout, the presentation of text, images, articles, headers, and so on are complementary to navigation. Bernard & Larsen (2001) found no significant differences between the layout conditions in terms of search accuracy, time or efficiency, although significant subjective differences were reported favouring a fluid layout – where contents of a web page fill the window. Interestingly, reading speed and comprehension were unaffected by layout, however the enhanced layout (using optimal white space with headers, indentation, and figure placement) was less fatiguing to read (Chaparro et al., 2005).

Layouts should be designed to reduce the cognitive burden associated with spatial visualisation and visual-motor coordination. Designers should focus their efforts on creating interfaces that appropriately group information by function and reduce overall information density to less than 50 per cent of the screen area (Bernard, Hamblin & Scofield, 2002).

Colour

Laurer and Pentak (2002) reveal two design principles that influence harmony–balance and colour, because when something is not harmonious, it becomes either boring or chaotic. They also found that balance is important in appeal because it provides users with a psychological sense of equilibrium. Nonetheless, Brady and Phillips (2003) report that user satisfaction is related more to successful navigation than aesthetic appearance although aesthetically pleasing sites were ranked the easiest to use.

The use of colour presents a number of issues relating to the development of graphics and text and how the primary and combinations of specific colours have a negative impact on a user's ability to interpret what is displayed. A plain background with either white on black ('positive text') has been reported as the easiest to read, while negative text, again on a plain background, rated second (Brady, 2003). Consistency of colour is also necessary and has a particular relevance in areas such as alerts: Are they always red or some other colour?

Consumer specific issues

Consumers are potentially the entire population and include those people who are disabled, visually impaired and so on. There are many devices that enable greater disabled access such as specially designed keyboards, 'mouseless' input and so on. Visually impaired users find that the online environment provides benefits not found with printed information (Nielsen, 2000 p.98). However, the choice of the right colour combination for graphics, font type and size are important considerations, particularly for the colour blind, and must be considered in the design if websites are to be useable and effective for these groups (Lynch & Horton, 2001).

There are also specific abilities and performance attributes that need to be addressed for the diverse health consumer group. For example, a fundamental guideline for developing reading materials for our ageing population is to provide enlarged and highly contrasted text. Older users are also slower (Czaja & Sharit, 1998), and on a web site investigate fewer pages (Liao et al., 2000). However, they are more patient and less likely to leave a website when experiencing long delay times (Hart, 2004) and spend more time selecting targets for tasks (Chaparro et al., 1999). A comprehensive set of guidelines to improve accessibility to Internet sites have been developed internationally and, in 2002, a checklist consisting of twenty-five empirically based guidelines for websites targeting users sixty and over was published (National Institute on Aging, 2002).

The focus on simplicity in designing websites cannot be overstated and makes incredible difference to useability. For example, 'a very simple technique such as inserting a white space can assist users in understanding the grouping of information' (Nielsen, 2000, p.18). Clean crisp websites and computer interfaces are much more useable than masses of cluttered images, flashing text, and popup screens.

All of these ergonomic and interface issues must be considered in the initial design of digital devices because they will have a major impact on the safety, useability and appeal to practitioners and consumers.

Conclusion

It is important to remember in designing an interface that accessibility means acknowledging the diversity of users, including the cultural, social and economic differences. In healthcare, the development of specific interfaces for the various groups is necessary and care must be taken not to exclude those who need accessibility the most. The concept of user-centered design expands the principle of knowing the user, and focuses on interactivity in the development stages of software application design. In Australia, the composition of the population is diverse and complex, as are the solutions in providing uniform, ergonomically safe, secure and efficient online health interfaces suitable for health workers and consumers.

Review questions

1. What are four issues involved in considering the human technology interface? Why are these important?
2. How is the layout affected by the size of a device display?
3. Why is it necessary for healthcare providers to have standard interfaces?

Exercise

*   Ease of use is directly related to the way that the user interfaces with the computer. Discuss this statement taking into account the various users and age groups in the health sector.

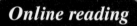

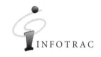
INFOTRAC

INFOTRAC® COLLEGE EDITION

For additional readings and review on ergonomics and the human technology interface, explore **InfoTrac® College Edition**, your online library. Go to: **www.infotrac-college.com** and search for any of the InfoTrac key terms listed below:

➤ Ergonomics
➤ Interface
➤ User centered design
➤ Navigation

References

Australian Bureau of Statistics (1996). *Australian social trends*. Retrieved 23 February, 2005, from http://www.abs.gov.au/Ausstats/.

Australian Bureau of Statistics (2001). *Australian national health survey*. Retrieved 28 February, 2005, from http://www.abs.gov.au/Ausstats/.

Australian Bureau of Statistics (2003). *Australian health trends*. Retrieved 24 February, 2005, from http://www.abs.gov.au/Ausstats/.

Australian Bureau of Statistics (2005). *Australian social trends*. Retrieved 18 February, 2005, from http://www.abs.gov.au/Ausstats/.

Badre, A. (2002). *Shaping web usability: Interaction design in context*, Addison-Wesley, Boston.

Bernard, M., Hamblin, C. & Scofield, B. (2002). Determining cognitive predictors of user performance within complex user interfaces, *Usability News*, 4(2), 1–24.

Bernard, M., & Larsen, L. (2001). What is the best layout for multiple-column web pages? *Usability News*, 3(2), 1–26.

Bernard, M., Lida, B., Riley, S., Hackler, T. & Janzen, K. (2003). A comparison of popular online fonts: which size and type is best?, *Usability News*, 5(2), 1–32.

Berners-Lee, T. (n.d.). *Web accessibility initiative*. Retrieved 25 February, 2005, from http://www.w3.org/WAI/.

Brady, L., & Phillips, C. (2003). Aesthetics and usability: a look at colour and balance, *Usability News*, 5(1), 1–28.

Chaparro, A., Bohan, M., Fernandez, J., Choi, S. & Kattel, B. (1999). The impact of age on computer input device use: psychophysical and physiological measures, *International Journal of Industrial Ergonomics*, 24, 503–13.

Chaparro, B., Shaikh, D. & Baker, R. (2005). Reading online text with a poor layout: is performance worse?, *Usability News*, 7(1), 1–32.

Cooper, A. & Reimann, R. (2003). *About Face 2.0: The essentials of interaction design*, Wiley Publishing Inc., Indianapolis, IN.

Czaja, S. & Sharit, J. (1998). Age differences in attitudes toward computers, *Journal of Gerontology*, 53B(5), 329–40.

de Groote, S. & Dorsch, J. (2003). Measuring use patterns of online journals and databases, *Journal of the Medical Library Association*, 91, 231–40.

Dey, A. (2002). *Empowering users through user-centred web design*. Retrieved 13 February, 2005, from http://www.its.monash.edu.au/.

Hart, T. (2004). Evaluation of Websites for Older Adults: How 'Senior-Friendly' Are They?, *Usability News*, 6(1), 1–28.

Hornbæk, K. & Frøkjær, E. (2003). Reading patterns and usability in visualizations of electronic documents, *ACM Transactions on Computer-Human Interaction*, 10(2), 119–49.

International Ergonomics Association (IEA) (2001). *The discipline of ergonomics*. Retrieved 21 March, 2005, from http://www.iea.cc/ergonomics/.

Lauer, D. & Pentak, S. (2002). *Design basics*. Wadsworth, Sydney.

Liao, C., Groff, L., Chaparro, A., Chaparro, B. & Stumpfhauser, L. (2000). *A comparison of web site usage between young adults and the elderly*. Paper presented at the IEA 2000/HGES 2000 Congress, San Diego, CA.

Lynch, P. & Horton, S. (2001). *Web style guide*, Yale University Press, New Haven, CT.

National Institute on Aging (2002). *Older adults and information technology: A compendium of scientific research and web site accessibility guidelines*, U.S. Government Printing Office, Washington, DC.

Nielsen, J. (2000). Designing web usability: the practice of simplicity, New Riders Publishing, Indianapolis, IN.

Rho, Y. & Gedeon, T.D. (2000). Reading patterns and formats of academic articles on the web, *SIGCHI Bulletin*, 32(1), 67–71.

Shaikh, D. (2004). Paper or pixels: what are people reading online?, *Usability News*, 6(2), 1–24.

Torre, D., Wright, S., Wilson, R., Diener-West, M. & Bass, E. (2003). Family physicians' interests in special features of electronic publications, *Journal of the Medical Library Association*, 91, 337–40.

24

Issues of ethics and law

Moya Conrick and Christopher Newell

> 'In a few minutes a computer can make a mistake so great that it would have taken many men many months to equal it.'
>
> Anonymous

Outline

As the healthcare system automates it has become apparent that many practitioners and consumers are significantly concerned about the introduction of electronic health records. This is directly related to ethical and legal considerations such as data security, privacy and confidentiality. Although some of the issues are dealt with by legalisation, this is not keeping pace with the current debate and technological change, and does not always adequately address deeper ethical issues. This chapter does not set out to recite law, as there are many publications that do this. Instead it looks at aspects of the ethical debate and deals with the salient issues of law contained in this debate.

Introduction

Whether or not we think about it consciously, we constantly make ethical decisions, as individuals, organisations, professionals and even countries. The decisions regarding the provision of electronic databases and how they are constructed and used may be seen as raising important ethical issues within the health system in terms of the age-old question: 'How are we to live?' We often look to law to provide the parameters for living the day-to-day realities associated with such broader philosophical questions.

For example, stopping at traffic lights may be seen as more than just a pragmatic desire to avoid a fine; it could be construed as being based upon consideration and respect for human life. It may also be the recognition of the interconnectedness of all of us in society. Often we refer to the broad concepts governing our behaviour as principles or even virtues. Law has a fundamental practical role of assisting us to live as part of a society rather than as autonomous disconnected individuals.

Whatever our terminology, when we discuss law and ethics we are talking about relationships: how we are treated in those relationships, and how we should treat others. Often we can see that our conduct can vary from the ideals that we uphold and for that reason is pertinent to pause here to consider briefly the principles of bioethics.

Bioethics

Bioethics (*bios* meaning life) involves the application of general normative ethical theories, principles and rules to medical practice, the allocation of health care resources and research. Within the ethical literature there are fundamental and derived principles that are particularly important:

Autonomy. This is derived from the Greek *autos* (self) and *nomos* (rule). It holds that a person has a right to non-interference, to make decisions for him or herself and to be self-determining. A very important way of giving autonomy is to ensure informed and valid consent. This involves giving adequate information that is understood, that the consent is free and voluntary, and that the person has the competence required. This is obviously a problem with regard to children and those of perceived lessened capacity.

Confidentiality. The principal rule of confidentiality is considered crucial in all health care and moral matters. Interpretations differ as to how much confidentiality should be observed but, for those who regard rules as important, absolute confidentiality of information imparted in a privileged way to a healthcare practitioner is fundamentally important, although exceptions do exist.

Non-maleficence. This is *associated* with the maxim *primum non nocere*, which means 'above all do no harm'. The duty of care owed to the principle of non-maleficence includes not only actual harm, but also the risk of harm. Its violation may be in terms of commission as well as omission.

Beneficence. This may be defined as active altruism or conduct aimed towards the good and well being of others. It is intimately related to the notion of above all doing no harm. One can see this as both a responsibility to patient and society. However, none of us have the time to do everything possible for any one patient and we also have to consider the allocation of resources.

Justice. There are several different ways of talking about justice:
- it generally refers to defacto standards and expectations held by society
- it is a fair or even distribution of power and jurisdiction (Locke, 1963)
- it can be comparative, for example, treatment for one person may only be assessed by weighing up the competing claims for treatment of others in society (Hume, 1969)
- it can be distributive, which strives both for an average or common good, but is also designed to ensure that this does not occur at the expense of the rights of the least advantaged (Rawles, 1999).

When we come to consider ehealth there are some very real tensions. For example, consumers can pragmatically see the real benefits associated with timely access to health records, especially in emergency situations or with unknown providers. There are some significant ethical benefits, but there are also recognisable costs. For example, personal information, which has deep significance to the consumer, may be more available or available in a way that has previously not occurred. The linkage of electronic health records (EHR) and the wider availability of these raises a familiar raft of ethical and legal issues associated with healthcare. The fundamental new issues relate to the power – negative and positive – that such technology potentially has to impact upon people's lives. One of the most contentious issues over the years has been that of ownership of health records and this is set to continue with EHRs.

Who owns the record?

The issue of who owns the record has long been contentious. Health*Connect,* the national summary electronic health record as distinct from the provider's medical records, brings with it some unique challenges.

Clayton Utz (2005, p.8) argues that 'Health*Connect* will not alter the legal ownership of the provider's physical files (paper or computer-based) or the provider's copyright in their records in those files'. They hold that in the absence of written agreement to the contrary, copyright is owned by providers who create and upload to the electronic system. Similarly, consumers have copyright over their inputs directly into databases. However, where the copyright is owned by one person and updated by another a complex mix of copyright ownership structures is created.

Exploring legal protection

In Australia, common law provides for the person who suffers damage because of a breach of confidence by another. This involves the use or disclosure of information, which is not publicly known, and which has been entrusted to a person in circumstances that impose an obligation not to use or disclose that information. It can only be released with authority of the person it has been (directly or indirectly) obtained from.

The legal duty of confidence may be based on the professional relationship between clinicians and the patient. Clinicians have a duty to maintain confidentiality, between themselves, their patient, and the patient's record. Information must be shared only with those within the system who need to know.

Medical practitioners' ethical obligations extend back to the Hippocratic tradition, with a continuing emphasis on the maxim that any information given to a physician must remain confidential. The Australian Medical Association (AMA) would like to see this practice extended to public policy regarding EHRs (McSherry, 2004). However, codes of professional ethics are not legally binding although infringement can lead to professional discipline (Tranberg, Rous & Rashbass, 2003; Commonwealth of Australia, 2003).

The implementation of electronic birth-to-death patient records has the potential to present many problems such as unauthorised access, loss of data and so on. However, it is argued by supporters that the advent of computerised patient records will not create security situations any worse than the present system.

Security

In many institutions, the current system consists of a centralised holding storeroom, accessed through the medical records staff during office hours and other designated staff out of hours. While the physical access to paper files is most often restricted by location, computerised records seem more accessible because of the proximity of the terminal to many users and, without doubt, the record is more legible than freehand writing. But, in fact, access to the computer record is more restricted and it is held in a central database which in many cases is also located off the hospital campus.

The involvement of many specialty areas and health personnel with a single patient has always had inherent problems of disclosure as well as lost and misplaced files. However, the community seems much less forgiving of computer error than human error and perhaps this is justified. We have been assured that technology advances practice and patient care, that errors should be reduced, and that the systems are more secure. This must be so as there seems little point in replacing one questionable system with another infinitely more expensive one that cannot be guaranteed. If we are to invest time, money and effort in automation, then surely it must be superior to the system it replaces in all respects.

It is vital that an information system used to collect patient data must keep faith with the consumer by securing data and that systems design must incorporate safeguards to protect patient records. The three major issues in relation to healthcare information are security, confidentiality and integrity. The Information Privacy Principles (see Table 24.1) used in healthcare agencies address these issues and provide a sound basis for the collection, handling and use of personal information in healthcare, although they are general and non-specific.

In a hospital or practitioner's surgery the design of databases may not be problematic. It is when data are shared outside that problems arise. For example, in the case of HealthConnect, Clayton Utz (2005) found that the design will impact upon liability, depending on whether it is just a passive database, provides alert summaries (such as known allergies), or whether it pushes information, warnings or follow-up by reminders by email, for instance. The more that the design undertakes greater responsibility for users, the more these systems move beyond just a passive database, the greater the potential for liability.

Data quality

Most organisations that hold personal information may be seen to be subject to privacy rules and/or legislation, meaning that the uploading of data will involve the taking of reasonable steps to ensure accuracy, currency, quality and completeness. Likewise, during the storage of such information, database and systems operators must take reasonable steps to maintain the integrity of data and prevent its corruption or deletion by accident or unauthorised access/amendment (Clayton Utz, 2005).

Access rights

One of the key issues introduced by systems such as HealthConnect is that a consumer's health record is not made available within one particular practice or even hospital, but to all providers across the country. Hence, the implicit consent associated with access to paper-based systems do not apply with HealthConnect. Such distributed systems have a need to allocate access rights to database records to different users according to different needs. This will include the need to directly authenticise the identity of an individual interacting with the database. Clayton Utz (2005, p.18) argues that:

> it is considered essential for consumer confidence and provider confidence in the integrity of the database and to comply with privacy laws that the *HealthConnect* database keep a robust audit trail of each upload of data, amendment of data, access to and download of a data view from the database.

Securing physical access

Securing computers also has its challenges. Data stored on one personal computer is user-specific and can be secured by the user. If the machine is used by more than one operator, the risks of security breaches increase. If the computer is linked to a system with multiple users, the risks to data integrity increase exponentially. Of course, the security of data becomes even more tenuous when telecommunications link the systems.

Security levels must ensure they are as inaccessible to computer hackers and unauthorised people as possible. Considerable attention has been given to securing electronic data with access restricted by passwords and elaborate encryption systems. Security of systems produces a vexing problem: the more secure the data, the more complex is the system needed to gain access. At the same time the user demands a 'friendly' system, that is, a system that is easy to access and use.

Hospital-based systems are usually maintained by a dedicated department and have security measures to restrict physical access and generally use multiple passwords. These factors combine to make the information more secure than in traditional written notes. However, security can never remain invulnerable as a knowledgeable and determined individual can breach any system whether it is computerised or paper-based.

Perhaps one way for the healthcare sector to circumvent many of the ethical and storage issues related to the patient records is for responsibility for the record to be given to the patient. An innovation has been the use of a smart card to hold the patient record, which is 'owned' and possessed by the patient.

Digital signatures

Another result of automation, which has many security implications, is the use of the electronic signature. The clinician's logon is a legal signature just as much as the signature at the bottom of a handwritten document. What if your colleague has forgotten their password – can they use yours, just this once? What are the implications? In the eyes of the law you are responsible for any data entered in your name. Because there is no handwriting to verify otherwise, whatever is written in the electronic record belongs to the person who has logged on to the system – you, if your password is used.

The legality of electronic signatures has still to be addressed. There is legislation that provides for paper-based or manually-signed prescriptions, however, in the *Electronic Transactions Act* of the Australian Government and each state and territory it is apparent that not all the issues are adequately dealt with. Accordingly, Clayton Utz (2005) recommends the convening of a national working party of regulatory authorities to amend relevant legislation and regulation to allow for electronic prescriptions and dispensing on electronic prescription, including the recording of electronic prescriptions. How this fits with digital signatures on other documents is not clear.

Point-of-care devices

Many security, privacy and confidentiality issues are raised by the use of point-of-care devices. If the healthcare worker is called away and leaves the terminal, can the patient's visitors gain access in the minutes before the computer shuts down? What are the implications of this, and is it worse than patient details and observations hanging from the end of the bed or charts filed in an open, unattended office?

In the community, the use of portable terminals and modems is also rapidly expanding. The most flexible and transportable technology would be a palmtop or notebook computer with pen-based data entry. However, the factors that make this technology appealing also add to the security risks. The small, portable notebook or palmtop can be easily stolen from the car or as happens – the car stolen from the health visitor!

Participation in local and national EHR

As individuals in society we often want the benefits of electronic health initiatives, but we will increasingly look to legislation and professional ethics to deliver the necessary safeguards. It is also apparent that a major ethical and legal consideration with regard to these recent developments is the area of consent – or, in its more active conceptualisation, informed decision-making. Specifically, should we ensure informed consent by all players or are the benefits associated with electronic health records so great, as has been argued by some commentators, that consent becomes a luxury that cannot be afforded, given problems in ensuring take up?

All patients who enter hospitals have either a paper or EHR and most private practioners operate under the same system. However, Health*Connect* (2003a, p.2) stresses that individuals must freely agree to participate in the network in the first instance and on a continuing basis after that. They also say that:

- a person could not be penalised or discriminated against for not participating in the system
- consumers would have access to their own information and be able to control who can see their information
- stringent security measures would be in place wherever health information was collected, stored or exchanged in the network
- consumers would know what information is being collected about them, the purposes for which it would be used, and who had accessed the information
- information collected and stored on the network could be used only for agreed purposes and would be restricted to the health sector
- any providers or health services participating in the network would be bound by legislation
- strong penalties would be in place to both deter and punish misuse of information on the network
- complaints and redress mechanisms would be in place to allow consumers or providers to take action in the unlikely event there were a breach of privacy or a breakdown in security.

Health*Connect* is adamant that the model should be opt-in, although NSW are trialing an opt-out model after considering cost implications. Debate still continues with clinicians and others pointing to the inadequacies of fragmented records. Opt-in, however, seems little different from the current system where consumers may deliberately or inadvertently withhold information. Yet, there is no doubt that systems such as Health*Connect* have the potential to increase the level of information available to health providers. Because of this debate, the major issues of 'Opt-in' or 'Opt-out' will be discussed further here.

For some, the arguments revolve around practicalities of how one signs up for an opt regime. Yet, it is apparent that many of the socio-economic inequities present in society raise factors in terms of whether or not people believe that they have adequate knowledge and know that they could opt-out of any arrangement. (For an overview of many ethical issues in primary healthcare see Newell & Nisselle, 2005.)

A major consideration is what to do about some of the most vulnerable in the healthcare system: for example, those people who cannot adequately consent for themselves because of intellectual or mental impairment, or people who may have episodic conditions impacting upon their ability to make decisions at times. Parents need to make decisions for their children that have implications on their future in terms of availability of medical records some years down the track. While to some such considerations seem overly precious, it is worth remembering that sensitivities expressed by groupings such as people with disabilities have revolved around the historical and current lack of making life choices and the way in which it is difficult to have privacy.

Another issue in the opt-in or opt-out debate is the ability to collect huge amounts of data about a person and what happens to this when they opt out. Under the current proposal, Health*Connect* event summaries are accessible while a person consents to participating in Health*Connect*. If they choose to opt-out, records are not removed from the system; they are no longer accessible by users. If the person opts-in again, the user regains access. If a person continues in the system, Health*Connect* will establish a life-long summary health record. This has implications for the retention and destruction of Health*Connect* data that needs to be resolved (Commonwealth of Australia, 2005).

Liability and indemnity

Legal liability is part of any professional activity or business these days. Rather than creating a new type of legal liability, systems such as Health*Connect* may affect the risk of a liability being incurred. Sometimes the operation of excellent electronic databases will actually reduce legal risk for providers such as when it involves the provision of more accurate and timely patient history. Likewise, some of the other benefits include better coordination of care, addressing drug interactions, the provision of a comprehensive lifetime record, and avoiding unnecessary triplication of tests. It should be remembered that legal responsibility is shared among stakeholders and can be seen to be situation-specific.

However, there are also other issues, such as the important difference between reliance on a Health*Connect* summary and a General Practitioner relying on a full specialist report. The General Practitioner might rely on the summary with regard to a treatment or condition but construe it quite differently from what the author of the event summary was meaning.

Clayton Utz (2005, p.23) elucidates health providers' duties in writing health summaries for Health*Connect* and stresses the importance of issues like:

- creating an inadequate event summary or failing to create an event summary
- failing to properly review the Health*Connect* record
- failing to bring something in the Health*Connect* record to a patient's attention and ask questions about it; or the unreasonable reliance by health provider on the Health*Connect* record in preference to information that is reasonably available or could be reasonably obtained by making appropriate enquiries of the patient or reviewing other relevant material that might cause injury to a patient.

Privacy

Australia's approach to the privacy of health information is affected by the disparate nature of the health sector. Separate legislation applies in the states, territories and nationally as well as between public and private sectors. There are established, consistent privacy principles across each legislative area that not only apply to health but to other areas of information collection. These principles are informing the development of privacy and access control principles in information systems.

Threats to privacy have existed with manual, paper-based records, just as they do with computerised records. The principles of trust and information protection do not change in an electronic environment. Additional privacy considerations are required because of the capacity to share information with a wider range of organisations more easily and quickly in a format that is easier to comprehend and use effectively (National Electronic Decision Support Taskforce, 2002).

The *Privacy Amendment (Private Sector) Act 2000* amendments to the Commonwealth's *Privacy Act (1988)* deals with the collection, use and disclosure, nature and security of personal information. The eleven Information Privacy Principles in this Act protect personal information and confer rights in the way Commonwealth and ACT government agencies handle personal information, while the ten National Privacy Principles in the Act (see Table 24.1) protect personal information and specify the way private sector organisations, including some small businesses and all private health service providers, must handle the information. It is also worth referring to the Federal Privacy Commissioner's website regarding this topic.[1]

The National Privacy Principles provide base-line privacy standards that some private sector organisations need to comply with in relation to personal information they hold. All health service providers in the private sector need to comply with these principles. Because of their central role, it is worth briefly considering those National Privacy Principles (NPP) not discussed earlier. Grain (Chapter 25) has also contributed to this discussion.

Table 24.1: The privacy principles

Principle	Information privacy principles*	National privacy principles**
1	Manner and purpose of collection of personal information	Collection
2	Solicitation of personal information from individual concerned	Use and disclosure
3	Solicitation of personal information generally	Data quality
4	Storage and security of personal information	Data security
5	Information relating to records kept by record-keeper	Openness
6	Access to records containing personal information	Access and correction
7	Alteration of records containing personal information	Identifiers
8	Record-keeper to check accuracy etc of personal information before use	Anonymity
9	Personal information to be used only for relevant purposes	Transborder data flows
10	Limits on use of personal information	Sensitive information
11	Limits on disclosure of personal information	

* Information Privacy Principles under the *Privacy Act 1988*.

** Summarised from the *Privacy Amendment (Private Sector) Act 2000*

National privacy principles

Principle 1: Information Collection – describes what an organisation should do when collecting personal information. In essence, information collected must be necessary, fair and lawful. The guidelines apply to all information except where the information would 'pose a serious threat to the life or health of any individual' (Privacy Commissioner, 1994).

Principle 2: Use and Disclosure – this requires that organisations not disclose personal information for purposes other than the reason for which that information was collected, and that a record is kept of any information that is *disclosed*. A health service may disclose information about an individual if the individual is unable to provide consent, provided that the disclosure is not contrary to a wish expressed by the individual or her or his carer.

The concept of 'collect once, use many times' applied to health information may pose difficulties to compliance with this principle. The electronic environment significantly *increases* the potential to use health information for many purposes other than those clear to the patient at the time of collection. However, Mulligan (2001) reports that almost 10 per cent of South Australians surveyed about EHRs raised the issue of lack of confidence in the appropriate storage and dissemination of personal information by healthcare providers.

A national survey undertaken by the Privacy Commissioner had similar results with 84 per cent of Australians trusting the health system 'to keep and use information in a responsible way' (Privacy Commissioner, 2001, cited in Mulligan & Braunack-Mayer, 2004, p.50). It would appear that Australians are not as sceptical as Americans where 54 per cent of consumers worried about privacy and felt threatened by EHRs (Smith, 2000).

Principle 3: Data Quality – this requires that an 'organization must take reasonable steps to make sure that the personal information it collects, uses and discloses is accurate, complete and up-to-date' (Privacy Commissioner, 1994).

Principle 4: Data Security – This principle sets the standards that organisations must meet for the protection of health information, including protection from misuse, loss and unauthorised access, modification or disclosure.

McDonagh (2002) feels that the more data that are collected, the greater are the number of organisations both public and private that will seek access to personal information. However, trading of information is of concern and reports of General Practitioners on-selling patient information to drug companies seems to be an unfortunate occurrence (National Nine News, 2005). However, the precedent has been set in America where marketing firms have obtained patient information to send patients reminder calls to repurchase drugs (Eisenberg, 2001) or to send them samples.

The Australian Privacy Commissioner revealed that the de-identified information traded by General Practitioners was being used within the bounds of privacy law while the AMA referred the issue to their ethics committee (National Nine News, 2005). The AMA is sceptical about the ability of the *Privacy Act 2001* to protect patient records from being on-sold (Bomba, Svardsudd & Kristiansson, 2004). Although audit trails can be put into place whereby all access to an individual's EHR can be tracked. When layered with patient identification and password, encryption, and authentication with digital certificates, security can be set at a very high level (Englebardt & Nelson, 2002).

Principle 5: Openness – this requires organisations to be open about how they handle personal information and to have established, documented policies on the management of health information (Privacy Commissioner, 2002). The advantages of active and open communication are outlined in the Australian Standard on open communication in public and private hospitals (Australian Council for Safety and Quality in Health Care, 2003).

Principle 6: Access and Correction – this ensures that clients have the right to access their personal information to correct inaccurate, incomplete or out-of-date entries (Privacy Commissioner, 2002).

Principle 7: Identifiers – this requires that Commonwealth Government identifiers (for example, Medicare or the Veterans Affairs number) can only be used for the purposes for which they were issued (Privacy Commissioner, 2002). Legislative amendment may change this principle, and the Australian Government now has this firmly on the agenda. At the same time McDonagh (2002) warns of the development of a National Identifier by default with the advent of electronic records, and the problems of function creep.

Principle 8: Anonymity – when practical, this allows for people to receive healthcare without identifying themselves. In Australia this is seen as vital in the provision of quality healthcare and the protection of the individual and the community. However, it becomes difficult with an automated system where identification is necessary (Privacy Commissioner, 2002).

Principle 9: Transborder Data Flows – this outlines guidelines to cover transfer of health information outside Australia (Privacy Commissioner, 2002). In an electronic health record environment this principle is especially important because any data transfer of personal information must be covered by contractual or legally binding rules. These ensure that where the transfer of information is for the benefit of the individual it is handled in a manner consistent with the national privacy principles.

Principle 10: Sensitive Information – this requires that certain information be considered especially sensitive and includes all health information. This principle requires health organisations to ensure that clinicians handling and collecting health information understand:

- the purpose for which they are collecting personal information
- how they are going to use it
- who they are going to give it to
- how consumers can access and correct the information held about them.

(Privacy Commissioner, 2002)

It should be noted that consumer reaction to the privacy issues listed above are discussed by Grain (Chapter 25).

Conclusion

In many respects the convergence of healthcare with information technology raises significant ethical and legal issues associated with affirming and managing relationships that are an integral part of healthcare. A vital component of that is dealing with issues of consent, security, privacy and confidentiality. In many respects it is how well we address these issues into the future that will determine the success of these developments and their ownership by consumers and health professionals.

Review questions

1. Should the imperative associated with health mean that, regardless of the consequences, we adopt health initiatives? What safeguards are necessary in order to deliver benefits of automation?
2. How does the automation of health records impinge upon the relationships that are an everyday part of healthcare?

Exercises

- Discuss the ethical, privacy and security issues for clinicians or your clinical practice in the electronic collection and use of a person's health data.

- Critically analyse the issues involved in the 'option' models of access to Electronic Health Records.

- Critically analyse this statement.

  Although some of ethical and legal considerations such as data security, privacy and confidentiality are dealt with by legalisation, this is not keeping pace with the current debate and technological change, and does not always adequately address deeper ethical issues.

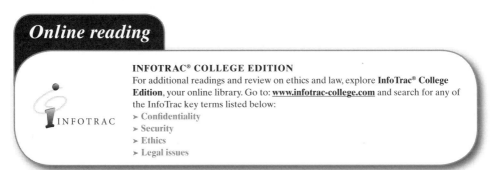

Online reading

INFOTRAC® COLLEGE EDITION
For additional readings and review on ethics and law, explore **InfoTrac® College Edition**, your online library. Go to: **www.infotrac-college.com** and search for any of the InfoTrac key terms listed below:
- Confidentiality
- Security
- Ethics
- Legal issues

References

Australian Council for Safety and Quality in Health Care (2003). *Open disclosure standard: a national standard for open communication in public and private hospitals, following an adverse event in health care,* Commonwealth of Australia, Canberra.

Bomba, D., Svardsudd, K. & Kristiansson, P. (2004). A comparison of patients' attitudes towards the use of computerised medical records and unique identifiers in Australia and Sweden, *Australian Journal of Primary Health*, 10(2), 36–41.

Clayton Utz (2005). *Legal Issues Report*. Retrieved 2 July, 2005, from http://www.healthconnect.gov.au/.

Commonwealth of Australia (2003). *National health privacy code*. Retrieved 2 March, 2003, from http://www.health.gov.au/.

Commonwealth of Australia (2005). *HealthConnect legal issues report,* Health*Connect* Project Office. Canberra.

Commonwealth of Australia (2003). National health privacy code. Retrieved 2 March, 2003, from http://www.health.gov.au/.

Eisenberg, J. (2001). Can you keep a secret? Measuring the performance of those entrusted with personal health information, *JG/M*(16), 132–4.

Englebardt, S. & Nelson, R. (2002). *Health care informatics: an interdisciplinary approach*, Mosby Inc., Sydney.

Wolff, R. (ed.) (1969). *The essential David Hume*. New American Library, New York.

Locke, J. (1963). *The works of John Locke,* Scientia Verlag (reprint, John Locke 1632–1704), Darmstadt.

McDonagh, M. (2002). E-Government in Australia: the challenge to privacy of personal information, *International Journal of Law and Information Technology*, 10(3), 327–43.

McSherry, B. (2004). Third party access to shared mental health records: ethical issues, *Psychiatry, Psychology and Law*, 11(1), 53–62.

Mulligan, E. (2001). Confidentiality in health records: evidence of current performance from a population survey in South Australia, *Medical Journal Australia* (174), 637–64.

Mulligan, E. & Braunack-Mayer, A. (2004). Why protect confidentiality in health records? A review of research evidence, *The Australian Health Review*, 28(1), 48–55.

National Electronic Decision Support Taskforce (2002). *Electronic decision support for Australia's health sector*, Department of Health and Aging, Canberra.

National Nine News (2005). GPs warned over on-sell of patient information, 25 May, Australia.

Newell, C. & Nisselle, P. (2005). *Ethical and legal issues in general practice in Australia 2004*, Department of Health and Aging, Canberra, pp.502–43.

Privacy Commissioner (1994). *Plain English guidelines to information privacy: principles 1–3*, Office of the Federal Privacy Commissioner, Sydney.

Privacy Commissioner (2002). *My privacy my choice: your new privacy rights*, Office of the Privacy Commissioner, Sydney.

Rawls, J. (1999). *A theory of justice*, Oxford University Press, Oxford.

Smith, S. (2000). Are you protecting your patient's confidentiality?, *Nursing Economics*, 18(6), 313–16, 319.

Tranberg, H., Rous, B. & Rashbass, J. (2003). Legal and ethical issues in the use of anonymous images in pathology teaching and research, *Histopathology* (42), 104–9.

25

Consumer issues in informatics

Heather Grain

'There is no reason for any individual to have a computer in their home.'

Ken Olson, President of World Future Society Convention (1977)

Outline

This is a world where people are making their own decisions about their healthcare. Often they will choose a combination of vitamins, herbal supplements, traditional western medicine, traditional eastern medicine, and other forms of healthcare. The picture of the 'paternal all knowing' health professional is changing to a provider of services who helps with healthcare choices and treatment. This chapter discusses the consumer issues in the adoption of healthcare technology.

Introduction

In ancient times people made choices about healthcare according to their preferences and beliefs; the Greek approach to healthcare originated from clinical observation of disease processes and treatment successes, and the Roman approach was based on the study of injuries occurring during battle. In medieval times, the general population might have called those practising 'medicine' witches, but, despite this, still sought them out when they needed help. During the Napoleonic wars, naval surgeons had skills not far removed from those of the barber or butcher, while the physician was seen as a 'scientific man'. Since the 1800s the community has increasingly seen medicine as a science. They respected those with the 'knowledge' of healing and medical practice developed into a revered profession, generally unchallenged by the patient who was expected to 'take their medicine' without question.

People seeking medical attention became increasingly aware of the fallibility of the health profession in the twentieth century. The unrealistic expectation that the health professional will always be able to 'solve' the problem has naturally led to disappointments. The emergence of the information age has meant that health consumers can obtain significantly more information about healthcare (verified and unverified). The availability of this information, along with the shrinking globe and greater availability of alternative treatments, mean that there is a health consumer society that is often highly informed and open to many different forms of treatments and healthcare modalities. Consider the following case study:

Case study 1:

Mary wakes up in the morning with a stiff neck and feeling as if she is getting a cold. She starts to self medicate with Echinacea for her cold and hopes that her neck will improve. She has a doctor's appointment today for follow-up after removal of an ingrown toenail last week. The doctor is happy with the progress of her nail bed, and suggests that she see a physiotherapist for treatment of her neck (which has not improved through the day). Mary decides to see her chiropractor on the way home from the doctor, rather than the physiotherapist, as she has had neck problems before and knows that she feels better after the chiropractor's treatment.

This is a common scenario and demonstrates that the position of the health consumer in healthcare has changed significantly, along with consumer expectations, provider expectations and responsibilities.

What are the human issues?

It is difficult to imagine that there is any aspect of healthcare that does not have human issues. Yet many people involved with information technology do not immediately see the relationship of computerisation and technology to healthcare. Human relationships with health information and the systems that collect, store, retrieve and present that information is an essential component for safe, quality healthcare. These systems and the information they provide support all clinical staff in the provision of healthcare and in undertaking research to improve healthcare delivery. They also support the health consumer as a partner in their healthcare.

Systems, patients and providers – the relationships

Information systems have always served a range of purposes for healthcare providers – aide-mémoire, legal record, communication tool and, increasingly, a system for knowledge management. The consumer, on the other hand, sees the information system from a very different position. This is information about them, personal, private, and important as a communication tool for those who are to advise and provide healthcare to them. Figure 25.1 illustrates the interconnectedness of the requirements at the clinician/consumer interface.

Figure 25.1: Clinician/consumer requirements of the health record and knowledge

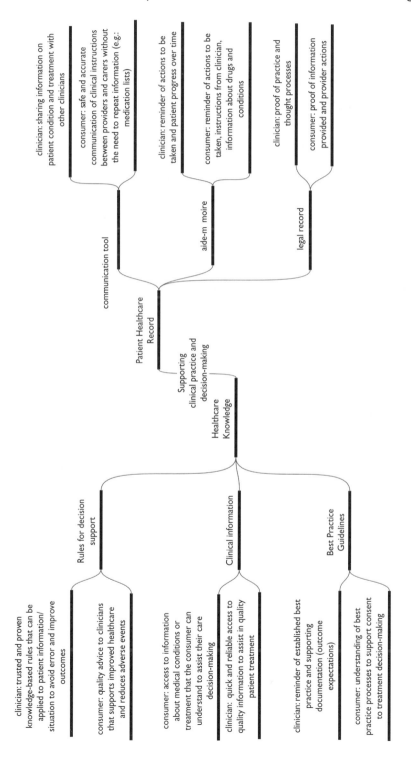

Consumers expect that information shared privately with one provider will not be automatically available to the next provider they see. However, they also expect that in today's electronic world, information will be made available across the continuum of care where appropriate. Consumers do not necessarily understand the different elements of the healthcare system and how these integrate.

Case study 2:

A patient feeling ill at home calls her GP and requests a home visit. The GP refers her directly to the hospital. After treatment in the emergency department, she is discharged home, and the district nurse and community services are organised to call. The patient is to see her GP the next day. Because this process appears to consumers to be a coordinated approach to care they are likely to expect that information about the emergency visit, and follow-up requirements will be shared and that each service provider will know exactly what is expected of them. Consumers today know that the technology can do this – and many find it odd that it has not happened.

Case study 3:

A patient attends the emergency department without consulting his GP. Last time he attended the hospital (two years ago) he was referred by his GP whose details are held in the hospital computer system. At this admission the GP is not mentioned. The patient is discharged. Some weeks later he attends his GP for a different condition and is surprised that the GP has been given details of his emergency visit to hospital. From the patient's perspective the GP was not involved in that episode of care in any way. This time the patient's expectation would not necessarily be that the information would be sent to their GP.

It is vital that healthcare professionals appreciate the consumer perspective. Consumers may or may not appreciate some of the processes that health professionals must complete. This following scenario accentuates this:

> 'Why are they writing a book about me?' was a query from an elderly patient, receiving district-nursing care. She became distrustful and eventually cancelled this service because of a perception that the nurses were recording inappropriate information about her. The situation could have been significantly improved if the nurses involved had shown the patient what they were writing and encouraged her to make entries in the record themselves – to see the record as a mutual tool.

Health practitioners should realise that patients may not be aware of all the health professionals' obligations. Practices that seem everyday and insignificant to the practitioner might be seen as reassuring, threatening, confusing or even annoying to the consumer. People may also behave quite differently from normal when confronted with illness and injury, the stresses of carers, or the sudden changes in life expectations and lifestyle.

Consumers' role in their healthcare

Consumers take many different roles in their healthcare – the 'supplicant', the 'wary' or the 'partner'. These roles are described below in a simplistic manner, but they serve to indicate some of the most common ways that health consumers interact with healthcare providers and their likely interaction with technology. The prevalence of each of these roles varies across different consumer groups.

The supplicant allows, encourages and sometimes is comforted by a paternalistic approach from their service provider whom they expect to assume all responsibility for their care. This attitude may also stem from a cultural view of the medical profession as ultimate authorities, with 'mystical' knowledge. This group rarely challenge the decisions and choices of the care provider, accepting with implicit faith the outcomes of their healthcare. Some people in this group demand solutions of their health service provider, any solution that will achieve the consumer's required health state. These patients do not actively seek information from the Internet or anywhere else. They prefer to allow their 'trusted clinician' to access and manage their health information with little input from them.

These patients are passive and unlikely to actively accept responsibility for their health state. Therefore, it is vital that healthcare providers serving people with this attitude do not abuse their faith knowingly or more commonly unknowingly and unintentionally.

The wary health consumer has usually been damaged or threatened by their experience of the health system. Most often this experience has been real and disturbing to the patient, though it may have seemed normal to the care provider at the time. It is possible for some events, which seem of little import to those busy with what they see as normal treatment and process, to cause significant distress to patients and their families. All healthcare involves communication as well as treatment and each of these activities may have less than optimal outcomes. The wary health consumer may fail to seek treatment and avoid contact with the system until there is no choice. This behaviour often results in poor health outcomes and a self-fulfilling view of the system.

These people are likely to seek treatment from many alternative sources, hoping to find a solution that they trust and find of value to them. They will turn to the Internet for information. They may refuse access to their health information in certain circumstances or fail to seek treatment if they feel threatened by the potential of computer systems to share or divulge information in a way that they consider inappropriate. This group accept responsibility for their actions, as they only trust themselves; the feeling that the system has failed them is strong and can result in a belief that the system should have been responsible for their healthcare. To expect this group to trust computer health information systems without proven safe and secure interaction is unrealistic. Health information system developments need to encourage participation from this group in a manner that will build their trust.

Partners on the other hand accept responsibility for their healthcare. They ask for guidance and treatment from healthcare professionals then willingly read the health information printed out and provided by them. They also seek information about health, disease and treatment from a wide range of sources including the Internet and chat rooms. Partners seek to understand their condition, in order to improve health outcomes.

The majority of health consumers tend to be 'partners', with a decreasing mix of 'supplicants'. However, there will always be a mix of consumer types, therefore systems and professional attitudes must accommodate this. Understanding consumer issues and needs requires an appreciation of the wide variety of different consumer perspectives.

Expectations

Health consumers have simple expectations of the health information system. These expectations may be realised in different ways according to the type of consumer, but the principles apply to them all. Consumers understand that:

- information about themselves will be treated with respect and confidentiality
- they have the right to make decisions about their healthcare (and generally should be responsible for those choices)
- the healthcare system provided by their taxes is available equally to all Australians
- healthcare will be safe and continually improving
- the introduction of change (information technology or other initiatives) will provide an improved healthcare system and interactions while preserving existing freedoms
- health information systems will support improved knowledge management, quality assurance mechanisms and best practice to improve health outcomes
- consumers are represented and their needs taken into account when system changes are being planned, designed and implemented
- consumers and/or their representative can participate in their healthcare by contributing to their own health record.

Issues of the individual

Individual health consumers, their information and care are the first issues that arise. The collection of 'de-identified' data is another issue. This information is grouped with other consumers with similar conditions, treatment or services to provide statistical information for healthcare planning and epidemiology. Health consumers are concerned that maximum benefit be gained from the health information collected and used to support improved healthcare and medical research. Nevertheless, they are also concerned that these activities be completed in a manner that totally protects their rights and privacy. To gain a greater insight into this, it is pertinent here to discuss the essence of de-identified data.

De-identified data

There is no established formula for the de-identification of health data. However, de-identification does not simply mean removing the patient's name, date of birth and address from the data. It must ensure that identifying an individual from the information provided is impossible. Consider this:

A child may have an unusual infectious disease causing her to miss school for three weeks. Publishing the fact that a seven-year-old living in a particular suburb is suffering from the unusual infectious condition would probably be sufficient to identify the individual to those at the school. On the other hand, a population of 500 children at the school may have 80 people within the given age group and 25 might be absent from the school with infectious diseases. In this case, the one student becomes one of 25 and much more difficult to identify.

The individual's information

Modern computerised health information systems have the potential to provide significant benefits to the individual. Systems that retain or improve the privacy of health information will encourage consumer participation in their healthcare. The availability of health information in a format that makes retrieval easier and more consistent offers the consumer improved continuity and consistency of care.

Consumer issues in privacy and security

Conrick and Newell (Chapter 24) have discussed the issues of privacy and security in some depth based on the National Privacy Principles (NPP). The same framework will be used here to elucidate the issues from the consumers' perspective.

Patients often regard the content of their health record as very sensitive but understand the importance of having relevant information available to support good healthcare. It is therefore important that health information remains both private and available for future retrieval. Research into consent processes for electronic health record access has been undertaken based upon consumers' expectation that 'at least the same level of confidence in their clinician's management of their confidential records' will be maintained (Primary and Coordinated Care Health Services Division, 2002).

Consumers expect that clinicians can be trusted with their health information. They also expect clinicians to use this information only for the purpose for which it was provided, and not to unilaterally transfer the information to anyone else for any other purpose. This is the consumers' response to the National Privacy Principles (NPP) briefly discussed below.

Response to National Privacy Principles

Principle 1: Information Collection – in this area consumers relate that although it may be clear to those working in the 'organisation' they do not always understand the 'fuzzier' limits of information collection.

Principle 2: Use and Disclosure – the electronic environment significantly increases the potential to use health information for many purposes other than those clear to the patient at the time of collection. This issue must be dealt with sensitively and with open communication. Health consumers expect that their information will not be linked to financial information, insurance or similar registries. Where patient consent is obtained, information may not need to be re-collected for future use, in fact it is more likely to be more accurate and less intrusive to the patient if data are obtained from existing, verified sources.

Principle 3: Data Quality – the consumer expects that relevant information will be shared, if consent to share *information* has been provided, but the giving of consent for one purpose does not imply consent to disclose unrelated information. For example, a patient with a broken leg would be unlikely to consider the provision of access to their mental health record a related disclosure of information.

This principle supports the consumer's right to contribute to their health record, including the notation of errors or misconceptions that might appear in their clinician-originated record. This is a point upon which consumers and their families/carers feel that they have the potential to significantly contribute to care and communication.

Principle 4: Data Security – health consumers look forward to the potential protection offered by an electronic healthcare system to be able to identify each individual who has looked at their record. Such systems have the potential to significantly increase trust in the systems managing information use and disclosure.

Principle 5: Openness – health consumers are entitled to know what sort of information is held about them, how it is collected, used and provided to others. This is part of the trust process, ensuring that health consumers understand what is being done to protect their information and feel that they can trust the systems – electronic or otherwise.

Principle 6: Access and Correction – while consumers look forward to actively accessing their information, they need to understand what is presented. This implies that consumer terminology, rather than terms only clinical staff would understand, are available to represent health concepts in the record viewed by the health consumer. Other issues that need to be further discussed and clarified are issues of access, authentication of identity, and how the electronic system will handle group information such as family discussion records.

Principle 7: Identifiers – the issue of identifiers used in the electronic health record is another trust-related issue requiring sensitive development and implementation to meet the privacy, trust and cost-effectiveness demands of the healthcare system.

Principle 8: Anonymity – anonymity is discussed in the previous chapter, however the issue must be debated more fully in the community because, without the ability to seek sensitive diagnostic and treatment services with anonymity, there are people who will not seek healthcare, thereby putting themselves and possibly the community at risk.

Principle 9: Transborder Data Flows – consumers expect that in an electronic health record environment any transfer of personal information will be covered by contractual or legally binding rules.

Principle 10: Sensitive Information – during the late 1990s and early 2000s computers were introduced more *broadly* into general practice in Australia. Research undertaken by the Consumer Health Forum identified concerns about the implications of computerisation in general practice. These reveal that many consider that the potential benefits of computerisation outweigh the potential risks. Despite that, some consumers were concerned that with electronic storage of health information there was a possibility that information could be disclosed and transferred without their knowledge.

This research also indicated that the simplest method to overcome concerns was for practitioners to 'explain to consumers how and why they are using the technology' (Consumer Health Forum, 2004) and to build systems that respond to consumer concerns about their information.

Access

Consumers in Australia have been involved in debate about what health information should be collected, stored and retrieved and how this should be managed. In an electronic health record the technology provides a mechanism to manage access to health information in a more controlled manner than in the paper-based record. The health consumer can control access to their record, but there are two general principles of access control to be considered. The first relates to *gaining* access and the second to *who has accessed* information.

Gaining access to health information

The ability for computer systems to manage access to health records with due regard to patient consent requires the establishment of a structure and process that is computer processable.

Early electronic health record systems took simplistic approaches with regard to accessing patient health information. A 'statement' required confirmation from the person accessing the record that they understood that their activity would be recorded and inappropriate access would have specified, serious implications. In America, monitoring systems are implemented and staff found inappropriately accessing information are threatened with dismissal. It should be noted that these systems were not sharing information outside the healthcare organisation. More consistent and constrained approaches are required to ensure appropriate access in the more extensive widely shared electronic health record systems being developed today.

Standards for managing access to health information are being developed. These include consideration of the functional role and the appropriate level of access to information required for the person to do their job. This gives a context to the information provided. Standards related to the sensitivity of information are also being developed. The combination of a functional role and a level of sensitivity of the information can provide an automated approach to the release of information. Systems also need to manage the situation where the patient (for their own safety) will not have direct access to their information. Here an agent may act as the patient.

The consumer and the system

Patients are the central focus of the healthcare system and their expectation is that systems will share information that is appropriate and necessary for care. The decision on what is appropriate rests with health consumers because they determine what information they will divulge in particular circumstances. However, there are circumstances today where consumers expect information to be shared and it is not.

Health consumers look forward to having common health information, particularly medication lists, readily and accurately available at all points of healthcare. This requirement is tempered by the need to provide only what is relevant and what is expected. Consider the following scenario:

> Consumer usually visits Doctor B (who is a family friend). They decide to visit doctor A in other city for consultation on their family situation and depression. The patient does not wish to share the details of this consultation with Doctor B. This episode is considered 'private' to the patient.

In the scenario above, the consumer would expect that Doctor A would not share details of the visit with Doctor B and that Doctor B would not know that the visit ever occurred. This is a great challenge to the health professional who feels that quality care requires complete health information. The consumer in this scenario takes responsibility for the information restriction from Doctor B.

The difference between this situation in a paper environment and this situation in an electronic environment is that, should an adverse health situation result from the non-disclosure, Doctor B is able to prove that he was unaware of the patient's visit to Doctor A and that the consumer chose not to disclose this information. This is called 'masking'.

Consumer representation

The Consumer Health Forum (CHF) represents over 800 health consumer organisations and many individuals. It has an advocacy role and increasingly informed representatives to participate in healthcare system developments. They insist on:

* consumer involvement in system design that aims to establish their perspectives at all stages of development. This reduces the development risks inherent in lack of consideration of consumer requirements and expectations.
* implementation strategies that suit consumer needs. This requires open disclosure at all points as to the intent and operation of the system. If people understand what is happening they are more likely to approve the system.

Education of consumer representatives in the last five years has been more extensive resulting in an increasing number of consumer representatives able to represent a wide range of consumer interests. They also understand the potential of information technology.

Conclusion

The healthcare system exists to improve health outcomes for Australians. Understanding the diverse needs and perspectives of consumers is essential to meet that goal. Consumers are hopeful of improved communication and the ability to contribute to, understand and control their information with the introduction of information systems and electronic health records.

The potential to increase consumer trust and to deliver clear, accurate information across the continuum of care is real, but so too are the challenges to those introducing these systems. The need to build belief in these new approaches is paramount, not only to health consumers, but also to healthcare providers who need to be convinced that these systems will benefit their patient's interactions and deliver the promised outcomes.

Consumers are keen to assist in developing and assessing systems and to find answers to the dilemmas of privacy, access control, and identification and information security for electronic health records because consumers are central to these developments.

Review questions

1. What is your personal reaction to the idea of having your information stored in a national database and do your concerns become greater if you have a stigmatising condition such as mental health, AIDS, etc?
2. How do you think the automation of health records impinge upon the relationships with the healthcare team?

Exercises

- Discuss the most common ways in which health consumers interact with the health system and the implications of these for automated healthcare.
- Critically analyse the issues associated with de-identified information.
- Choose a health issue for example, diabetes or chronic pain. Critique 4 online, consumer focused health sites that are dedicated to this issue. Take into account issues such as those discussed in Chapter 23 as well as the focus, validity and reliability of the resources.

Online reading

INFOTRAC® COLLEGE EDITION

For additional readings and review on consumer informatics explore **InfoTrac® College Edition**, your online library. Go to: **www.infotrac-college.com** and search for any of the InfoTrac key terms listed below:

INFOTRAC

➤ Consumer informatics
➤ De-identified data
➤ Privacy
➤ Consumer access
➤ Consumer advocates

References

Australian Council for Safety and Quality in Health Care (2003). *Open Disclosure Standard: A National Standard for open communication in public and private hospitals, following an adverse event in health care*, Commonwealth of Australia, Canberra.

Consumer Health Forum (2004). *Consumers use of computers in General Practice*. Retrieved 29 September, 2004, from www.chf.org.au/projects.

Primary and Coordinated Care Health Services Division (2002). *Electronic consent research: summary of final reports*, Department of Health and Aged Care, Canberra.

O'Connor, D. (1996). Health consumer issues, in E.J.S. Hovenga, M. Kidd and B. Cesnik (eds), *Health Informatics an Overview*, Churchill Livingstone, Melbourne, pp.251–60.

Part 6

Health informatics supporting practitioners

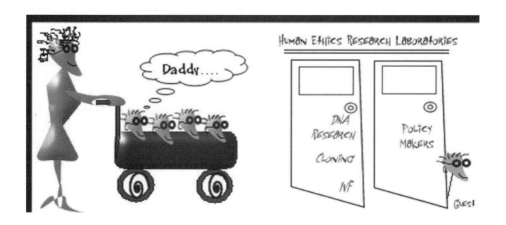

26

Health education

Moya Conrick and Joanne Foster

'Home computers are being called upon to perform many new functions, including the consumption of homework formerly eaten by the dog.'

(Bill Gates, 1955-)

Outline

In recent years, the drive to augment curricula with technology-based solutions while maintaining the contemporary principles of androgogy has been at the forefront of the major developments in tertiary and continuing education. This chapter discusses education and instructional design as well as the human factors that affect learning in these environments.

Introduction

Futurists have been warning for decades that the twenty-first century will bring great change to education and healthcare. Technology, accessibility of information, and new understandings of how human beings learn from experience will shape future educational practices. Additionally, students immersed in high end technology education settings will be better prepared to practise in the future (Nelson, Sadler & Surtees, 2005; Vozenilek et al., 2004). These factors have made this an extremely exciting and challenging time to be involved in education.

> Soon ... 'see one, simulate many, do one competently, and teach everyone' may become reality.
>
> (Vozenilek et al., 2004, p.1153)

The core responsibility of the faculty in education has always been the implementation of curricula and the teaching and preparation of students. However, the world of market economies constantly reminds us that we live in a consumer society and that students are consumers of educational services (Conrick, 2000). These types of economies have dictated the ways in which education is delivered and how individuals behave. In recent years, attempts to implement innovative and theoretically sound curricula have been tempered by the need to marry educational theory with the social constructions of education to attract and retain students while balancing the needs of the professions. This has led to the recent catch cry of implementing flexible learning into programs.

Flexible learning

Although teaching has included some elements of flexibility in the past, flexible learning as a concept has attracted much attention over the last few years. Sometimes it is loosely used, referring to education delivered via the Internet, but it is an approach to education that provides choice and options for the learner. Instead of expecting students to adapt to fixed methods of teaching, learning is adapted as far as practicable to their requirements.

Flexible learning environments encourage students to take more control over learning and provide opportunities for them to develop increased responsibility and independence. They provide students with:

- choice about how, when and where they learn
- choice about the content and sequence of learning activities
- support systems that meet the needs of those from different backgrounds and countries
- access to a range of learning materials presented in a variety of ways that enhance independence and control
- flexible assessment procedures.

Eclectic and often multiple strategies, particularly practices that enable increased access, independence, choice and life-long learning, are incorporated into flexible learning strategies. For example, a flexible learning environment might provide face-to-face delivery (teacher-student, student-student) or a range of resources like print-based materials, audio and video materials, conferencing, CD-ROM, and materials delivered via the Internet.

Although the flexible learning environment is not totally dependent on the technology, there is no doubt that it has a large part to play in the delivery of materials in various formats at any time, anywhere in the world.

Technology-based solutions are prevalent and range from stand-alone packages integrated into face-to-face courses, to fully online programs. Many of these strategies depart quite markedly from traditional curricula in delivery and therefore from the students' social construction and expectations of education. This is particularly so when online courses require students to use virtual groups and cooperative learning.

The terms 'flexible' and 'online' should not be interchangeable as they are not the same thing. Online learning is a strategy used in flexible learning and can be either flexible or inflexible!

Differences between traditional and online learning

There are many differences between traditional and online learning and these are explored in Table 26.1. Here it can be seen that online learning demands sophisticated approaches, as there is an expectation that students will participate in educational decision-making and become autonomous, self-directed learners. In a study of students' transitions to a course using contemporary approaches to learning, students who expressed passive approaches to learning were more dependent on the teacher and preferred the more formal, structured and detached atmosphere of lectures. They did not change this philosophy when faced with contemporary, constructivist approaches to learning. On the other hand, students employing more active approaches and who seemed to hold more relativistic educational conceptions responded well (Conrick, 2000).

Table 26.1: Contrasting approaches between traditional and online curricula (based on Conrick, 2002)

Dimensions	Traditional curricula	Online learning
Method	A pre-established learning environment is expected. Students are presented with material and engage in mostly face-to-face learning.	A process method that expects students to: – be self-directed and autonomous learners – be motived to access material in a timely fashion – respond to direction from technology as a proxy for their teacher – acquire knowledge and information from knowledge bases – participate in physical isolation from their peers.
Learning approach	– teacher centred (Knowles, 1975) – large group learning – more likely to cause surface approaches (Gibbs, 1982) – subjects studied in finite depth (Dahlgren, 1993) – passive (Dahlgren 1993).	– can be both student or teacher centred – students may engage in forced small learning groups where they are expected to work cooperatively, share ideas, brief each other and solve problems with people they may never see.
Cognitive aspects of approach	Able to reproduce knowledge (Dahlgren, 1993).	– expects the development of reasoning skills, self-directed learning strategies – expects self discipline.
Motivation	Fosters extrinsic (Ramsden, 1992)	Fosters intrinsic
Teacher roles	– impart knowledge – present information	– guides, questions, probes and supports student inquiry – facilitates acquisition of learning skills – relinquishes much responsibility to the students.
Student role	Passively receive knowledge (Barrows, 1986)	– actively construct knowledge, autonomous, collaborative learning – responsible for own learning – time management skills and planning.

The students who had strong negative reactions to contemporary learning responded well when they were presented with different learning options and provided with scaffolding, support and the opportunity to negotiate the change at a rate they could accommodate.

Learners' responses to flexible and online learning

A student's transition to flexible or online learning can be a complex process because initially they are taken out of their educational comfort zone. The transition to a completely different way of learning challenges their social construction and expectation of education that can cause significant levels of disequilibrium and anxiety. These experiences are interconnected and interwoven.

It does not seem to be so much the environmental change that students resist, but the largely unseen psychological transition brought by the changed learning environment. The transitions are complex and arise from disorientation and loss caused by the contextual, affective and cognitive change to the method of delivery. Affect is central to much of this and should not be treated as incidental to the process because it is fundamental to a successful transition.

There is an expectation that, if change is imposed, transition will follow (Bridges 1991). However, the reality is somewhat different. Transition has to be managed carefully so that the change does not become unmanageable, producing negative student outcomes and high attrition rates as they exercise their right to an education they perceive as more relevant to their needs (Conrick, 2000).

Contemporary approaches to learning including online strategies can facilitate the development of problem-solving abilities, diagnostic and clinical reasoning skills and nurture self-direction. Some of the principles and assumptions about learning that are relevant here come from the work on self-management and adult-learning principles (Knowles, 1970).

The adult learner

The notion of learner empowerment through self-determination and self-direction is reflected in the work of the pioneers in adult education, although some claims seem largely untested. Knowles (1950) began to identify the strategies that he thought would work best for adult learners. He considered social interactions important and that adult learners were self-directed, basing their learning on self-identified needs. This work on adult learners underpinned constructivism that has been the dominant learning philosophy over the last decade or so.

These researchers claim that learning is enhanced when learners:

- perceive that the learning process and outcomes are relevant to their own purposes
- are treated as self-directing, responsible people who are encouraged to take an active role in decision-making, planning and implementation of learning activities
- discover their preferred learning styles: when people become more aware of how they learn and become exposed to other ways of learning they can redefine and modify their own styles as they seek ways of becoming more competent and responsible learners.

Educational theory as a basis for technology-assisted learning

New technology and non-traditional teaching methods are becoming commonplace in education and must be supported by theory and validated by research. Although there are multiple theories and philosophies in education, most techniques applied to the use of computers in education have their foundations across the continuum – from behaviourism, cognitive theory to its later evolution, constructivism. These are discussed below.

Behaviourism is based on the principle that instruction should be designed to produce observable and quantifiable behaviours in the learner and has the goal of producing behavioural change (Simonson & Thompson, 1990). So, when using technology-based learning, behaviourists would expect to change the student in some obvious and measurable way.

In behaviourism, instruction material is organised from the simple to the complex. It uses the strategy of breaking the content into chunks (chunking) and frequent practice activities followed by immediate feedback. Positive reinforcement is also used, as is the practice of keeping the learner informed of progress and success in a lesson (Simonson & Thompson, 1990). This theory was the design basis for many computer packages such as Drill and Practice as well as being the impetus behind the development of other teaching methods.

Strength – the learner is focused on a clear goal and can respond automatically to the cues of that goal.

Weakness – if the stimulus for the correct response does not occur, the learner may not be able to respond.

Cognitive theory is a shift from behaviourist theory to the internal processes that influence learning. Cognitive psychologists describe the importance of the combination of external stimulus, response behaviour and internal cognitive activity in learning. These theorists focus mainly on the way in which learners receive, organise, retain and use the information. They emphasise the more complex intellectual process such as thinking, language and problem-solving, seeing these as important aspects of the learning process (Snelbecker, 1985) and needed for the performance of actual tasks (Montague, 1988).

Strength – the goal is to train learners to do a task the same way to enable consistency.

Weakness – the learner learns a particular way to accomplish a task, but it may not suit the learner or different situations.

Knowles' (1975) work on adult learning underpinned many of the developments in educational theory towards the more experiential approaches including constructivism, which is the most visible of instructional designs over the last decade.

Constructivism theorists believe that learners actively construct their own knowledge; that knowledge is not transferred from the mind of one knower to the mind of another (filling the empty vessels). This means that learning and teaching are not synonymous (Conrick, 2000); one might teach, but students do not necessarily learn. Constructivists also take into account the learner's prior knowledge in terms of cognitive processes and self-reflective skills (Vrasidas, 2000).

Constructivist theories of learning have a number of assumptions:

- learning is an active process of constructing rather than acquiring knowledge
- there should be a learner-centred approach to instruction
- instruction is a process of supporting that construction (scaffolding) rather than communicating knowledge
- individuals impose meaning on their world (what they are studying/learning)
- knowledge construction is collaborative and meaning is constructed socially.

(Jackson & Fagan 2000; Winn 1997)

Rather than stepped processes and chunking, constructivists believe that knowing is an adaptive process that organises the individual's experiential world (Hendry, 1996). Constructivism requires design that provides problems, which may be solved in different ways, and leave students to struggle with problems of their own choice (Von Glasersfeld, 1993). In this way students actively construct knowledge.

The teacher, facilitator or the instructions assist the student to identify the problem, the knowledge required to understand the problem, and the skills needed to resolve it. Perkins (1991) points to the need for discovery learning using two approaches of constructing knowledge: 'Without the Information Given' (WIG) and 'Beyond the Information Given' (BIG). These processes foster deep, transformative approaches to learning and they also present a unique challenge to instructional designers.

Classical instructional design has continued for many years because it was much less difficult and less costly when compared to the more open constructivist approaches. Over the last few years, technological advances have made constructivist approaches to learning more possible. 'Hypermedia environments that allow for non-linear learning and increased learner control are frequently mentioned in the literature as particularly useful for the constructivist designer' (Mergel, 1998, p.20). Multimedia and the Internet are also alternatives to linear structure and facilitate data-gathering techniques supportive of constructivist learning principles. As an experiential learning tool, virtual reality also offers an active environment for knowledge creation.

It seems that the emergence of environments – such as toolkits and phenomenaria, multimedia, socratic dialogues, coaching and scaffolding, role-playing games, simulations, story-telling structures, case studies and holistic psychotechnologies could promote instructional strategies that also facilitate more active construction of meaning (Wilson, 1997). Moreover, microworlds and virtual reality simulations could stimulate authentic learning while the World Wide Web in general and Web Quests as innovative teaching strategies in particular can offer multiple representations of reality (Cey, 2001).

Strength – because the learner is able to interpret multiple realities, they may deal with real life situations more effectively. If a learner can problem solve, they may better apply their existing knowledge to a novel situation (Schuman, 1996).

Weakness – in a situation where conformity is essential, divergent thinking and action may cause problems.

In any educational program design, planning the environment in which the learning takes place is as important as the content itself, and must be underpinned by educational theory. Some of those environments are discussed here.

Technology-assisted learning

When a technology-assisted course is being planned, four specialised areas are readily identified in design: instructional design, content specialist, graphic design and programming. The content specialist must work closely with instructional designers as the framework developed must meet course objectives and be underpinned by sound educational principles. This in turn gives direction to the rest of the team. As Guest and Conrick (Chapter 23) discussed many of the principles of graphic design that can be applied to computer-aided technology, only instructional design will be pursued here.

Instructional design organises thinking and ideas, ensures the inclusion of important steps in the developmental process and ultimately helps to produce instructional products. Many different methods of technology-assisted learning have evolved and the most prevalent are discussed here. These include the more basic and evolutionary developments, followed by discussion of the contemporary and constructivist approaches of Virtual Reality.

Computer-assisted learning

Computer-assisted learning (CAL) grew rapidly in the 1960s and, despite money and research, by the mid-seventies it was apparent that it was not going to be the success that people had believed. Most computer-assisted instruction was drill and practice and the program developer rather than the learner controlled learning. Little branching of instruction was implemented. CAL fosters surface approaches to the learning task in which students are rich with information, but do not increase their knowledge or understanding.

Drill and practice has many of the limitations associated with behaviourism, including the loss of motivation and rote learning. However, quality packages do hold student attention much longer than the traditional methods and there are some instances when rote learning can be effective.

> ### *Case study*
>
> A student is having a problem learning medications calculations. Drill and practice allows students to stay with the same type of problem until a level of proficiency is attained, before progressing to problems of a more difficult nature. The packages can be individualised allowing students to work at their own pace with the computer determining mastery before more complex questions are posed.

Tutorials

Well-designed tutorial programs can offer one-to-one, individualised instruction, which is impossible in the large classroom. The student, by having to drive the package, becomes an active participant with some control over the rate of advancement and of his or her own learning.

Self-teaching tutorial programs present short passages of information, then ask questions about the material that has been presented. The program may adjust to the level of knowledge in line with the knowledge level exhibited by the student and in this way provides a degree of individualised teaching. However, other tutorial packages behave like an electronic page-turner. They are repetitive and students soon become bored. Both programs reward surface approaches to learning.

These packages were fairly good at doing what they were set up to do, and that is to augment teaching and learning and release teachers from the repetitive aspects of teaching. They were also boring after the first few uses and students were much more motivated by games that allowed them to be part of the action.

Drivers and developments for advancing instructional design

Health professions require practitioners to develop basic clinical skills prior to actual patient encounters and these skills were often 'learnt by doing', but this practice is now under pressure because of societal and financial pressures (Vozenilek et al., 2004; Kneebone et al., 2004). Other issues that impact on clinical education are the increasing acuity of patients, the changing contexts of care, an ageing population, nursing and medical shortages, lack of clinical resources for placements, and lack of access for students to experience all aspects of healthcare.

There is clearly a need for some form of educational technology to support a clinical practice format that replicates reality. This would allow students to undertake multiple attempts at clinical skills in various contexts to enable competence to be achieved in a safe setting prior to their placements at healthcare agencies. Virtual reality and simulation (to a lesser extent) are technologies that support this (Vozenilek et al., 2004; Kneebone et al., 2004).

Simulation, virtual reality and inquiry-type database searches linked to case studies are experiential strategies that support constructivist principles of education. There have been varied simulation developments undertaken in health education that are often referred to as virtual reality, but are often simply computer-based simulations.

Simulation

Simulation is a representation or model of an event, an object or some phenomenon. In clinical terms, it refers to the verbal or pictorial description of a real-life patient care situation, but in reality it is generally an incomplete model that contains only the essential elements of what is being simulated. Nevertheless, simulation is recognised as an effective method of managing clinical teaching. It encourages the student to become an active participant, to think more deeply, and to become part of the educational environment.

Case study

Queensland Health Skills Development Centre (SDC) at Herston in Brisbane acts as a hub for a wide variety of training programs for healthcare professionals. It features state-of-the-art procedural skills laboratories, sophisticated simulation models, a communications laboratory and a versatile training ward that can be adapted to meet the training needs of doctors, nurses and other health professionals (Queensland Health, 2004). The Skills Centre has medium to hi-fidelity automated training manikins and an endo-vascular virtual reality trainer. This enables training from basic to advanced level for proficiency in a range of interventional radiology, invasive cardiology and vascular surgical techniques. The centre has two Haptica trainers that allow for assessment of the motor skills of surgeons. This system uniquely combines both real tissue and virtual reality.

Virtual reality

Virtual reality (VR) on the other hand can be defined as the simulation of a real or imagined environment that can be experienced visually in the three dimensions of width, height and depth. It may additionally provide an interactive experience visually in full real-time motion with sound and possibly with tactile and other forms of feedback (http://whatis.techtarget.com).

VR can be delivered as either a fully immersive experience using CAVE's Immersive Desks devices such as goggles, gloves and tactile interface devices that enable the person to see, hear and touch virtual objects, or non-immersive delivered via conventional desktop computers (Nelson, Sadler & Surtees, 2005; Simpson, 2002). Examples of this would include many of the current computer-based games (such as Medal of Honour; Unreal Tournament, The SIMS).

Constructivism supports the design and implementation of VR as it enables multi-participant activities where collaborative learning can occur. Immersive VR can provide beneficial educational experiences unobtainable from any other means if they focus strongly on the specifics of the technology such as presence, interaction, autonomy, rich visual, audio and tactile metaphors, scale, time, distance and safety (Jackson & Fagan 2000). There are many other examples of the use of VR in education and the health professions and include areas such as haptic surgical skills, rehabilitation, mental health, trauma, airway management and emergency skills to name a few.

VR is also used in pilot training, mine safety, astronaut training, manufacturing systems, police and armed services for educational purposes. In the United Kingdom, a virtual reality community that consists of homes, shops and other facilities found in a normal community environment has recently been developed. It introduces students to eight families/individuals who explore how social and environmental issues impact on their health (Nelson, Sadler & Surtees 2005).

Interest box

A fun web site is Welcome to Froguts! – Virtual Dissection Software. The demo is short but fun, and gives some insight into the use of one type of VR. It also saves frogs!

http://www.froguts.com

Educational blogs

Weblogs are now part of mainstream social communications. They are powerful, intuitive and easy to use; they nurture, foster and enable community, and are now emerging as a popular educational tool (Glogoff, 2005; Maag, 2005; Skiba, 2005; Rosenbloom 2004).

A weblog or blog is a web page similar to an online journal or diary.

(Ferdig & Trammell, 2004; Skiba, 2005)

Educational blogs provide social interaction in teaching and learning as well as knowledge construction. They provide space for students in the blogosphere (a collective term encompassing all weblogs (Wikipedia, 2005)), where they can write, reflect, publish their thoughts and understandings, and receive comments and feedback that enables scaffolding for knowledge construction (Maag, 2005; Ferdig & Trammell, 2004; Rosenbloom, 2004).

Ferdig and Trammell (2004) suggest that there are four benefits to using blogs in education:

1. Blogs assist students to become subject matter experts:
   * the processes involved in blogging are scouring, filtering and posting, which expose students to vast amounts of information on their given topic. It empowers them to build an ever-increasing knowledge base based on the repetitive nature of the processes and regularity of blogging (Blood, 2002).

2. Blogs increase student interest and ownership:
   * as a new technology and as topics are relevant to their learning, students direct their own learning while receiving feedback and comments from others, which motivates ongoing research and learning.

3. Blogs give students legitimate chances to participate:
   * provides a legitimate way to communicate and interact with an authentic audience in a community of practice by opening blogs to the virtual learning community.

4. Blogs provide opportunities for diverse perspectives, both inside and outside the classroom:
   * enables all students to share their thoughts, ideas and knowledge, not just with those attending the class, but to a broader community, enabling more

diverse interactions and communications in the learning process, which ultimately empower all participants (Glogoff, 2005; Ferdig & Trammel, 2004).

Blogs differ from online discussion forums in that they provide an environment more advanced and open, whereby students establish personal and intellectual ownership and control of their learning, something not available in a structured hierarchical topic-based discussion (Ferdig & Trammel, 2004). Other uses of blogs include vlogs, which includes video/multimedia in a blog, and moblogging, which is using a mobile phone to blog (Maag, 2005).

This type of tool promotes critical thinking, synthesis and provision of information as well as written communication in real time. It fosters self-directed versus teacher-directed learning, enables self-reflection as a model of social experience and self-identity, enriching the process of learning and according to Maag (2005) should be supported for future learners.

Conclusion

Work on developing ways to use innovative technologies in education is ongoing and strategies vary. However, the human issues involved indicate that proceeding with these developments requires some caution and a well-planned strategy. At all stages of development this must be underpinned by the principles of theory and instructional design appropriate to the strategy used.

Review questions

1. Discuss the possibility of using VR in clinical education and include some examples.
2. Do you think it is feasible to undertake a clinical health degree completely online with clinical practice undertaken in a VR environment? Discuss the advantages and disadvantages.

Exercises

- Critically analyse technologies that would best support clinical skills development.
- Critique the use of any online education included in your undergraduate course on the basis of its underlying educational theory.

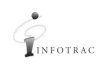

Online reading

INFOTRAC® COLLEGE EDITION
For additional readings and review on education, explore **InfoTrac® College Edition**, your online library. Go to: **www.infotrac-college.com** and search for any of the InfoTrac key terms listed below:
> Educational philosophy
> Computer based learning
> Virtual reality
> Simulation

References

Barrows, H. (1986). A taxonomy of problem-based learning methods. *Medical Education*, *30*, 481–6.

Blood, R. (2002). *The weblog handbook: practical advice on creating and maintaining your blog*, Perseus Publishing, Cambridge, MA.

Bridges, W. (1991). *Managing transitions: making the most of change*, Addison-Wesley Publishing, New York.

Cey, T. (2001). *Moving towards a constructivist classroom*. Retrieved 2 July, 2005, from http://www.usask.ca/.

Conrick, M. (2000). *Students transitional experiences of problem based learning*, Unpublished thesis, Griffith University, Brisbane.

Dahlgren, L. (1993). *Problem-based learning*. Experiences from the Health University Linköping.

Dewey, D. (1944). *Democracy and education: an introduction to the philosophy of education*, McMillan, New York.

Engum, S., Jeffries, P. & Fisher, L. (2003). Intravenous catheter training system: computer based education versus traditional learning models, *The American Journal of Surgery* 186, 67–4.

Ferdig, R. & Trammell, K. (2004). Content delivery in the 'Blogosphere', *T.H.E. Journal* 31 (7), 12, 16–17, 20.

Gibbs, G. (1982). Twenty terrible reasons for learning. *SCEDSIP* (Occasional Paper 8).

Glogoff, S. (2005). Instructional blogging: promoting interactivity, student-centered learning, and peer input, *Innovate* 1 (5). Retrieved 12 May, 2005, from http://www.innovateonline.info/.

Hendry, G. (1996). Constructivism and educational practice, *Australian Journal of Education*, 40(1), 19–45.

Jackson, R. & Fagan, E. (2000). *Collaboration and learning within immersive Virtual Reality* in Proceedings of the third international conference on Collaborative virtual environments, San Francisco, California, CA, pp.83–92.

Kneebone, R., Scott, W., Darzi, A. & Horrocks, M. (2004). Simulation and clinical practice: strengthening the relationship, *Medical Education* 38, 1095–1102.

Knowles, M. (1950). *Informal adult education: a guide for administrators, leaders and teachers*, Associated Press, New York.

Knowles, M. (1970). *The modern practice of adult education: androgogy versus pedagogy*, Associated Press, New York.

Knowles, M. (1975). *Self-directed learning: a guide for learners and teachers,* Associated Press, New York.

Maag, M. (2005). The potential use of 'Blogs' in nursing education, *CIN: Computers, Informatics, Nursing* 23 (1), 16–24.

Mergel, B. (1998). *Instructional design and learning theory.* Retrieved 5 July, 2005, from http://www.usask.ca/.

Montague, W. (1988). Promoting cognitive processing and learning by designing the learning environment, in L. Jonassen (ed.), *Instructional Design for Microcomputer Courseware,* Lawrence-Erbaum, New Jersey.

Nelson, L., Sadler, L. & Surtees, G. (2005). Bringing problem based learning to life using virtual reality, *Nurse Education Today* 5, 103–8.

Perkins, D. (1991). Technology meets constructivism: do they make a marriage?, *Educational Technology,* 31(5), 19–23.

Queensland Health (2004). *Annual Report.* Retrieved 3 March, 2005, from http://www.health.qld.gov.au/rbwh/profile.asp.

Rosenbloom, A. (2004). *The Blogosphere,* Communication of the ACM 47 (12), 31–3.

Schuman, L. (1996). *Perspectives on instruction.* Retrieved 12 May, 2005, from http://edweb.sdsu.edu/.

Simonson, M. & Thompson, A. (1990). *Educational computing foundations,* Macmillan Publishing Co., New York.

Simpson, R. (2002). The Virtual Reality revolution: technology changes nursing education, *Nursing Management* 33 (9), 14–16.

Skiba, D. (2005). People of the year: Bloggers, *Nursing Education Perspectives,* 26 (1), 52–3.

Snelbecker, B. (1985). *Learning theory, instructional theory and psycho-educational design,* University Press of America, Lanham.

TechTarget (2005). *What is?com,* The Leading IT Encyclopaedia and Learning Centre. Retrieved 16 April, 2005, from http://whatis.techtarget.com/.

Von Glasersfeld, E. (1993). Questions and answers about radical constructivism, in K. Tobin (ed.), *The practice of constructivism in science education* (pp.23–38). Lawrence Erlbaum, Hillsdale.

Vrasidas, C. (2000). Constructivism versus objectivism: implications for interaction, course design, and evaluation in distance education, *International Journal of Educational Telecommunications,* 6(4), 339–62.

Vozenilek, J., Huff, S., Reznek, M. & Gordon J. (2004). See one, do one, teach one: advanced technology in medical education, *Academic Emergency Medicine,* 11 (11), 1149–54.

Wagner, C. (2003). Put another (B)Log on the wire: publishing learning logs as weblogs, *Journal of Information Systems Education* 14 (2), 131–2.

Wikipedia (2005). *Wikipedia: the free encyclopaedia.* Retrieved 2 June, 2005, from http://en.wikipedia.org/.

Wilson, B. (1997). Reflections on constructivism and instructional design, in C. Dills and A. Romiszowski (eds.), *Instructional Development Paradigms,* pp.63–80, Educational Technology Publications, New Jersey.

Winn, W. (1997). *The impact of three-dimensional immersive virtual environments on modern pedagogy.* (Technical Report R–97–15), Human Interface Technology Lab., Seattle. Retrieved 2 June, 2005, from http://www.hitl.washington.edu/.

27

Research and evidence-based practice

Evelyn Hovenga

'Research is four things: brains with which to think, eyes with which to see, machines with which to measure and, fourth, money.'

Albert Szent-Gyorgyi (1893–1986)

Outline

The application of evidence-based practice is dependent upon one's ability to correctly interpret research studies and their findings as well as the ability to locate the most appropriate evidence to suit the area of practice. Both research and evidence-based practice are complex topics that may be explored or described from various perspectives. This chapter provides an overview of these issues from a health informatics perspective.

Introduction

Research methods may be defined as forms of inquiry or methods used to seek 'truth' or new knowledge. They are generic, although their applications will vary to suit context and data types. Research methods may be categorised as being either quantitative or qualitative, although qualitative data can be converted to quantitative data in some instances. However, it is appropriate in many instances to adopt a number of different methods concurrently.

Research design is about samples, distributions, data collection, organisation, observation, measurement and analysis methods. Research conclusions are based on either inductive (from particular to general), or deductive (from general to specific) reasoning. The context in which the research is undertaken and the data collected are discipline specific. The results of all data analysis must include evidence that demonstrates scientific rigour to add to the body of knowledge of a particular discipline. This is where it is critical to consider the number of variables that can be controlled, interact with one another, or which are not controllable, as this determines the most desirable sample size and the extent of statistical sophistication required.

All research involving people is subject to ethical rules such as 'no harm to subjects', 'voluntary participation' and 'informed consent'.

There are essentially three distinct types of research along the continuum from qualitative to quantitative research as shown in the following table:

Table 27.1: Types of research

1. Qualitative	2. Explorative – Applied	3. Quantitative
Hypothesis or theory generating. To gain understanding – inductive reasoning.	Modes of observation/data collection and measurement methods vary.	Hypothesis or theory testing. To test knowledge and understanding – deductive reasoning.

There are many types of research methods, all of which can be classified into one of these three main categories; although individual research designs may fit anywhere along the continuum or may adopt multiple research methods. The most commonly used research methods that fit in each of these categories are listed in Table 27.2.

Table 27.2: Research methods by type of research

Qualitative	Explorative – Applied	Quantitative
• Grounded theory • Phenomenology • Ethnography • Delphi studies • Field work • Case studies • Action and interpretive research • Archival research	• Operations research – modelling & simulation • Correlational methods to study relationships between variables • A variety of observational studies such as cross-sectional, longitudinal, cross-sequential and trend studies. • Field research • Work sampling • Surveys (questionnaires, telephone) • Participant and non-participant.	• Experimental research • Quasi-experimental, randomised controlled trials • Population and cohort studies • Time series that are field or laboratory-based.

As there are many texts written in this area, only the fundamentals associated characteristics of these research methods are described here.

Qualitative research methods

Qualitative research methods are based on the view that knowledge has a social construct and that multiple realities co-exist. These research methods have a broad focus and are context bound. They are used to explore feelings, perceptions, attitudes, depth of knowledge and thoughts from informants. Qualitative research uses semi and unstructured interviews, focus groups, documents, free text, photographs, videos, audiotapes or direct observation as data collection methods. It is characterised by the use of unstructured data that may be structured through data organisation and coding. Validity is described in terms of trustworthiness, authenticity, credibility or confirmability, representativeness, or transferability or dependability and meaning.

Explorative and applied research

This type of research is characterised by the methods of observation and data collection used. It may be predominantly qualitative or quantitative or a mix of both. It is used to research everyday events in controlled or uncontrolled environments to explore, describe, predict, explain or quantify phenomena or to categorise and compare it. These methods may be used to examine relationships between variables, their strengths, the amount of variation attributable to an association or the amount of variation. They may be descriptive or analytical, and when measurement is used this is in terms of quantity, intensity, frequency of occurrence and dimensions. These are measured in terms of nominal, ordinal, interval, ratio or relative values. Either primary or secondary data sources may be used.

Quantitative research

Experimental research is characterised by its use of controlled variables. It represents the extreme quantitative end of the research methods continuum. Other research methods in this group are quasi-experimental, which uses independent and dependent variables, control groups, randomised controlled trials, population and cohort studies, and time series. They may be either field or laboratory-based. Other characteristics are a narrow focus, free of context to avoid bias, and an interest in cause and effect. Sampling techniques, sample size and selection are very important. These research methods rely on statistical inference and statistical analysis determines reliability and validity.

Designing a research proposal

As a starting point the *aims* of the research must be considered. Different researchers, either consciously or unconsciously, make any number of assumptions that influence the methods chosen. These assumptions are of a philosophical nature and concern the nature of reality and knowledge and the means by which knowledge can be acquired. Therefore, the assumptions concern *ontology* and *epistemology*. Ontology concerns the nature of the world, what things exist and the nature of reality. Epistemology is concerned with the means by which we obtain valid knowledge about the world.

Health service evaluation

Research that evaluates health service outcomes requires the study of performance at both a clinical and organisational level relative to treatment options and chosen healthcare delivery methods. Underlying these simple statements are difficult and sophisticated issues coming from attempts to define such fuzzy concepts as quality and outcomes and to measure them in a quantitative way.

Quality and positive healthcare outcomes have different meanings and implications to clinicians, health service management, government agencies, third party payers and patients – the actual consumers or subjects of healthcare. Each of these groups defines quality in a different way and none of these viewpoints can be ignored when developing policies and methodologies concerning health service evaluation.

What is evidence-based practice?

The knowledge used as a basis for clinical, management and policy decision-making to support healthcare varies in terms of quality, accuracy and soundness. It is often clouded by values, opinions and other people's views, and consists of or comes from:

- tradition – 'we've always done it this way'
- authority, position power and perceived expertise
- borrowing from other disciplines
- what was learned during professional education and from textbooks
- reasoning, trial and error – 'let's try this and see'
- experience – 'this worked for me the last time'
- rules, regulations, procedures and protocols
- a role model or mentor, someone perceived as having expertise
- journal articles, popular press, the Internet, sales representatives
- processed data collected routinely, systematically, such as trend data
- research, both qualitative and quantitative and including randomised clinical trials usually conducted by others.

Evidence-based practice is about less reliance on the above and a greater reliance on the best possible evidence available about what works and what does not. This requires an ability to look for, retrieve and assess what is good evidence and what is not. Evidence-based practice may be defined as a practitioner's ability to process critical evidence that supports their practice/activity to achieve an optimum outcome at least cost within the circumstances that such care is provided. It requires every person working in the health industry to identify the best available evidence for every intervention and to use this as the basis for all decisions. Furthermore, it requires the ability to question plus the skills to search out, retrieve, interpret and apply the evidence. Evidence is needed to inform health policy development as well as to support all health service management and clinical decision-making.

Patient-determined factors influencing outcomes (independent variables) include, but are not limited to, initial health status including mental state, expectations, socio-economic status, cultural affiliations, age, sex, geographic location, and more. Community factors would include morbidity and mortality patterns, availability of and access to healthcare services including primary care, community expectations, and so forth. Other factors influencing outcomes include availability of staff and specialists, level of staff training, co-morbidities, and rates of iatrogenic complications and nosocomial infections.

Evidence-based practice is a process through which clinicians and other decision-makers use the best available evidence integrated with their expertise to make decisions regarding clinical care, resource allocation, or other areas that can ultimately have an impact on health. The process applies to a broad range of healthcare areas, including diagnosis, prognosis, therapy and other interventions. It answers questions such as:

- Do we get the best value from our investment in healthcare?
- What is known about the outcome of various interventions?
- To what extent does clinical practice use the best available scientific evidence?
- Are health service managers effective?

The Cochrane collaboration is one of the leading organisations promoting the adoption of evidence-based practice (EBP). It is an international organisation that supports people to make well-informed decisions about healthcare by preparing, maintaining and promoting the accessibility of systematic reviews of the effects of healthcare interventions. Its focus is on the conduct of systematic reviews of randomised clinical trials.

Interest box

In 1972, Archie L. Cochrane published *Effectiveness and Efficiency: Random Reflections on Health Services.*

A coding and classification group was registered with the Cochrane collaboration centre in 1995 and many discipline-focused groups are also registered.

Systematic reviews, using meta-analysis, are replacing 'expert opinion' reviews as a basis for guidelines and healthcare decisions. Journals like *Evidence-based Medicine*, and *Evidence-based Nursing* report clinically useful research and are useful resources. The Australian National Institute of Clinical Studies (NICS) was also established to assist clinicians to bridge the gap between what clinicians know and what they do.

What constitutes evidence?

The 'gold standard' of evidence is that which results from rigorously conducted randomised controlled trials (RCT). These are undertaken to establish whether a preventive screening, diagnostic, therapeutic, rehabilitative, educational or administrative intervention does more good than harm, but the emphasis of RCTs is more on efficacy than on clinical effectiveness. However, it is still very difficult to introduce new methods into practice, even when the evidence is clear in the literature. Furthermore, not all interventions lend themselves to the conduct of such trials, nor have trials been conducted to provide evidence for all interventions. In such cases, the use of evidence of lesser quality is still regarded as better than little or no evidence.

Individual clinicians find it impossible to keep track of all clinical literature. Moreover, it is not clear how to distinguish good and useful clinical research from badly done studies that are irrelevant to clinical practice. Much of the time the evidence is conflicting. According to Allen, Arocha, and Patel (1998), the results of investigations of medical decision-making found that:

- hypothesis generation and clinical reasoning differ as a function of expertise
- the gathering, interpretation and use of evidence against hypotheses depends on the prior knowledge of the clinician.

This led these researchers to investigate how clinical evidence is gathered and evaluated during diagnostic reasoning. Their results showed that:
- the ability to index and use adequate evidence by physicians, residents and students is a function of the early generation of accurate hypothesis
- strategies for resolving inconsistent evidence differ as a function of medical expertise.

This knowledge suggests that it is important for all clinicians to learn how to frame the right question for which evidence is needed to inform clinical decision-making. Skills needed are as follows:
- convert a decision to answerable questions
- find the best evidence from a variety of sources
- critically appraise the quality of the evidence obtained in terms of validity and usefulness
- decide what outcome is to be achieved
- apply the evidence to support practice
- evaluate performance against target outcome.

The results from RCTs are held with the highest regard in some circles. They provide strong evidence, provided they were rigorously conducted in accordance with sound scientific principles such as random sample selection, sufficiently large sample size, and appropriate statistical analyses. Other evidence, in descending order of strength, can be obtained from cohort studies, case control and descriptive studies, or consensus of opinions and expert panels. The National Health and Medical Research Council describe six levels of evidence (NHMRC, 2000). In addition, one needs to assess the size of the effect and the relevance or usefulness of the evidence in clinical practice.

Unfortunately, most healthcare decisions are not based on any of this evidence. However, if evidence is obtained the decision-maker needs to first decide if it applies to the situation for which a decision needs to be made. Are the circumstances the same or sufficiently similar?

Collecting data as evidence of practice

An alternative to these methods of collecting evidence is the use of knowledge networks, which are less research but more practice oriented. This method was adopted by the European funded Wisecare Project conducted between July 1997 and December 1999 and presented as a case study below. The main objective of this was to exploit the mass of everyday clinical data, stored in patients' records for clinical and management decision-making. The project partner was 'the European Oncology Nursing Society', an established network of oncology centres throughout Europe (Sermeus et al., 1997; Sermeus et al., 2000).

However, despite the rigour and evidence found in clinical studies, it is how this is used that makes the difference at the end of the day. This is dependent on the reasoning foundations of the clinician. Ledley and Lusted (1959 reprint 1999) described three reasoning foundations used to formulate a medical diagnosis. These were symbolic logic, probability and value theory: all mathematical disciplines. Value or utility theory is also found to be particularly relevant when making decisions regarding treatment options.

Case study

In September 1999, fifteen centres in nine countries (United Kingdom, Finland, Belgium, the Netherlands, Greece, Denmark, France, Slovenia and Sweden) participated in the Wisecare project. All centres agreed that, as part of the clinical process, they would collect data routinely on a selected list of clinical indicators, using standardised scales and data collection design. The project focused on pain, nausea and vomiting, fatigue and mouth problems.

A WiseTool program was developed to collect the data that were sent regularly to a shared database that also provided regular feedback on clinical practice. Two feedback mechanisms were used. First, there was instant feedback for each clinical indicator on the level of an individual patient and second, there was global feedback, derived from the shared database.

Standardised clinical indicators for each site were developed. For reasons of comparison, adjustments were made for toxicity levels of chemotherapy and for clinical time. The global feedback served as benchmarks for the sites and could be used by a local feedback tool as an expected value.

What is the relevance of the Wisecare project for supporting evidence-based practice?

Sermeus and Vanhaecht (personal communication, 1 July 1999) reported the following:

> The most important effect was that by describing outcomes and sharing these results with other centres, feelings of dissatisfaction were created. This was due to not being the best, when compared with other sites, or from not being as perfect as they had always thought. Dissatisfaction acted as the main trigger for change; clinicians consulted the literature, contacted the other sites, exchanged guidelines and protocols and started to change practice. To enable this, a WiseNet web site was developed to communicate between sites, list evidence-based websites on cancer care and to update and evaluate clinical guidelines for the duration of this research project. The role of nurses has been enriched by the broader network and having more control over their work and results.[1]

The adoption of EHRs around the country potentially enables their use for data collection to serve secondary functions such as producing evidence of practice. This serves as a reporting function and is used for health planning and policy development. Of great importance is the need to maintain individual patient or client confidentiality, yet include data from all healthcare consumers, for this purpose. This requires data consistency, reliability and accuracy, irrespective of the data source. It is also important to collect only the data that suits specific and useful purposes, but who decides what data are needed to enable the discovery of new knowledge?

Making good use of clinical information systems

Clinical data can be used for statistical analysis to provide new knowledge regarding the impact of practice in the real world. Such an automated process can simulate randomised controlled trials provided the data are organised and structured appropriately. Systems must be designed to enable such use.

The adoption of the clinical practice improvement (CPI) methodology (Horn, 1997) permits the use of any number of variables representing the process of care while controlling statistically for patient factors to ensure homogeneity in the form of a virtual controlled trial protocol as an alternative to the conduct of conventional clinical trials. On admission, a patient's health status, demographic and environmental data, must be incorporated as a foundation for all clinical data collected.

This enables the researcher to include a risk adjustment of evidence obtained and provides better insight regarding causes of events like falls, pressure ulcers in hospitals, nursing homes or at home, for example. Several layers of time-based evidence are required: for example, an immediate outcome following a healthcare activity; outcomes at the point of care or discharge; later outcomes such as at one week or three months post-discharge.

Outcomes are time sensitive, but the relation of pre-existing conditions and/or processes of care to the occurrence are not always very clear. Furthermore, outcome indicators and the timing of such data collection need to be based upon the results of empirical research or established by consensus for well defined case-types of interest.

The International Severity Information Systems and the Institute for Clinical Outcomes Research (ICOR) conduct clinical practice improvement studies to develop and implement protocols that increase the quality and decrease the cost of healthcare. They perform data definition, data collection, statistical analyses and provide state-of-the-art patient severity of illness software and data collection tools. This permits clinicians to ask and answer questions about associations among patient types, process, and outcome variables. Given the state of current health information systems, much of the work undertaken by ICOR still involves manual data extraction. Effective EHRs should change that.

Knowledge discovery

Knowledge discovery requirements are similar to those necessary for the adoption of evidence-based practice. The emphasis is on the production and use of existing and new knowledge. Informatics provides an essential foundation for and supports the building of evidence related to practice, the accessing of evidence for practice, and the application of evidence to practice across the continuum of care. Informaticians must ensure that EHRs facilitate such use.

What should also become apparent is that the data terminology in use, together with the identification of data requirements to suit any number of purposes and the means to extract the desired data, can lead to the discovery of new knowledge. Much work is underway in a number of countries including Australia to develop minimum data sets to suit specified purposes. Each data element included in these data sets is defined in a data dictionary.

The standard data elements available to be extracted from EHRs, the system architectures and database design determine how well these systems can be used for knowledge discovery. In many instances this is also needed to provide information and knowledge for use for some decision support systems; others use knowledge that is discovered elsewhere. There is a variety of different types of decision support systems and they all need to access knowledge data however derived. This might include knowledge of known drug interactions, best practice guidelines, clinical guidelines, or results of systematic reviews on healthcare as undertaken by organisations such as the Cochrane Collaboration or the Joanna Briggs Institute for evidence-based nursing and midwifery.

Legacy systems often do not readily facilitate data retrieval to provide the desired evidence or evaluation of actual practice. To make sense, data must be structured and standardised in such a way that information can be connected to and compared with other data sources. Standardised coding and classification in healthcare is essential to enable this. There is already a vast amount of healthcare data in existence from hospitals, clinicians, insurers, employers and the government. These data do not have to be duplicated, but their use needs to be carefully planned. They need to be standardised for analysis, verification and comparison purposes. In addition, the systems supporting the data need to be flexible and compatible with other systems.

Interest box

Research involves all people with an interest in healthcare. For a more in-depth understanding of this, there are many general research and statistical texts, which include coverage of experimental design, randomised controlled studies and hypothesis testing topic.

A valuable information source is the NHMRC website, which has a number of publications that can guide you to review and use evidence based on definitions. Explanations are also provided about the strength and relevance of evidence as well as ways to assess the clinical importance of the evidence.

Conclusion

This chapter provides insights into the difficulties encountered in actually capturing reliable evidence of practice. Health professionals from every area of the sector must begin to think about the data needed to enhance decision-making at the point of care. Consensus is needed about the critical or minimum data requirements to enable the use of EHRs to make meaningful comparisons and to facilitate research and knowledge discovery endeavours. This does not restrict individual organisations that may well decide to include more than the minimum data in their system to suit specific purposes that they value.

Review questions

1.   What are the most common methods for research in informatics?
2.   What are the difficulties in using evidence based practice?
3.   How does one find the evidence for evidence based practice?

Exercises

- Discuss ways that technology might enable clinicians to keep abreast of evidence based literature.

- Choose a health or informatics issue then critique 3 online evidence based sites that are dedicated to this issue. Take into account the information focus and target audience as well as the validity and reliability of the site.

Online reading

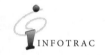

INFOTRAC® COLLEGE EDITION
For additional readings and review on research and evidence-based practice, explore **InfoTrac® College Edition**, your online library. Go to: **www.infotrac-college.com** and search for any of the InfoTrac key terms listed below:
- Research
- Qualitative research
- Quantative research
- Evidence-based practice

References

Allen, V., Arocha, J. & Patel, V. (1998). Evaluating evidence against diagnostic hypotheses in clinical decision making by students, residents and physicians, *International Journal of Medical Informatics*, 51. 91–105.

Australian Council for Safety and Quality in Health Care. Retrieved 18 January, 2005, from http://safetyandquality.org.

Clinical Practice Improvement (CPI) methodology. Retrieved 28 April, 2005, from http://www.isisicor.com.

Cochrane, A. (1999). *Effectiveness and efficiency: random reflections on health services*, Royal Society of Medicine, UK. Retrieved 28 April, 2005, from http://www.rsm.ac.uk/.

Cochrane Collaboration Centre's Strategic Plan. Retrieved 28 April, 2005, from http://www.cochrane.org.au/.

Horn, S. (1997). *Clinical practice improvement methodology: implementation and evaluation,* Faulkner & Gray/Institute for Clinical Outcomes Research. Retrieved 28 April, 2005, from http://www.isisicor.com.

Ledley, R. & Lusted, L. (1959). Reasoning foundations of medical diagnosis, *Science* No. 130, pp.9–21, reprinted in *Yearbook of Medical Informatics 99,* 'The Promise of Medical Informatics', eds, J. van Bemmel and A.T. McCray, pp.65–77.

National Health and medical Research Council (2000). *How to review the evidence: systematic identification and review of the scientific literature.* Commonwealth of Australia, Canberra. Retrieved 28 June, 2005, from http://www.nhmrc.gov.au/.

National Health and Medical Research Council (NHMRC) (2000). *How to use the evidence: assessment and application of scientific evidence,* Commonwealth of Australia, Canberra. Retrieved 30 June, 2005, from http://www.nhmrc.gov.au/.

National Health and Medical Research Council (NHMRC) (n.d.). *NHMRC additional levels of evidence and grades for recommendations for developers of guidelines.* Retrieved 30 June, 2005, from http://www.nhmrc.gov.au/.

National Institute of Clinical Studies (NICS) (n.d.). Retrieved 1 July, 2005, from http://www.nicsl.com.au/.

Sermeus, W., Kearney, N., Kinnunen, J., Goossens, L. & Miller, M. (2000). *WISECARE workflow information systems for European nursing care,* IOS Press, vol. 73, Amsterdam.

Sermeus, W., Hoy, D., Jodrell, N., Hyslop, A., Gypen, T., Kinnunen, J. et al. (1997). The WISECARE project and the impact of information technology on nursing knowledge, *Nursing Informatics: The Impact of Nursing Knowledge on Health Care Informatics,* IOS Press, pp.176–84.

Endnote

1   More information about Wisecare can be found at the University of Stirling in Scotland, http://www. cancercare.stir.ac.uk/projects/wisecare.html.

28

Case studies from clinical practice

Outline

This chapter consists of case studies written from clinicians and health professionals. They were asked to write a short case study or story about the impact of HI technology on their practice. These stories are from:

1. *Allied Health* by David Rhodes
2. *General Practice* by Peter Adkins
3. *Nursing* by Paul Donaldson
4. *Pharmacy* by Ron Natoli
5. *Public Health* by Stella Stevens
6. *Rural and Remote* by Bruce Roggiero.

1. Allied health

David Rhodes

Allied health includes diverse professions including dietetics, occupational therapy, physiotherapy, podiatry, psychology, social work, and speech pathology.

Case study

To facilitate information management across these professions, the National Allied Health Casemix Committee has developed and updated the Health Activity Hierarchy Version 1.1 (NAHCC 2001)[1]. The hierarchy categorises all allied health activities into a standard framework so that there is a common language across professional groups and workplace settings.

---

[1] National Allied Health Casemix Committee (2001). Health Activity Hierarchy, Version 1.1, School of Management, RMIT University, Melbourne.

Most software systems servicing allied health professions have incorporated the hierarchy into local and state developed products. With all clinical, service, management, teaching and research activities collected in the same way, a wide range of state and national projects have been supported through information technology. These have included the National Allied Health Service Weights Study, national and state hospital cost data collections, and a number of national benchmarking consortia, including participation from New Zealand. Two consortia utilise the methodologies developed by the Australian Health Roundtable to compare practice and examine opportunities for improvement in services, for example, the management of stroke and hip replacements.

Until late in the twentieth century, the focus had been on standardising data collections on activity. In recent years, the focus has shifted to technology supporting clinical management through provision of electronic clinical notes and decision support tools. Developments have included the CHIME system (Community Health Information Management Enterprise), various point-of-care clinical systems, electronic medical record systems, and the national HealthConnect projects. The objective is to provide multiple user same-time access to clinical documentation, development of care plan templates, and incorporation of other clinical decision support components. Clinical activity data is to be largely a by-product of clinical service delivery and non-clinical activities are derived from electronic scheduling/diary entries. When operational, these systems should generally supersede stand-alone allied health systems.

With the utilisation of data warehousing technologies, it is feasible to analyse allied health service delivery across the full continuum of a client's journey – community-based and hospital-based services. This provides a very rich environment for collaborative quality improvement and research activities.

Telehealth is utilised increasingly to support allied health management and practice and, currently this supports case conferencing, meetings and professional development. However, there is a need for improved performance of systems to support substantial expansion into more innovative clinical service delivery.

With the development of a plethora of software, allied health professionals have recognised a need for standardising code sets to ensure that there is consistency and robustness of clinical and management information. Currently, there are multiple code sets that are often locally developed and are generally software specific. The push for standardisation will need to be enhanced to ensure quality data extraction. There is a high risk of compromising data mining capacity if this issue is not addressed as part of the emerging clinical management systems.

2. General Practice

Dr Peter Adkins

Information systems in general practice assist the practitioner to better manage patients' healthcare, allowing issues beyond the presenting complaint to be identified (for example alerts for vaccination and health assessment) and facilitating access to information to modify patient behaviour (such as statins and memory loss). They also generate efficiencies in patient care (referral letter and prescription generation), which allows more time to be spent on health promotion issues.

Case study

Mrs Dorothy K, widowed, aged 76 years, presents for a repeat prescription for two of her medications, namely Atorvastatin and Amlodipine tablets. Dorothy also has some concerns regarding Atorvastatin after watching a recent television current affairs program linking this medication to memory loss. She also requests a referral letter to her cardiologist.

On opening the patient's electronic record, alerts for influenza and pneumococcal pneumonia vaccination are displayed, as is a prompt for a Health Assessment.

The current medication page is accessed and this indicates that Dorothy may not be taking her daily aspirin and that her Atenolol tablets are due to run out. Dorothy admits that it is cheaper to buy her aspirin over the counter than on prescription and this is noted in her electronic record.

The product information on Atorvastatin is accessed and post-marketing data mentions that 'amnesia' may be a problem. This is done via the Internet as broadband has made access to non-practice-held electronic information feasible during the consultation. An Internet search engine highlights a number of information sources regarding this matter. A URL to the National Prescribing Service is located and a perusal of a Fact Sheet, 'Statins and Memory Loss', provides a summary of the evidence in this area. A copy of the brief report is provided to the patient to take home, as are the repeat prescriptions.

A subsequent appointment is recommended to see the practice nurse for the initial part of a health assessment followed by completion of the health assessment and vaccination at the next surgery visit. A clinical reminder is set regarding this visit.

Communication with specialists has also been assisted greatly through the use of an electronic health record to generate legible, comprehensive referral letters. A word processing template allows the population of a form letter with relevant patient information, for example, medical history, medications, allergies and relevant investigations (pathology and radiology). Currently most GPs print a copy of the referral letter and hand this to the patient to take when visiting the specialist. Some practices are now generating referral documentation, electronically signing and emailing this information to the specialist using Public Key Infrastructure to ensure security and confidentiality.

3. Nursing

Paul Donaldson

Nurses spend considerable time entering clinical information and updating condition and location lists in both acute and community care. It is important that this information is entered into clinical information systems once and in a manner that facilitates multiple uses. The general rule of thumb for data entry is that the more specific the data, the more likely it will have many uses in reports. In nursing, manipulating these data allows the calculation of acuity, time and resource use and so forth.

Case study

When providing care, the time-value consists of the minutes spent with the patient, plus a portion of the indirect minutes spent during the day. This is distributed based on the percentage of total client contact time spent during the period. In acute settings, where a nurse or a nursing team cares for numerous clients, performing planned interventions and attending to ad hoc needs, measuring the exact minutes spent with each patient is difficult. However, an average value for these clients can be determined by categorising them into groups, based on their relative use of resources. While inexact, it provides a useful and total picture for measuring acuity.

Patient acuity can be determined by entering the patient dependency triggers, or as nursing tasks performed during the course of care and client attributes that significantly impact on their ability for self-care and so require nursing time. These data are mainly used to apportion nursing costs to individuals. They are based on the relative value of time spent by particular nurses, as a portion of the client population managed, during the period of time being rated. The local finance system combines the acuity summary data with roster information and payroll data, to cost the direct patient care provided for each period rated. As it accumulates, the cost of care for an episode is calculated.

When clients with the same Diagnostic Related Group (DRG) are costed, an average labour cost per DRG is determined along with average length of stay (ALOS) and Separation weightings. The state government remunerates the facility per patient DRG, based on these figures. Facilities use remuneration data to determine activity targets for a financial period and to provide appropriate staffing to meet budget targets. Therefore, the data entered by nurses about the care provided during a single shift ultimately determines the number of nurses necessary to provide care within a facility.

Because dependency entries require the identification of tasks performed and client attributes on a shift-by-shift basis, the elemental data can be used in developing a framework for clinical pathways. Logically, clients admitted for the same condition and undergoing similar treatment should have a similar course of treatment and nursing interventions throughout the episode of care. Grouping clients in this manner can identify which interventions are occurring during each shift and each day across the episode of care. This enabled a draft pathway framework to be built from this data.

While not the definitive solution, it saves much time, as the framework does not have to be built from scratch. It is based on the history of care in the patient group and refined to include adjustment for changes in care and for what should occur. Adherence to the pathway and the identification of where variance occurred in individual clients' care can be determined by auditing the DRG against the pathway.

Another use of the data is to develop a skills profile because Registered Nurses can only perform certain interventions and Assistants in Nursing could not perform others. Grouping tasks into these areas provides the manager with the skillmix required for providing safe care. These data can also apportion the annual total hours of care in a unit across all levels of nursing. Each unit manages specific client populations and, unless the unit's core business changes, this provides a good indicator of skillmix requirements. When a change in business is proposed, the historical data can be combined with DRG data and used for gap analysis that can drive staffing changes and professional development requirements for the unit.

State budgets, clinical standards, pathways, skillmix criteria and education plans are developed from the data used to cost patient care. The multiple uses of the data increased its value because of the economy built into its collection. Although the initial data collection may appear tedious, it provides details not available by other means.

4. Pharmacy

Ron Natoli

Pharmacists were initially at the forefront of utilising technology in their practices. However, ten to fifteen years later, areas remain where the implementation of IT systems would provide for better clinical outcomes and further enhance the pharmacist's professional role.

Case study

State Health Departments regulate the control of drugs and poisons through various Schedules. Schedule 8 (S8) regulations cover the prescribing, dispensing, possession and consumption of medications that are considered drugs of addiction. These drugs include opioids, pyschostimulants, or drugs that have a propensity for dependence.

State instrumentalities may collect information on the prescribing and dispensing of these products, yet centralised databases of S8s to ensure appropriate monitoring of their distribution is non-existent. For example, at present data collection of opioid use is confined to the TAMS (Treaties And Monitoring System) at wholesaler level.

Pharmacists as custodians of medications are concerned about evidence indicating diversion, misuse, non-medical (especially injecting) use of S8s and some Schedule 4s (S4s) such as benzodiazepines. Added to this is the issue of medication misadventure and prescribing errors and the potential for greater risk to the individual and the community increases exponentially. The daily dispensing and administration of Pharmacotherapies for Opioid dependence by pharmacists requires involves further recording and monitoring, imposing an extra cost burden on the taxpayer.

Pharmacists dispensing S8s must ensure the safe and optimal use of these agents. They must account for all drugs, maintain a hard copy register and retain all prescriptions and records for two years. Approved persons can inspect registers and copy records in pharmacy computers at any time. S8 medications can be prescribed and dispensed for a particular patient for a maximum of 60–90 days (depending on the state), again necessitating further monitoring.

While the dispensing process in the majority of pharmacies is electronic, most state authorities still require the use of hard copy S8 Registers, necessitating double processing. S8 Registers are stock records and do not support patient use monitoring. Although a system already exists for electronic pharmacy records, the dispensing data records held in pharmacy computers are not collected or utilised, except for HIC issues/use under the Prescription Benefits Scheme. Although most S8 medications are listed on this scheme, prices charged to recipients are below the patient contribution level (except for pensioners etc) and therefore these data are not forwarded to the HIC.

Generally, state health departments do not maintain central databases on Schedule 8 usage; as a result prescribers and pharmacists cannot access current medication information, except that held in their own systems.

All healthcare professionals' 'Duty Of Care' responsibilities require review and monitoring of medications when prescribing and dispensing. Yet, in the case of Schedule 8 drugs, the process is not optimal. The implementation of electronic recording and a National Central Database for these medications would overcome the deficiencies of the present system. However, privacy and consumer concerns would need to be accommodated in any new electronic recording system.

5. Public health

Stella Stevens

Public health depends on data and is the domain of 'big' data sets with upwards of seven million data entries per year. Because of the nature of public health data, and the long timeframes for projects to mature, it tends to attract the stayers interested in the big picture.

Case study

Jennifer Muller is excited by data because it makes such a difference in health outcomes and her unit exploits its capacity to the full.

Evidence emerged in the mid to late 1980s via the World Health Organisation's International Agency for Research in Cancer that screening was a public health initiative with demonstrable outcomes for the health of populations. The Queensland Cancer Screening Services were established as a response to this and Jennifer has managed the service from its initiation, not for want of other opportunities, but because it takes at least five years for exciting results to emerge.

The unit captures point-of-care data on patients undergoing cervical, breast and, shortly, bowel cancer screening. It also collects outcome data electronically from GPs via pathology laboratories and uses that data to perform several functions. Firstly, and most importantly from the patient's perspective, is to identify cases of cancer that can be acted upon by various health professionals and which is a functional clinical tool in the treatment of breast cancer. Secondly, data are provided to stimulate research into clinical improvements for treating early stage cancer: at this stage more possibilities for effective treatment become identifiable and testable. The third function is to provide reliable quality information for health professionals involved in early detection, which they can use to measure their success rate in identifying cancers and benchmark this against their colleagues. Lastly, the unit provides information on cancer rates for government.

The result of using data this way has been that 89 per cent of people diagnosed with cancer in the early stages now survive more than five years. The unit's success depends upon the quality of the data supplied and is in turn impacted upon by work practices of the treating clinician whose prime concern is not collecting data for secondary purposes. The unit needs clean, quality data from clinicians, or perhaps automatic electronic prompts that fit into the workflows of specialists.

The unit is also involved nationally in attempting to coordinate data so that a more comprehensive picture can be obtained, but failure to agree on definitions and the continuing absence of a unique patient identifier are major obstacles to success. One thing is sure though, in public health large data sets produce substantial outcomes for both individuals and populations.

6. Rural and remote healthcare

Bruce Roggiero

Information technology has made a great deal of difference in remote area nursing and this is an example of seamless continuity of care over great distances without one phone call.

Case study

It is 1994: I'm a remote area nurse walking back from the bakery in the township of Dargargu, an eight-hour drive south west from Darwin in the Northern Territory. Dargargu was once called Wattie Creek, famous in the Australian Aboriginal Land Rights history as the setting of the first ever 'Walk Off', commonly known as the 'Wave Hill Walk Off', and granting of land to Aboriginal people. An 'Old Man' (a man of cultural knowledge) from this historic time approaches me. 'Hey Youngfella' (a man of limited cultural knowledge), 'I need to see you!' 'No worries Old Man, what's the problem?' 'I want to see you in the clinic.' We walk to the clinic in silence. I am concerned, as Old Men do not do this unless there is a real problem.

At the clinic I somehow know to close and lock the door. The Old Man drops his pants and shows me a deep crater partially healed in his right groin. I observe debris of gauze dressing in the wound and look up at the Old Man. 'What's the story Old Man, looks like you have had some trouble there and been having some treatment?' He looks at me with serious eyes and tells me a story of being in hospital in Darwin for around three weeks being treated for this sore that would not go away. I surmised from his story a peripheral inserted catheter and large doses of drugs being administered several times a day.

I find his chart. There is no discharge summary or information about this admission. The hospital medical records department was called and a worker kindly faxed several sheets of paper to the clinic. The discharge summary told of a fungal infection being treated with specialist drugs, dressings, and a discharge to home when slow improvement had set in. There was also a note about an Outpatient appointment that was not attended.

This Old Man was discharged on a Thursday to travel on Friday with an Outpatient appointment arranged for the following Monday. The trouble for this Old Man was that using the normal travel meant that he did not arrive home till the day after his Outpatient appointment was due and was lost to follow-up! No further treatment. Remote Area Nurses are expert at this situation and after several more phone calls and another day or two he was admitted to a closer hospital receiving appropriate treatment and made an uneventful recovery.

It is 2004: The clinic I'm working in is six hours drive south west of Darwin. The computer is a normal feature in every clinical area. We are on a network using a combination of ISDN, ADSL landline, and satellite Internet VPN. Two concepts are being used. HealthConnect connected to health facilities in Katherine and a centralised server under the jurisdiction of the Katherine West Aboriginal Health Board.

There is a large number of people moving to our area to attend a Land Claim meeting from all over. Some from the north, some from the south, as the Aboriginal Ceremony Song line dictates in these matters. The people from the north are not part of the area covered by our Network. The people from the south are within our domain.

A young woman comes to the clinic with a four-month-old babe in her arms. The baby has diarrhoea, febrile and on examination severe otitis media. We open our software package and search for the babe's name. They live four hours' drive away from this community. We establish the babe was seen at the other clinic four days earlier with an URTI, was put on antibiotics and that the weight was stable. We established with the mother that the antibiotics had been given as instructed. We give Panadol and change the antibiotic. Over the next few days, review sees the babe improving and the weight rising. All details were entered into the software with notes on progress and the child placed on their home clinic's review list for the week after return, as per the protocol for ear disease. None of this would be possible without the use of information technology.

29

Management decision-making

David Evans

> One day Alice came to a fork in the road and saw a Cheshire cat in a tree.
>
> 'Which road do I take?' she asked.
>
> 'Where do you want to go?'
>
> 'I don't know,' Alice answered.
>
> 'Then,' said the cat 'it doesn't matter.'
>
> (Lewis Carroll, *Alice's Adventures in Wonderland*)

Outline

Modern healthcare services are constantly collecting and analysing information to allocate limited human and financial resources to meet the increasing needs of health services. The pressure is unremitting and managers face this every minute of their day. This chapter uses a range of clinical issues and case studies to demonstrate the nuances of healthcare management decision-making.

Introduction

Some decisions are made with little thought – what tie to wear or what to eat – while others impose enormous intellectual demands. Decisions are made individually or in groups; they may be conscious, with varying levels of effort, or reflex actions based on subconscious analysis. Decision-making is an activity common to all living organisms, but naturally the complexity between species varies. It may range from simple instinct and autonomic effects through to complex cognitive processes that share knowledge, make assumptions, undertake analysis and calculations, and rely on learnt experiences. However, common to all decision-making is the need for quality information to underpin effective processing.

Information management, using appropriate technologies, can assist decision-making in many ways. It can provide large amounts of information, aggregate and classify individual data elements, apply mathematical algorithms to difficult problems and enable communications activities such as group decision-making. It also improves the ability to monitor trends and changes following the implementation of decisions.

Individual and group decision-making models

Many models of management decision-making are discussed in the literature and they usually include debate on how individual managers use variants of a rational approach that may include:

- monitoring the environment
- defining the problem
- specifying objectives
- diagnosing the problem
- considering and evaluating alternative solutions
- choosing a solution
- implementing the chosen change process.

Individual managers use elements of the rational approach as they apply intuition, judgement, inspiration and experience daily and to varying extents.

Healthcare organisations require many decision-making processes running parallel or sequentially. They require managers with diverse skills in areas such as finance, human resources, legal, engineering and clinical, and often need to include patients and their carers in the process. Organisations apply many decision-making strategies and structures; the management science approach, for example, utilises mathematics supported by tools such as linear programming, Bayesian statistics, Program Evaluation Review Technique (PERT) charts, and increasingly complex computer simulations and decision support.

The Carnegie Model of Simon (1958) and Cyert and March (1963) however, acknowledged the uncertainty of information and the diverse conflicts within organisations. It also established that these factors led to coalitions of managers who resolved ambiguity, inconsistency and intrinsic limitations within large organisations by seeking out alternatives that were acceptable and satisfactorily in achieving the goals of each manager (satisficing). This model maintains that managers do not expect perfect solutions in situations with poorly-defined definitions, internal conflict or ambiguity. The difficulty for this model is creating and maintaining a working coalition.

In 1976, Mintzberg, Raisinghani, and Théorêt revealed that major decisions made in organisations tended to result from sets of smaller decisions and the Incremental Decision Process Model was born. It consists of many loops or decision interrupts that enable the organisation to learn, but the eventual outcome is often quite different from what was initially anticipated. Combinations of the Carnegie and Incremental approach are seen when either problem identification or problem solutions are uncertain.

The Garbage Can Model (GCM) of Cohen, March and Olsen (1972) appears to be the evolutionary development of these models. It does not regard decision-making as a sequential stepwise process from problem to solution. Rather, it describes an organised anarchy, where problem and solution are not necessarily related. Solutions may emerge before a problem is specified, choices may be made without solving the problem, and the problem may persist without solution. In general, however, the organisation ultimately moves toward problem reduction.

Rational and management science approaches are successful when the nature of the problem is agreed and when the possibility of achieving a solution is high. When both problem definition and solution knowledge is low, the GCM emerges. Certainty and agreement on a problem's definition leads to trial and error or incremental decision-making, while high quality information about solving a problem but uncertainty about the problem itself leads to coalitions forming and satisficing behaviour, as in the Carnegie Model. A typical healthcare organisation employs all these processes in its decision-making activities.

Decision-making in a health organisation

Healthcare organisations are dynamic, the problems they face are often poorly defined, and the information available for decision-making may be incomplete. In this climate, managers and clinicians, at each level of the health organisation, must make decisions about the most efficient use of available funds and resources. Planning provides a structured process to prepare for challenges and to take advantage of opportunities as they arise. It is about anticipating change and making decisions before crises occur.

> ## Case study
> The focus of this case study will be the increasingly ageing population and the associated increase in chronic diseases that dictate their quality of life and functioning. Disabling pain and reduced mobility leads to less social activity, falls and subsequent prolonged hospital care from head injuries or fractures. Many of these processes can be mitigated with expensive surgical interventions, costly medications and significant long-term contact with healthcare services.

How should managers or clinicians think when making decisions?

The Chief Executive Officer (CEO) in this case study has the task of ensuring that problems are defined accurately and information to underpin solutions is available. The CEO might benefit from critically evaluating how she applies her thought processes to dealing with the problems.

The application of a 'systematic way to form and shape one's thinking' is critical thinking (Paul, 1993, p.20). It incorporates the 'intellectually disciplined process of actively and skilfully conceptualising, applying, analysing, synthesising, or evaluating information gathered from or generated by observation, experience, reflection, reasoning or communication' (p.110). These processes demand rigour and a controlled structure that includes evaluating the weaknesses and strengths of conclusions reached.

When evaluating future directions and the most appropriate resources to allocate, the CEO needs to examine how she is to approach the problem. This includes the quantity, value, extent and quality of the thinking (Facione, 1998) and her critical thinking approach might include some of the attributes in Table 29.1.

Table 29.1: A critical thinking approach to decision-making

Intelligibility	Will the problem or concern actually be resolved by the decisions to be made? Is the data being applied in an unambiguous, understandable and clear manner? Are all the implications of all discussions easily understood?
Accuracy	How reliable is the information? Do the facts accurately reflect the real situation? What are the biases in the information? Is there adequate preciseness in the questions asked and solutions proposed?
Significance	Is the information the right information? Is other information needed? How much reliance is there on personal opinion and assumptions?
Depth	How superficial was the assessment on which the decisions will be based? Will a more in-depth examination of the problem expose other possible decisions or improve understanding of the problem?
Breadth	Have all potential sources of information been examined? Is there related material that might assist the decision-making?
Logic	Could another person follow the line of reasoning used in reaching the decision? Is the decision based on the facts available?

Drucker (1998) recommends that managers consider what information is required for the task, when they need it, the form it should take, and from whom they should acquire it. Dealing effectively with information is a foundation skill for all decision-makers; it is complex and crucial for quality health outcomes.

How do you determine what to think about when making decisions?

Managers often become aware of information that at first may appear peripheral to the goals of the organisation but which may impact later. For example:

The CEO in our scenario notes, while collecting information, that nursing student registrations at universities have dropped dramatically this year. Believing that she and her organisation have little direct impact on universities and vice versa she returns to her more immediate problems. After further consideration, our CEO realises that the reduction in student numbers will have an impact on the maintenance of services of her organisation. If the pool of skilled staff drops, she will have to compete on the open market. She may have to consider financial reimbursements to attract people that will reduce the funds available for providing care. She may need to consider longer-term strategies such as educating existing staff or up-skilling semi-skilled staff from other countries.

In her initial planning, she becomes aware that the health workforce will not be able to cope with the predicted number of elderly patients seeking care for multiple chronic diseases, because of a forecast shortfall of clinician numbers and inadequate skills levels. Developing a skilled workforce may take many years. Extensive and accurate information must be collected to analyse these trends and enable predictions. Our manager must be aware of the nature of the information required, how best to acquire it, and how to use it most efficiently.

How much should or can you know before making decisions?

The CEO needs information about surgical procedures and the future needs of the aged to inform her decision-making. For this she searches the Internet, only to be flooded with thousands of articles and commentaries. Not surprisingly, as it is said that surfing the Internet is like putting your mouth over a fire hose and turning it on to drink! The consequences of a decision are impossible to predict in the absence of 'good' information, and most information on the Internet is somewhat conflicting and difficult to correlate. Seeking information requires care and planning because a rush of unstructured information can totally overwhelm the decision-making process ('infoglut').

The enormous expansion of biological and health-related information enabled by technology has made evaluating the effectiveness of different treatment options challenging for specialised groups and a formidable task for individuals. Decisions in healthcare are generally made under some uncertainty because of incomplete patient information, poor observations and accuracy limitations in testing, misinterpretation of results, limited communication, cultural misunderstandings and insufficient time to evaluate material.

Information validity

Further down our organisation in a large metropolitan hospital, another manager is deciding whether to fund additional complex surgical procedures to alleviate the suffering of many ageing patients or to spend that money expanding the hard pressed aged care support services on which the ageing population is steadily increasing its demands. He needs valid data to guide his decision.

Over many years medical and surgical specialities have developed terms to describe concepts such as conditions, procedures or syndromes that affect people under their care. These terms are often complex, descriptive and usually unique, or may be aggregations of other terms (for example 'left toe' or 'index finger').

In our large speciality hospital a dedicated group of surgeons (clinical managers) have decided to create a database to store the details of their operations, methods used, complications and long-term outcomes for the types of prosthetics or devices used. After many months of entering information they are happy with the well-printed and clear reports the database provides on request. Management, however, were concerned at the patients' length of stay following procedures in that speciality. Knowing the surgeons had collected this information they asked which operations were taking the most time.

The surgeons discovered that when analysing an aggregated set of the data there were many anomalies. Each surgeon had entered a description or set of terms they believed best described the procedure they had undertaken. In addition, the terms were entered as free text with little regard to the terms they used earlier and they had no agreed definitions for the use of each term. Gradually the specialists had also changed how they described procedures and took shortcuts in typing; 'L' for Left or 'L' for Lateral. Sometimes they described the procedure by the prosthetic used, other times the procedure was defined by the anatomy site operated upon; Smith's prosthesis or L Knee replacement.

The surgeons realised that the words often differed between them, so they decided to collaborate to create an agreed list of all terms that they all authorised for use. Other rules were introduced so that abbreviations and acronyms were controlled and had only one meaning when used in the database. In other words, they developed an interface terminology. Data cleaning occurred every week and incorrectly entered material was kept out of the analysis until it could be corrected.

This improved the comparability of the information between the surgeons, but they realised that often they used different terms to describe the same health concept and at other times they used the same terms to describe different concepts. In other words a Reference Terminology was required to ensure validity. This was achieved by ensuring that each type of procedure was uniquely described in one set of definitions and linked back to terms in the interface terminology. Then, even if different terms were used when entering data at the interface, those terms would map to one and only one member of the reference terminology.

Despite long hours of discussion and frayed emotions in reaching a common set of definitions for each element or data item in the reference terminology, once finished the reports were meaningful and useful. To ensure that the system remained stable, a committee was established to examine any new candidates for the reference terminology and ensure the criteria for uniqueness was maintained.

The relevance, accuracy and validity of a term leads to improved data quality while the completeness, timeliness and clarity of information impacts on the quality of a decision, its consequences and, ultimately, the harm or benefits for patients or providers. The challenge for managers and clinicians is recognising that the information on which they are relying may be weak in one or more of those aspects.

Once information is received, decision-makers rely to a varying extent on the relevance and validity of that information to define the problems. The better the quality of information the better the definition of the problem, and the list of possible interventions.

Knowing what you do not know is as important as knowing what is known; it also assists in determining approaches to decision-making.

In our scenario, the surgeon's database was a good outcome for the hospital because when they compared the length of stay for a particular procedure they could agree that they were comparing the same factors. However, the funding bodies and quality assessors wanted to compare 'like with like' across organisations and countries.

Such benchmarking is a major challenge and impossible with 'in house' software unless it complies with recognised standards. Managers need to be aware of all data items and their definitions to enable consistency and improve the comparability of data within the health domain. The definition allows users of data to understand if the data is appropriate to the purpose to which it will be applied.

This case study demonstrates the health organisation's dependence on data, information and knowledge. Standards Australia (2004, p.6) agrees, saying that 'Safe, effective and efficient care is dependent upon accurate and detailed clinical information being reliably communicated, unambiguously interpreted and accurately transformed into data and knowledge.' It is crucial for health organisations to be certain that material is unambiguous and describes what it is that they wish to describe.

How do you know that what you know is true or valid before making decisions?

Our organisation now has considerable information about the relevant surgical procedures that can be benchmarked internationally and locally. However, decisions are only required when there is a set of alternative actions to choose from.

Decision-makers must seek an exhaustive list of possible decisions, be aware that if 'good' decisions are to be made, each decision should be as independent of others or as 'exclusive' as possible. This is not simple – it provides a challenge to progressing the decision process. In healthcare very few decisions can be based on exhaustive and exclusive choices. For example, if there are five different types of prosthetics for five different problems, then the decision on which to use is relatively easy based on five exclusive and exhaustive choices. However, this is not so if two devices can do the same task but are made of different materials. If one is quicker to use than the other, is the speed and ease of operation more important than the longevity of the material? What if the device you favour and are skilled in using is very expensive and a cheaper alternative is available?

Making decisions involves applying a cognitive process in a systematic or structured way that identifies alternatives, evaluates them, makes a conclusion and selects the appropriate action. However, there is no certainty that all factors on which the decision will be based are known. This level of uncertainty confounds decision-makers and makes this an interesting and challenging area of management.

Decision-making is involved in most aspects of healthcare and is applied across the health system, affecting individuals, wards, hospitals and policy-makers. While sound economic decision-making is crucial, the public is increasingly focusing on clinical governance or quality management decisions.

Discussion point

There are many non-financial decisions that can confront healthcare managers.

How will our manager react to ethical issues such as abortion, circumcision, involuntary detention, medication side effects, children giving consent, elective versus acute service provision, preventative versus acute treatment management, workforce roles and restrictions etc?

In this institution, the manager has made a strategic decision about the future surgical direction for the hospital and implements changes to progress this. One of the clinical staff, a supervisor, advises our manager that staff are complaining of significantly increased workloads and, unlike last year, there is a budget shortfall. The finance department is also questioning why the hospital is facing a budget deficit for the first time. The CEO confronts the manager querying why activity is down but the budget has been expanded.

There are many factors for the harassed manager to consider in analysing the impact of previous decision-making (see Figure 29.1) and all of these factors require the collection and analysis of large amounts of information. Each impacts on the hospital's performance and bottom line to a greater or lesser extent.

Figure 29.1: Factors affecting the analysis of previous decisions

- the nature of the work that staff undertake may have changed
- the patient mix may have altered in a way that is not reflected in admission activity data, for example, the age of the patients may have increased necessitating greater levels of supervision by staff because of dementia, postoperative delirium or confusion and perhaps increased assistance with daily living activities
- the operative mix may have changed; there may be less minor surgical cases and complex cases such as an increase in complex joint revisions
- there may be less experienced clinical staff resulting in less efficient work practices
- new quality initiatives may have been introduced, requiring changes to existing work practices, with less patient contact time
- the cost of resources, drugs, pathology tests or prosthetics etc may have increased
- work practices may have changed resulting in less uniformity and greater wastage.

Have these decisions had an effective outcome?

Our manager undertakes a clinical audit, a process in which patient care is reviewed by benchmarking against some agreed and desired standards. It allows changes in clinical and non-clinical processes to meet these standards and is repeated to understand the impact of any changes and their impact on the quality of patient care. The focus is to improve care outcomes by improving the service of organisations and professional practice of clinicians. Active audits form the basis of monitoring and evaluation in healthcare.

Advances in medicine and surgery are changing the way that health services are delivered and, more importantly for our manager, they are also changing funding models. Consider this example:

One of the newer innovations in orthopaedic surgery is the use of computerised guidance devices that improve the surgeon's abilities to judge angles when cutting through bone prior to implanting joint prosthetic replacements. The importance of this is evident because patients live longer, moreover, prosthetics inserted at less than optimal angles fail earlier due to uneven forces on joints and need revision more often. Revision is often more complex due to the presence and removal of the existing prosthetic and, more importantly, patients are older and often frailer than when the original procedure was undertaken.

Our managers and clinical staff can use computer technology to balance the increased cost and time for the initial operation against the benefits in years to come from reduced total expenditure on future revisions. These decisions require extensive and ongoing monitoring of the literature, clinical auditing, good records of the types of prosthetics used, and patient data such as activity, weight, nutrition and coexisting illness. All this requires accurate and well classified long-term storage of information.

Conclusion

Decision-making always depends on the availability of quality information before the manager commits to a particular course of action. This information is essential, given that the decisions made by managers have far reaching ramifications and are crucial for the ongoing viability of health organisations and the healthcare industry itself. If data are unavailable, the effectiveness of decision-making is compromised. The tools and skills of the health informatician in making clean, quality information available to managers and clinicians are critical in any health-related decision-making.

The health informatician's role is to enable managers to look 'outside the circle' of information that is easily available and seek knowledge so that they advance rather than constrain the provision of healthcare.

Review questions

1.   What are the implications of trying to collect an 'exhaustive' list of decisions? Consider cost, time and complexity in your discussion.
2.   What are some of the non-financial decisions that can confront healthcare managers?
3.   What impact will the problems of ageing and chronic disease have on the workforce?
4.   What are the costs involved in collecting information?
5.   Where does information for decision-making come from?

Exercises

- Explore the impacts on decisions of the 'doing nothing' option and considering the 'opportunity cost'.

- Foundations built on valid information improve the decision-making outcomes. Discuss this issue for the manager in this situation. Include the style of decision-making that is most appropriate.

- Discuss the following statement: 'Planning for an unknown outcome (for example, will the new technology deliver the postulated benefit?) is a common dilemma in healthcare.'

References

Cohen, M., March, J. & Olsen J. (1972). A garbage can model of organisational choice, *Administrative Science Quarterly*, 17 March, 1–25.

Cyert, R. & March, J. (1963). *A behavioural theory of the firm*, Englewood Cliffs, Prentice Hall, NJ.

Drucker, P. (1998). The coming of the new organisation, *Harvard Business Review on Knowledge Management*, Harvard Business School Press, Boston, MA, 1–19.

Facione, P. (1998). *Critical thinking: what it is and why it counts*. Retrieved 27 January, 2005, from http://www.insightassessment.com/.

Mintzberg, H., Raisinghani, D. & Théorêt, A. (1976). The structure of unstructured decision processes, *Administrative Science Quarterly 21*, 246–75.

Paul, R.W. (1993). *Critical thinking: how to prepare students for a rapidly changing world*, Foundation for Critical Thinking, Santa Rosa, CA.

Simon, H. & March, J. (1958). *Organizations*, Wiley, New York.

Standards Australia (2004). *The language of health concept representation*, DR 04114 (Draft), Standards Australia.

30

Policy decision-making

Sheree Lloyd and Helen Cooper

'There are few things wholly evil or wholly good. Almost everything, especially of government policy, is an inseparable compound of the two, so that our best judgement of the preponderance between them is continually demanded.'
(Abraham Lincoln 1809–1865, Sixteenth President of the USA)

Outline

Policy-making in health is complex and dependent upon a range of issues, however one constant is the need for quality and timely information. The availability of information to support policy-making is critical in a modern health system. This chapter examines the ways in which policy is made and used in the health policy-making process and the fundamental role that health information and informatics plays in policy decision-making.

Introduction

Health information is an important tool that is used by policy-makers to inform decision-making, enable the establishment of research priorities, plan for healthcare delivery, identify emerging health trends, monitor and allocate resources, identify clinical best practice and facilitate the management of health services. This chapter examines the relationships between information, and the making of policy decisions in healthcare.

To demonstrate the use of information and its role in policy formation, the example of one of the national health priority areas in Australia – cancer – will be used as a case study where relevant in the chapter.

The nature of policy-making in health

'Policy is the translation of government's political priorities and principles into programmes and courses of action to deliver desired changes.'
(The Comptroller and Auditor General, 2001)

Palmer and Short (2000, p.23) affirm that 'generally, the term "health policy" embraces courses of action that affect that set of institutions, organisations, services and funding arrangements that constitute the healthcare system'. While, Hanney et al (2003, p.3) observe that policy-making:

> can include people making the policy as government ministers and officials, as local health service managers, or as representatives of a professional body. Policy-making involves those in positions of authority making choices that have a special status within the group to which they will apply. The results take many forms ranging from national health policies made by the government to clinical guidelines determined by professional bodies.

The overall objective of health policy is to improve health outcomes. In turn, health policy development can be influenced by 'events', for example, disease outbreaks such as SARS, political agendas – like the provision of universal health coverage through Medicare, professional bodies – representation by medical specialities to have medications added to the Pharmaceutical Benefits Scheme and lobbying by individuals (Hanney et al., 2003). Since 1996, the Australian Government has set a number of health priorities and targets with the aim of either disease prevention or health status improvement for the Australian population (Commonwealth of Australia, 2005). These priorities influence and inform health policy directions and strategy. One of the National Health Priority Areas is cancer and this disease will form the basis of the examples in this chapter.

Case study

In 1996, Australian Health Ministers announced cancer as a National Health Priority because of the major burden it places on the community. Statistics from the Australian Institute of Health and Welfare (Commonwealth of Australia, 2002) show that in Australia:

- about 345 000 people are diagnosed annually with cancer, and approximately 270 000 of these are non-melanocytic skin cancers
- cancer accounts for 30.2 per cent of male deaths and 25.2 per cent of female deaths annually
- the most common cancers are prostate cancer in males and breast cancer in females
- in 2000 there were 35 628 deaths from cancer
- lung cancer in males and breast cancer in females most commonly caused death
- at the current incidence rates, cancer might affect one in three men and one in four women by the age of 75.

From this data eight 'priority' cancers have been targeted:

1. Lung cancer
2. Melanoma skin cancer

3. Non-melanocytic skin cancer
4. Cancer of the cervix
5. Breast cancer
6. Colorectal cancer
7. Prostate cancer
8. Non-Hodgkins lymphoma.

Requirements for using information in a policy environment

In order to use information for policy-making it needs to be timely and broad enough to inform strategy, planning and service delivery configurations. The information used for policy-making must be able to be aggregated to provide a strategic 'big picture' view. This information should also enable the performance of the health system and its components to be measured, compared and managed in an environment of continuous improvement (Boston Consulting Group [BCG], 2004, p.31).

In short, policy-makers need information that is comprehensive and complete and that provides an overall system perspective. This information should also provide details of expenditure and sufficient detail to support quality management activities (BCG, 2004 p.33). The information should 'enable resources to be focused on the areas of highest priority and provide the ability to track health outcomes and identify continuous improvement opportunities, as well as change policy and funding as required' (BCG, 2004, p.33).

Recognising that policy-makers require good quality data and information, the Australian Government has undertaken a number of strategic activities. These include the formation of the Australian Health Information Council (AHIC) and the development and implementation of national health info- and infrastructure through the National Health Information Group (NHIG). AHIC was established to provide strategic advice on national directions and reform for information management and information and communication technology (IM&ICT) in health. The role of AHIC is to provide independent advice to help inform Australian Government jurisdictions about national priorities and the requirements of end users of health information technology. NHIG has been established 'to provide advice on national health information requirements, related technology planning and management requirements. NHIG manages and allocates resources to health information projects and working groups where joint Commonwealth/state and territory resources are involved' (Australian Government, 2004).

While both AHIC and NHIG have a major focus on information management and information and communications technology (IM & ICT) infrastructure development in Australia, both groups have also brought focus to the *infostructure* that underpins health information collection in Australia. This is evidenced by the development of standards, data dictionaries and minimum data collection sets coordinated by the

Australian Institute of Health and Welfare (AIHW). The work of these agencies serves to highlight and advance the quality of health data collections and thereby provide informed advice and evidence-base to health policy-making.

Interest box

You can learn more about Australia's work in the management of health information IM & ICT at: http://www.ahic.org.au/ and http://www.aihw.gov.au/.

There is a number of specific requirements for information used to make policy. The information must be high quality, timely, relevant, valid and available.

Quality

Unless data are of high quality, the information and knowledge that result from them have little value. For example, the value of a cancer registry is diminished if the histology of the cancer is incorrectly or incompletely reported. Poor quality data can undermine the benefits of the policy it contributed to making.

Timeliness and relevance

Information to enable effective policy-making must be timely and relevant. However, there are a number of issues, associated with this, including:
* the information lifecycle – it can take time to accrue data to evidence the issue or for trends to emerge to identify a health issue or problem
* information usage – information collected today may have uses in twenty years not anticipated today
* data cleaning – to ensure high quality data there may often be delays in data receipt due to data 'cleaning' processes.

Validity

Evans (Chapter 29) identified validity as an important factor in using information. Valid information is needed to ensure that the decisions made are appropriate.

Availability/accessibility

At times data needed to make policy might not be available or easily accessed. This includes data not collected at all or when a long lead-time is needed to gather data to evidence the issue, for example, asbestos-related cancers. Palmer and Short (2000) also acknowledge the paucity of information available to describe the quality and outcomes of healthcare treatments.

Stages in the health policy-making process

Information is needed at all stages in the health policy-making process. The Comptroller and Auditor General (2001, p.31) accentuate this, saying:

> Drawing on quality information from a variety of sources helps to establish 'what works' and to identify optimum opportunities for intervention. To be effective,

information needs to be provided and/or interpreted by experts in the field working closely with policy-makers.

Figure 30.1, adapted from the report written by the Comptroller and Auditor General in the United Kingdom, shows a typical government department's policy-making function. The involvement of information in each step of the model should be noted.

Figure 30.1: A policy-making model (adapted from the Comptroller and Auditor General, 2001)

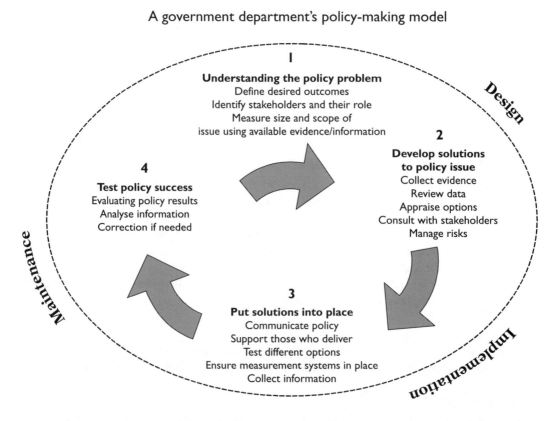

A government department's policy-making model

1
Understanding the policy problem
Define desired outcomes
Identify stakeholders and their role
Measure size and scope of
issue using available evidence/information

2
**Develop solutions
to policy issue**
Collect evidence
Review data
Appraise options
Consult with stakeholders
Manage risks

4
Test policy success
Evaluating policy results
Analyse information
Correction if needed

3
Put solutions into place
Communicate policy
Support those who deliver
Test different options
Ensure measurement systems in place
Collect information

Design

Implementation

Maintenance

Palmer and Short (2000, p.32) describe a number of steps in the health policy-making process:
- Problem identification and agenda setting – key policy problems are defined and the agenda set.
- Policy formation – policies are created or changed.
- Adoption – policy is enacted, or brought into force by state or federal legislation.
- Policy implementation – the actions and mechanisms that bring policy into practice – the policy document is turned into a reality.

Each of these steps uses information for different purposes. The table below shows these stages and examples of the types of information needed. The example below is based on the steps leading to establishing a new cancer-screening program:

Table 30.1: Establishing a cancer screening program – information needed at different stages of policy-making

Stage	Information needed
Problem identification and agenda setting	• Morbidity • Mortality
Policy formation	• Screening options • Best practice and evidence • Resource (financial and human) implications
Adoption	• Treatment options
Policy implementation	• Utilisation information • Trend data on morbidity and mortality

Evaluation of policy is also an important part of the health policy-making process. The ability to monitor and measure performance and evaluate policy against the objectives established during the formulation stage is critical to effective policy-making. Ensuring that the information needed to undertake this evaluation process will be available should be considered during the adoption and policy implementation phases.

Identifying and disseminating information about good practice, reviewing policy effectiveness and communicating the lessons learned from policy experience have also been identified as key activities in the policy-making process (The Comptroller and Auditor General, 2001).

Levels of policy and decision-making

In Australia, there is a number of governing and decision-making levels within the healthcare system. On an international level Australia contributes information that is used by the World Health Organisation (WHO) and other organisations to inform their decision and policy-making processes. Table 30.2 below shows the types of information needed at the different levels of policy and decision-making.

Table 30.2: Types of cancer-related information used at different levels of policy and decision-making

Level	International	National	State	Organisational	Departmental/ Sectional
Types of Information	Morbidity Mortality Alert, e.g., Kaposi's Sarcoma in HIV/AIDs	Morbidity Mortality Health Status Alert, e.g., Kaposi's Sarcoma in HIV/AIDs	Morbidity Mortality Screening Morphology	Morbidity Mortality Treatment Technology available	Clinical expertise Caseload Morbidity Mortality Treatment efficacy

Although there are various points of accountability for policy and decision-making in the Australian healthcare system, the information used at the various points can be drawn from many sources including hospital information systems and specialised registries such as those established for cancer. Frequently, this information is analysed in aggregate through the layers in the system from point-of-care to national database. For example, cancer incidence data are drawn from a number of sources including hospital admission data, pathology databases and death registries. This information is collected by cancer registries at state level and used to drive local policy issues. It is then aggregated to form a National Cancer Statistics Clearing House (NCSCH).

Interest box

Overview of the National Cancer Statistics Clearing House (NCSCH)

The NCSCH fosters the development and dissemination of national cancer statistics for Australia specifically to:

- enable computation and publication of national statistics on cancer
- allow tracking of interstate movement of cancer cases via record linkage
- facilitate exchange of scientific and technical information between cancer registries and promote standardisation in the collection and classification of cancer data
- facilitate cancer research both nationally and internationally.

In 1982 the NCSCH commenced to collate statistics from registries from individual states and territories. The data items provided enable record linkages and the analysis of cancer by body site and behaviour.

The NCSCH reports national incidence and mortality data. Periodically, analyses of specific cancer sites, cancer histology, differentials in cancer rates by country of birth, geographical variation, trends over time and survival are undertaken on an accumulation of data which permits examination of the data in greater depth. The NCSCH also makes a broad range of statistical data available to researchers after a strict scientific and ethical review process.

(Australian Government, n.d.)

How is information used to support policy and decision-making in health?

Health policy can be implemented to prevent disease and injury, to correct problems using 'best clinical practice' interventions, to treat patients by providing access to care, or to manage the use of resources (such as the availability of drugs listed on the Pharmaceutical Benefits Scheme) in line with government policy and direction.

Policy-making involves a number of stages. Decisions about current and future policy are likely to embrace a range of routine activities performed as part of the policy-making process. Information is an important component of all stages of the policy-making process and Table 30.3, adapted from the BCG, shows the ways in which information can be used in policy applications, again using the example of cancer as a disease entity.

Table 30.3: Examples of data used to meet varying policy applications (adapted from Boston Consulting Group, 2004)

Policy applications	Types of Information
Performance monitoring	• Cancer trends • Benchmarking
Survey	• Health status
Research	• Epidemiology of cancer
Registries and Screening	• Collection of cases • Screening of the community • Incidence • Survival • Morphology • Risk factors
Management and Administration	• Morbidity • Mortality • Costing data • Safety and quality of treatment for cancer
Resource allocation (e.g. high cost drugs, funding of linear accelerators)	• Cancer trends • Health status • Treatment efficacy • Evaluation

In 2005, the Australia Government released the National Sexually Transmissible Infections Strategy 2005–2008 to control sexually transmissible infections. One part of this strategy is aimed at better identifying and treating Chlamydia infections. This was based on evidence demonstrating an increase in infections (Commonwealth of Australia, 2005). The information system was able to trend data that showed a marked increase in notifications of Chlamydia. This document is freely available from the Internet and provides another example of how data have been used to inform this strategy and the policy-making process.

Ensuring that services provided are of a high quality and safe is an emerging issue in healthcare systems around the world. Hovenga and Lloyd (2005) relate that increasingly agreement is being sought on the type of data items that need to be reported in order to assess the health system performance, particularly in relation to the safety and quality of healthcare services. These data will inform and influence the policy that is made in order to ensure the safety and quality of healthcare systems.

Types of information and information systems needed to inform policy and decision-making

Healthcare organisations use data and information derived from their information systems to manage the clinical and administrative aspects of their business. These information systems form the basis of reporting used for many different purposes including policy-making. At each level of the health system key stakeholders have different data requirements. Figure 30.3 below shows examples of these requirements.

Table 30.4: Health stakeholder data requirements

Key stakeholders	Data requirements	Example data types
Policy-makers	Fitness for purpose for example:	Performance monitoring
		Surveys
Administrators and Health Service managers	• Detail level	Patient history
	• Anonymity when needed	Registries and screening
Providers	• Aggregation	Case series
Patients/consumers	• Linkages to other data sets	Case studies
Researchers	• Ability to supplement from other sources if needed	Administrative
		Financial
		Management
		Indicators of safety
		Quality measures

Adapted from: Boston Consulting Group (2004, p.33)

Health information systems and processes have developed and evolved to support the increasingly wide range of uses, including policy-making, through progressively more comprehensive data collections.

Clinical

Clinicians collect a range of data and are supported by information systems that report on patient history, status, movement and results. Clinicians also use research databases and clinical monitoring systems that provide information to support and make policy concerning their domain.

Operational and administrative systems

Operational systems have been widely used to support decision-making to inform the policy-making process and were among the first systems deployed in healthcare. These:

- register and track patients
- record morbidity and mortality information
- manage financial, human and physical resources.

These systems play an integral part in providing information used in the policy-making process.

Research databases

Hanney et al. (2003, p.23) relate that research in health policy-making:

> should eventually lead to desired outcomes, including health gains. Research can make a contribution in at least three phases of the policy-making process: agenda setting; policy formulation; and implementation.

Research data in health may source new or existing data and study it in purposeful ways to answer particular issues or problems. The study may be in response to a possible policy issue or lead to 'new' policy. For example, studies into the benefits of bowel cancer screening programs may lead to a national policy for a bowel cancer screening program or alternatively to best practice clinical guidelines.

Alert systems

Disease outbreak notification systems are a prime example of alert systems. Due to experiences of infectious disease epidemics (for example, polio in the 1950s), the international community has recognised that alert systems operating from local through to international levels are vital to the early detection of serious disease outbreaks. The experiences of SARS and avian influenza are examples of how alert systems can motivate and dictate policy in the health system.

Performance monitoring and utilisation

Performance monitoring and using information systems in health are both influenced by and can influence policy. The monitoring of the incidence of various cancers in the community has been influenced by the listing of Cancer as a National Health Priority Area. In turn, the list of cancers of particular focus (see case study) within that policy arena has been influenced by the monitoring of the incidence of particular cancers in the population.

Financial management and resource allocation

It is well documented that the Australian healthcare system continuously struggles to afford the level of health services and care that the community demands and expects. Implementing certain types of treatment and care increasingly requires evidence of outcomes and benefits to society and the consumer. Finance and resource use are integral to these debates (see Edwards, Chapter 12). Financial systems that cover the public and private health services and the costs of care are both subject to policy as well as influencing policy. One example that demonstrates this is the use of financial data in conjunction with clinical data to determine cancer treatments that deliver the best outcomes and are economically sustainable.

The knowledge of how resources other than financial are used is important to health policy-makers. In particular, how human resources are allocated in the health system is an issue. The changing age profile of the Australian population is reflected in the health industry, for instance, in 2001 the average age of the nursing workforce was 42.2 years (Australian Government, 2001). Human resource management databases in the health system provide part of the information used to determine the profile of the health workforce and to determine workforce issues for the health sector. They are also the basis of ongoing health workforce issues research and analysis and many of these are publicly available on websites.[1]

Financial data are essential for health policy-makers to distribute or redistribute health resources. Casemix funding models are one example of where data has been integral to a particular policy direction. In Victoria, in the 1990s data were used to formulate, implement, monitor and refine a casemix funding policy.

Interdependencies that can affect information management

Policy-making is a complex process and is unable to be developed in isolation. It is dependent upon and influenced by a number of interdependencies including legal/legislative issues and societal expectations.

Legal/legislative

Policy can 'make' law and legal precedent can influence policy. One example of this might be privacy policy becoming Privacy Law or the development of informed consent policy to address medico-legal issues within healthcare settings.

Societal expectations

Policy is informed by demands and expectations of healthcare consumers and society. An example here is the introduction of a national health identifier. This has been identified as a pre-requisite to an electronic health record that will enable better health outcomes and linkage across the different points of healthcare. However, a national health identifier is a policy direction that has been unpalatable to some parts of the community. As a consequence, governments have been reluctant to pursue this strategy.

Influence of other government agencies

Health policy can be informed by other agencies and vice versa; examples of this are injury prevention and road safety initiatives. This type of interdependency has seen the introduction of seatbelts and child restraints in cars as well as pushbike helmets.

Obstacles to using information in the policy-making process

> The extreme complexity of the policymaking process is compounded by '... many genuine obstacles to evidence-based policy-making'.
>
> (Hanney et al, 2003, p.2.)

Political agendas

Health policy-making is often influenced by the priorities of particular governments and the profile of 'hot topics' in health. Political support for a problem has the potential to redirect limited resources to that issue. This may also drive new information requirements, for example, the establishment of the National Cost Data Collection in Australia arose from the emphasis of the government of the day on casemix measurement. This costing information is now routinely collected and is used for benchmarking, budget allocation and performance monitoring.

Financial

Information is needed to justify how resources can be best allocated in line with policy. The plight of the health system and its inability to cope with demand is consistently highlighted in the media and, although research and data support this, there simply may not be enough financial resources to implement the solution (or the solution may come at a cost to other issues). An example here is where resources might be allocated to developing screening programs for prostate cancer, but this in turn could mean reduced funding to meningococcal immunisation. Policy-makers must constantly balance the need for policy with the cost of its implementation.

Advocating agencies

Often a health issue will be brought to political and community focus through advocating agencies based in the community, for example the Country Women's Association (CWA), Rotary and Lions. While the issue might have merit, developing and implementing policy to address it may come at a cost to addressing other equally urgent concerns. Policy-makers need to be able to analyse the concerns of these community groups and explore options through the use of a number of strategies that might include information analysis.

Flexibility and suitability of information technology systems

Independent institutions and providers largely deliver healthcare in Australia and, as discussed in earlier chapters, this leads to information silos. There are many initiatives underway aimed at integrating information systems and providing better information. One of the difficulties is the lack of standardisation of systems and environments. According to the Boston Consulting Group (2004), '... policy-makers often struggle to locate, interpret and validate the information they need to manage the system and enhance outcomes for consumers'. The National E-Health Transition Authority (NEHTA) initiatives (discussed in previous chapters) will lead to the developments of standards and enabling infrastructure to counter this. Improved information systems and flexibility will facilitate policy-making into the future.

The United Kingdom has identified that information and criteria to review, evaluate and measure performance should be built into the policy implementation process, because if 'information is not available then the success of policy implementation may be unclear' (The Comptroller and Auditor General, 2001 p.3).

Volume of information

The vast size and rapid increase in new information every day poses challenges to its use in the policy-making process. As reported by Hovenga and Lloyd (2005), one of the challenges for healthcare organisations is the assimilation and management of new knowledge and its availability to managers and clinicians in real time. This is no less a challenge for policy-makers and raises the issue of balancing information assimilation with timely policy-making.

Presenting information to policy-makers

One of the important issues in using information to inform and set policy is presenting information in ways that identify the relevant issues, alert policy-makers to possible problems, and enable monitoring.

Healthcare organisations collect vast amounts of data to satisfy a range of needs. However, there can be a temptation to gather large amounts of information from a variety of sources to ensure informed decision-making, and more is not always better. The risk is of long delays in policy-making for issues that are affecting the population now and that might have wide-ranging effects on the entire community.

It is also important to present information in ways that enable policy-makers to identify trends. Health researchers must present data to policy-makers as useable information, to enable them to quickly identify issues that are in line with policy and that provide the information necessary to address those issues. A classic example is where research demonstrated the benefits of cancer screening programs in the early detection and therefore treatment of cancers.

The benefits of Cancer Registries led to improvement in the quality of the data collected and to policies and government funding for cancer prevention campaigns (such as 'Slip, Slop, Slap').

Hanney et al. (2003) also explain the importance of using health research, noting that research and other information should contribute to policies that may eventually lead to improved health gains. These authors provide an excellent overview of the issue of integrating research information into the policy process to illustrate this point.

While aggregate information is essential, the ability to 'drill down' through the layers of data when needed is also an important requirement. Presenting information in a meaningful way greatly assists in its understanding, while enabling users to examine and draw appropriate conclusions from it. A number of different techniques and methods that effectively achieve this, for example, the use of tables and graphs clearly depicts trends or outcomes.

The role of information, knowledge management and evidence in policy-making

The information processing cycle discussed in Chapter 6 is also seen here, where data are analysed becoming information and then applied becoming knowledge, which is used to develop and evaluate policy and drives the need for more data. Put simply, quality information from centralised computer systems can drive or initiate policy. Examples of data are provided in Figures 30.2 and 30.3 to demonstrate this point.

Figure 30.2: How information can initiate policy in health

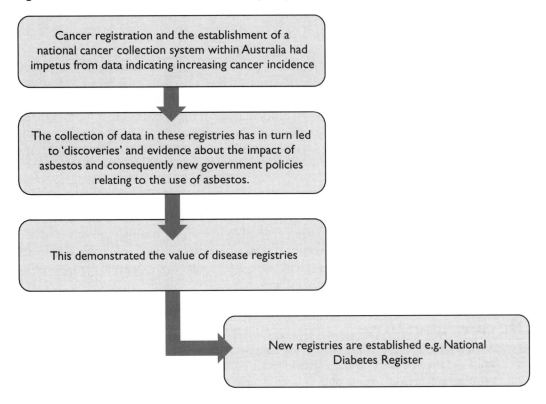

The National Injury Surveillance Program is another Australian example, and an adapted model for policy-making is shown below as Figure 30.3.

Figure 30.3: Example of how data can lead directly to policy in health

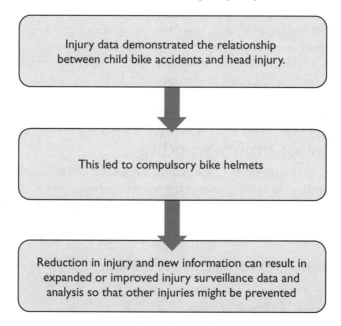

Injury data demonstrated the relationship between child bike accidents and head injury.

This led to compulsory bike helmets

Reduction in injury and new information can result in expanded or improved injury surveillance data and analysis so that other injuries might be prevented

The Australia Government (2005, p.4) observes that 'evidence-based policy ensures improved efficiency and effectiveness through adoption of and continuous evaluation of proven interventions and knowledge'. Information and its analysis are integral to this process. Investment in information management and technologies will improve 'the collection, management and dissemination of health information boosting administrators' and policy-makers' ability to undertake informed, system-wide planning' (BCG, 2004).

Conclusion

The ultimate aim of health policy is to ensure that the health system improves health outcomes and that services provided are acceptable to the community, are safe and are of a high quality. Good quality information is required to support policy development because implementing reasonable, logical and cost-effective policy must also consider and be sensitive to societal values and beliefs.

Review questions

1. What are the sources of information for policy-making?
2. What are the barriers to using information for policy-making?
3. What do you consider some of the key challenges are for policy-makers when using health information?

4.   What are some of the key issues for managers of health information, if appropriate policy is to be developed and implmented in health care?

Exercise

- In healthcare, does policy-making influence data collection, or does data influence policy-making? Discuss this in relation to the National Health Priority Areas and the National Health Information agenda.

Online reading

INFOTRAC® COLLEGE EDITION
For additional readings and review on information in policy decision-making, explore **InfoTrac® College Edition**, your online library. Go to: **www.infotrac-college.com** and search for any of the InfoTrac key terms listed below:
- Evidence-based policy-making
- Knowledge management
- Performance monitoring
- Policy
- Policy-making
- Trends

References

Australian Government (2001). *Labour force – nurses*. Retrieved 30 June, 2005, from http://www.aihw.gov.au/labourforce/nurses.cfm.

Australian Government (2004). *About NHIG*. Retrieved 26 June, 2005, from http://www.ahic.org.au/nhig/.

Australian Government (n.d.). *Overview: National Cancer Statistics Clearing House*. Retrieved 1 July, 2005, from http://www.aihw.gov.au/.

Boston Consulting Group (2004). *National health information and communications technology strategy report*. Retrieved 23 March from http://www7.health.gov.au/.

Commonwealth of Australia (2004). *Year book Australia, number 86,* Australian Bureau of Statistics, Canberra, ABS Catalogue no.1301.0.

Commonwealth of Australia (2002). *Australia's health*. Australian Institute of Health and Welfare, Canberra.

Commonwealth of Australia (2005). *National sexually transmissible infections strategy 2005- 2008,* Canberra.

The Comptroller and Auditor General (2001). *Modern policy-making: ensuring policies deliver value for money* (No. HC 289 Session 2001–2002). House of Commons, London.

Hanney, S., Gonzalez-Block, M., Buxton M. & Kogan, M. (2003). The utilisation of health research in policy-making: concepts, examples and methods of assessment, *Health Research Policy and Systems*. Retrieved 24 June, 2005, from http://www.health-policy-systems.com/.

Hovenga E. & Lloyd, S. (2005). Working with information and knowledge, in M.G. Harris and Associates (eds), *Managing Health Services: Concepts and Practice*, 2nd edn, Elsevier (in press).

Palmer, G. & Short, S. (2000). *Healthcare and public policy: an Australian analysis,* 3rd edn, Allen and Unwin, Sydney.

Endnote

[1]   http://www.aihw.gov.au/publications/.

Part 7

Pushing the boundaries

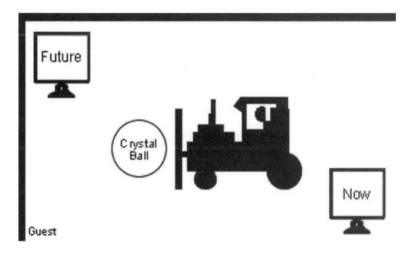

31

Genomics and biotechnology

David Mitchell

'This structure (DNA) has novel features which may be of considerable biological interest.'

(James Watson and Francis Crick, 1953)

Outline

This chapter will explore the relationship between molecular genetics and health informatics. It will provide a historical context against which to view the current position in molecular genetics and show how that is likely to impact health informatics.

Introduction

We stand at a healthcare crossroads. In one direction healthcare costs are spiralling out of control: expensive drugs, designer therapies, chronic lifestyle diseases and bloated informatics projects driven by entrenched interests. In another direction, we can see a high standard of care for the privileged and an increasingly lower standard of care for the rest, as the public/private divide in healthcare grows. Finally, we can look down a road where healthcare information is used to drive evidence-based programs to reduce healthcare costs, the latest technologies are available when needed, and there is a high quality of care for all Australians.

We now have a plethora of detailed genetic information that we are able to integrate with the clinical information collected as a patient interacts with the healthcare system. If we assume that health informatics will seamlessly integrate all this information and make it available at our fingertips, how will that change our lives?

What is a genome?

Genomics is the study of an organism's genome, that is, how its DNA is arranged, how many genes it has and their function and expression. Starting with the elucidation of the structure of DNA in 1953 (see 'Interest box'), and finishing with the complete sequence of the human genome in 2001, the study of molecular genetics has exploded over the last fifty years.

Interest box

The structure of DNA

In 1953, in the Cavendish laboratory, Cambridge, James Watson and Francis Crick elucidated the structure of DNA. The second sentence of their seminal paper in the journal *Nature*, 'This structure has novel features which may be of considerable biological interest', must be one of the scientific understatements of all time. Many people view this as the beginning of the modern era of molecular genetics. The story of this discovery is told in Watson's own words in the somewhat controversial book *The Double Helix* (Watson, 1968).

Humans have forty-six chromosomes. There are twenty-two pairs (think, socks) and two sex chromosomes, X and Y (think, odd socks). Each parent contributes one chromosome from each pair and one sex chromosome. Females are XX and males XY. So your mother always gives you an X. If your father gives you an X, you are a girl, if he gives you a Y, you are a boy. Chromosomes are made up of DNA wrapped round special proteins called 'histones'. But the DNA is the real story. This is the code that determines what we will look like, how fast we can run 100 meters and, to a certain extent, how smart we will be and how long we will live. Of course, there is a fair bit of environmental influence, but just how much is genes and how much is environment is a great discussion.

DNA is written in a code of four bases, adenine (A), guanine (G), cytosine (C) and thymine (T). The actual molecule is a double strand of these bases on a backbone. Think about slicing a ladder down the middle, the backbones are at the edge and the bases pair up in the middle. The genome is made up of 'expressed' DNA (genes that code for proteins) and 'non-expressed' DNA, which is essentially everything else. The non-expressed DNA is often referred to as 'junk' and is actually about 95 per cent of the genome. Junk DNA contains all sorts of things, repeat sequences, bits of leftover viruses, old genes, control sequences, and so forth, but it seems that junk DNA might be the most interesting part of the genome. The more it is examined, the more its important functions are discovered.

The rise of sequencing

Initially research focused on the function of genes. One of the first genes cloned was for human insulin, which had previously been purified from pigs. This had immediate and direct benefit for diabetics. More and more expressed genes were cloned with sequence information deposited in a number of newly established databases. GenBank® (see 'Interest box') has become the worldwide repository of sequence information.

Interest box

NCBI – National Center for Biotechnology Information (NCBI)

Established in 1988, the NCBI (http://www.ncbi.nlm.nih.gov/), part of the National Institutes of Health (NIH) in the USA, is home to the world's largest database of publicly available DNA sequence, GenBank®. Researchers from all over the world use it to deposit gene sequences. From modest beginnings in 1982 when it had just over 600 sequences containing 680 000 base pairs, in 2004 it catalogued 40.5 million sequences containing 44.5 billion base pairs of information.

Throughout the 1980s, more and more genes were sequenced from many different organisms and by 1988 there was a vigorous discussion about tackling the sequencing of the whole human genome. At that stage, sequencing anything greater than 100 000 base pairs was a major undertaking and the thought of sequencing three billion base pairs of the human genome was hotly debated (after all, most of it was junk!). After much discussion, the sequencing of the human genome was started more or less simultaneously in the United States, Italy, the USSR, Canada, Japan and the European Union (Cook-Deegan, 1994). It is interesting to note that Australia was a glaring omission.

The Human Genome Project (HGP) was launched in 1990 (with significant funding from the NIH and the US Department of Energy) and initially concentrated on mapping activities in mice and humans and the sequencing of several smaller genomes, including the bacteria *Escherichia coli* and the nematode worm *Caenorhabditis elegans*. This latter effort served to refine sequencing methods and, in the mid-1990s, it became clear that it would be possible to actually sequence the human genome.

The International Human Genome Sequencing Consortium (IHGSC) was a publicly funded collaboration of twenty groups in six countries dedicated to sequencing the human genome. They were committed to making public all data and, as such, raw sequence data was uploaded into public databases every night. By March 1999 they had about 10 per cent of the genome completed. But, despite all these efforts, in the end the complete draft genome of humans was completed, from scratch, in only nine months by a private company, Celera Genomics based in Rockville, Maryland (Venter et al., 2001) – if only the story were that simple!

The sequence of the human genome

Ultimately, the effort to complete the sequence of the human genome became a race, and like all good stories was a mix of politics, power and personalities. Part of the difference between the two groups was a difference in strategy. Celera Genomics, led by Craig Venter, believed that the whole genome could be cut up randomly into small pieces, sequenced piece by piece and the complete sequence assembled using powerful computer programs. This approach, called 'whole genome shotgun', relied on significant computing power. However, Venter had already trialled the approach on smaller bacterial genomes (around four million bases) when he was Director of

The Institute for Genomic Research[1] (TIGR). The IHGSC, on the other hand, believed that the genome should be cut up into large pieces, and then ordered in a series of overlapping segments to make complete chromosomes. Each segment would then be shotgun sequenced and the genome assembled in a hierarchical way.

February 2001 saw the simultaneous publication of the complete draft sequence of the human genome. IHGSC published in the journal *Nature* on 15 February (International Human Genome Sequencing Consortium, 2001) and Celera Genomics in *Science* on the 16 February (Venter et al., 2001). This achievement attracted significant attention on the world stage and there was even a joint statement and press conference by America's President, Bill Clinton, and Great Britain's Prime Minister, Tony Blair, on 14 March. There was a great enthusiasm for the project with Celera Genomics raising nearly one billion $(US) in March 2000 on the stock market. Interestingly, Celera Genomics completed their sequence in nine months (compared to IHGSC's fifteen) and it was of significantly better quality. However, they were also able to use the data from the IHGSC's effort as it was made publicly available in real time.

The 'final' sequence of the human genome was published by the IHGSC in October 2004 (International Human Genome Sequencing Consortium, 2004). While there are still things to be resolved (341 gaps for example), for all intents and purposes, this finished sequence will provide a complete picture of our genome. Some summary statistics of Build 35 of the Human Genome are summarised in Table 31.1.

Table 31.1: This is as close as we will get for now. The highlights from Build 35 of the human genome (International Human Genome Sequencing Consortium, 2004)

The Human Genome – the stats	
Length	2 851 330 913 bp
Gaps	341
Coverage	99%
Error rate	1 in 100 000
Expressed genes	20 000–25 000

February 15, 2001 was the day when the pre-conceived notion of our species superiority was dealt a severe blow. For the latter part of the 1990s, a vigorous debate ensued about the number of expressed genes in humans. Initial work sequencing expressed genes suggested that humans might have as many as 120 000 genes (Liang, 2000) – 100 000 also had a pleasing ring and was often quoted. Essentially two major schools of thought emerged. One school believed that humans were 'superior' to other species and hence we would have more genes (language was often cited as a reason) and the other school believed that we are basically the same as other organisms and would have about the same number of genes. The latter school was right – humans have around 21 000 genes, more than fruit flies, but less than rice.

The Human Genome Project and bioinformatics

One of the more interesting things about the human genome project (apart from the actual sequence of course) was that it took biology out of the laboratory and into the factory. Some of the earliest debates about sequencing the genome was about the philosophy of how it should be done. Venter et al. (2001) favoured a large-scale factory approach, pioneered at TIGR and perfected at Celera Genomics. Others believed that the physical sequencing would be distributed to many laboratories and the data integration and analysis carried out at a central location. At the beginning, everyone felt that some, as yet undiscovered technology, would mostly sequence the genome. In the end, it came down to industrialisation, automation and optimisation of existing technologies (used by both groups). The factory won. Biology had become a 'discovery' science where the application of fairly straightforward technology on a massive scale generated interesting and important results.

Bioinformatics played three crucial roles in the sequencing effort. The first was in moving from manual to automated sequencing, the second was in the assembly of genomic sequence, and the third was in the data analysis.

> Bioinformatics is the collection, organisation and analysis of large amounts of biological data, using networks of computers and databases.
> (www.abc.net.au/science/slab/genome2001/glossary.htm)

Initially bioinformatics became important as more and more sequence was deposited into sequence databases. Even though most of the sequence was generated manually, the sheer numbers of entries threatened to overwhelm database curators. The European Molecular Biology Laboratory (EMBL) sequence database (established in 1982) employed a small army of curators to assign accession numbers to incoming sequence and incorporate them into the growing database. Every so often the database was 'frozen' and two to three months later a release was distributed on magnetic tape. As the volume of data increased, there became very real limitations around the amount of processing power available to run similarity searches over the entire database. This drove a demand for centralised biological computing facilities as well as more efficient search algorithms.

As sequencing moved from a manual to a fully automated process, many things that had been done manually had to be automated. Sequence data was read directly from automated sequencers, trimmed of extraneous sequences and deposited into databases. This in turn increased the amount of data in databases, exacerbating problems of analysis. However, arguably the most significant contribution of bioinformatics to the Human Genome Project was the development of methods (and the harnessing of enough computing power) to assemble whole genome sequences from a series of individual runs. Craig Venter at TIGR pioneered this with the sequencing of *Haemophilus influenzae* (Fleischmann et al., 1995).

TIGR chopped up the whole chromosome (bacteria only have one) into short fragments and sequenced them at random. Then they used a bank of networked computers to assemble the pieces into a single sequence. Celera Genomics also used this technique in their draft of the human genome. They had the added advantage of being able to take the data from the public project, shred it into short fragments and add it to their own data, thereby generating a better draft. Without the advances in bioinformatics (and an inexorable increase in computing power) made by a number of large-scale sequencing projects, the human genome project would have been a different story.

Finally, bioinformatics has become an entirely separate discipline. There is a massive amount of sequencing, expression and genetic data in the public domain and a great deal in private hands. There is a push to extract information from this data for a wide range of applications, including the development of pharmaceuticals, diagnostics and selection of beneficial traits in agribusiness. With the integration of clinical, lifestyle and genetic data, bioinformatics/health informatics will play a crucial role in future healthcare.

Single nucleotide polymorphisms (SNPs)

SNPs (pronounced 'snips') are single base changes in our genomic sequence. Think of comparing two identical books, but every so often a letter has been changed. You can still read the book and understand the text, but not all words are spelt the same. SNPs are what makes you, you and me, me. For a change to be considered a SNP, it must occur in at least one per cent of the population. It is estimated that there is a SNP every 1200 base pairs along our genome. So we anticipate human variation can be attributed to around 10 million SNPs.

SNPs are very useful for tracking regions of our genome. They do not vary much from generation to generation, and while they are not usually the cause of disease, they move with DNA that may be associated with disease (even if we do not actually know what that particular piece of DNA does yet). As a consequence, a number of companies and research institutions are very interested in developing technology to measure thousands of SNPs at once for individuals. One of these companies is Affymetrix[2], who have developed an array-based platform that measures 100 000 different SNPs (using two arrays). These are evenly spaced over the genome so they provide a 'map' with a resolution of just over 23 000 bases. Eventually they hope to be able to measure 500 000 SNPs at once.

Researchers have long linked specific mutations with predisposition to disease. The BRCA1 and BRCA2 mutations for breast and ovarian cancer are particularly well known (Miki et al., 1994), if only because Myriad Genetics patented them. However, in these studies they surveyed a large number of families with a limited number of markers. With the advent of 'genome scanning' technology for SNPs, it should be now possible to link so-called 'non-causative' SNPs with disease by association studies. Not only does this open up new possibilities for genomic molecular diagnostics and prognostics, but it also opens up the possibility of linking drug efficacy to a person's genetic makeup.

Figure 31.1: an Affymetrix SNP array

(Image courtesy of Glenn Brown, CSIRO.)

In this Affymetrix SNP array, each square (feature) has a different DNA sequence (oligonucleotide) and currently there are over 2.6 million features per array. However, a number of oligonucleotides are needed to measure each SNP and so the number of SNPs measured per array is around 50 000.

The HapMap project

Having sequenced the human genome, researchers are now interested in individual genomic variation and how that might be linked to health and disease. In a similar vein to the IHGSC, the international community established the haplotype mapping project (The HapMap[3], 2002). The HapMap will look at genetic variation in 270 individuals from four populations, the Yoruba in Nigeria, Japanese, Han Chinese and the USA (northern and western European ancestry). Over one million SNPs will be genotyped and all the results made publicly available. It is anticipated that this will provide the basis for linking individual variation to the genes responsible for predisposition to disease or lifestyle factors such as obesity and responsiveness to drugs as well as linkages to environmental factors.

Progress in human molecular genetics has been looking at the human genome in greater detail. Initially interesting expressed genes were sequenced on a case by case basis, then the expressed sequences were looked at wholesale and finally sequenced the complete genome. Now we are looking at the *variation* between whole genomes.

Studying individual genes has increased our understanding of disease and disease control enormously and leads to a range of new medicines. However, it is the study of variation between individuals that will lead to medicines that act specifically on groups of individuals. This is now called 'personalised medicine'.

Pharmacogenomics and personalised medicine

There has been increasing recognition that medicines act differently on different patients and under different conditions. It has been well documented that medicines can interact, either with each other or with environmental factors, especially diet. However, there is an increasing body of evidence to suggest that our genotype can play a significant role. A recent study published in *The Lancet* (Israel et al., 2004) found that people with a particular genotype (representing about one sixth of the American population) had adverse responses to a common drug used to treat asthma. While this genotype change was within a gene, it is reasonable to assume that genotype variation in non-expressed regions of the genome may act as 'markers' for different conditions.

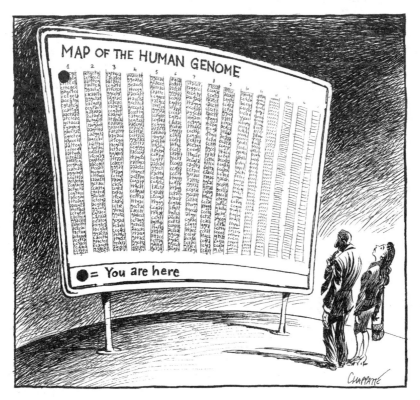

The idea that new medicines approved may be only able to be prescribed to a subsection of the population has split the ethical pharmaceutical industry. On one side are those who believe that this will in fact lead to more drugs approved, as they will be able to be shown to be effective. On the other are those that believe that the era of the 'blockbuster' drug is finished and that the pharmaceutical industry will become unviable. Only time will tell.

Case study
– SNPs and the Pharmaceutical Benefits Scheme (PBS)

The PBS subsidises the cost of medicines for Australians. The PBS is a very effective mechanism for controlling the costs of medicines by using the government's bulk purchasing power. Currently, medicines are not available through the PBS unless they have been shown to be more effective than existing treatments. However, we know that some medicines are not effective on all people, with part of that being due to genetic differences. Imagine if we could prescribe medicines based on the knowledge of a person's individual genetic makeup – it might not be as far away as we think.

Currently, all children born in Australia are tested for a number of metabolic genetic diseases by screening a blood sample taken when the baby is under 10 days old. This is done by pricking the heel of their foot and absorbing some blood on a card. This was pioneered by Guthrie in 1961 to detect phenylketonuria, hence the name, 'Guthrie Cards'. There is currently a vigorous debate about who can have access to the DNA contained in the blood sample stored on Guthrie Cards. In Western Australia, Guthrie Cards are only kept for two years to prevent possible 'misuse' later in life.

A modern day Guthrie card might be a standardised 500K SNP chip (measuring 500 000 SNPs). The information from this chip (the individual genotype) would be securely stored in a centralised database and linked to the patient's (your) Medicare number. When a doctor wants to prescribe a drug on the PBS they type in the patient's name, Medicare number, and the drug to see if the PBS will pay for it. The PBS would only decline to prescribe a particular drug if it had been shown to be ineffective for the patient's particular genotype.

The impact of genomics on health informatics

Genomics has clearly already had a significant impact on healthcare. There are many new drugs in clinical development that owe their origins to genes discovered as part of the human genome project. However, it is now with the advent of large-scale genotyping that the interplay of individual genotype information with individual lifestyle and clinical data will add an extra dimension to health informatics.

The fundamental difference about genotype data is that it does not change (ever). So if genotyping data is collected it can be archived and accessed whenever needed. So long as the same panel of SNP markers is used for example, the genotyping data collected when you are a child could be useful for a drug that will not be invented for fifty years. The question becomes: How is the data, such as that collected on Guthrie Cards, archived and stored for life without compromising privacy, but at the same time always remain available for access when needed? In an ideal world, it would be part of the personal health record accessible at any time by healthcare practitioners to provide better healthcare outcomes.

Conclusion

At the beginning of this chapter there were a number of alternatives for healthcare in the future. Combining genomic data with other healthcare data in a single seamless integrated system could provide improved outcomes for patients through more effective treatments, early intervention for some diseases and less adverse incidents – and all at a lower cost.

Review questions

1. What does SNP stand for, what are SNPs and how many do you have? How many does your best friend have? (If you don't have a best friend you can skip this part of the question.)
2. How many expressed genes are there in the human genome? Is this more or less what was previously thought? What percentage of our DNA codes for expressed genes? What is the rest of the DNA commonly called?

Exercise

The National Center for Biotechnology Information (www.ncbi.nlm.nih.gov) contains GenBank, the repository of DNA sequence information. The site contains statistics for the number of base pairs of information deposited from 1982–2004.

Estimate the number of base pairs of information that GenBank will contain in 2025 if we continue to increase our rate of sequencing at the current rate.

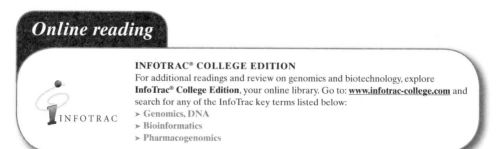

Online reading

INFOTRAC® COLLEGE EDITION
For additional readings and review on genomics and biotechnology, explore
InfoTrac® College Edition, your online library. Go to: **www.infotrac-college.com** and
search for any of the InfoTrac key terms listed below:
➤ Genomics, DNA
➤ Bioinformatics
➤ Pharmacogenomics

INFOTRAC

References

Cook-Deegan, R. (1994). The origins of the human genome project, *Risk: Health, Safety and Environment* 5, 97.

Fleischmann, R. et al. (1995). Whole-genome random sequencing and assembly of Haemophilus influenzae Rd, *Science* 269(5223), 496–512.

International Human Genome Sequencing Consortium (2001). Initial sequencing and analysis of the human genome, *Nature*, 409, 860–921.

International Human Genome Sequencing Consortium (2004). 'Finishing the Euchromatic Sequence of the human genome', *Nature*, 431, 931–45.

Israel, E. et al. (2004). Use of regularly scheduled albuterol treatment in asthma: genotype-stratified, randomised, placebo-controlled cross-over trial, *The Lancet*, 364(9444), 1464–6.

Liang, F. et al. (2000). Gene index analysis of the human genome estimates approximately 120 000 genes, *Nature Genet*, 25, 239–40.

Miki, Y. et al. (1994). A strong candidate for the breast and ovarian cancer susceptibility gene BRCA1. *Science*, 226(5182), 66–71.

The HapMap (2002). Retrieved 15 August, 2005, from http://www.hapmap.org/.

Venter, J.C. et al. (2001). The sequence of the human genome, *Science*, 291(5507), 1304–51.

Watson, J. & Crick, F. (1953). A structure for Deoxyribose Nucleic Acid, *Nature* 171, 737.

Watson, J. (1968). *The double Helix – a personal account of the discovery of the structure of DNA*, Touchstone.

Endnotes

[1]   https://www.tigr.org.

[2]   http://www.affymetrix.com.

[3]   http://www.hapmap.org/.

32

Gazing into the crystal ball

Moya Conrick with contributions from Bob Ribbons, Sisira Edirippuligé and Richard Wootton

'Prediction is very difficult, especially of the future.'

(Niels Bohr, Danish physicist 1885–1962)

Outline

This chapter allows us to gaze into the future where 'bleeding edge' technology, genomics and advanced robotics underpin the utopian vision for many health workers, of equitable healthcare for all … or we can come back to earth and consider where we are now and where we might reasonably be headed.

Introduction

In the current healthcare systems we have winners and losers and the winners are not always those people for whom the system operates. Choice allows consumers to select caregivers or other providers based on their own criteria. They usually see more than one practitioner a year and this leads to fragmentation of care with its inherent problems of error, duplication, lack of coordination, and so on. Consumer-focused collaborative care delivery models must be central to any system and technology has the power to enable this with integration and interoperability holding the key to future services and service development.

In this book many authors have referred to the silos in the current health system, most discussed ways to negate these, and all referred to the interoperability of systems. Technical barriers and a lack of standards have cultivated the silos until recently, but advances in these areas mean that health can become truly interoperable and consumer-centric.

Interoperability has the capacity to offer a global health system where there are no boundaries and all people are able to access quality resources and healthcare, no matter their means, continent or country. Innovative technologies can help us to realise some of that dream, but sadly that will not be enough. It requires much commitment, leadership, a skilled workforce, and adequate funding for research and development to make it a reality, and perhaps we need to begin closer to home in our own under-serviced rural and remote communities.

Case study

Think of an information-rich, consumer-centric healthcare sector where patients' health information seamlessly and securely follows them across geographic boundaries and between multiple healthcare providers. This system stores a patient's complete health and medications history, health records, a current medication list, laboratory results, scans and x-rays, and all other information relevant to the person. These data are available to clinicians with appropriate access at the point-of-care in fractions of a second.

All medication orders are processed by computerised systems that automatically check for correct doses and send alerts about allergies, a dose too high or too low or likely drug interactions. In this system, decision-making is informed and guided by current, timely and evidence-based practice guidelines and information tools. The consumer has a partnership with clinicians. They hold and annotate their own health record, and only essential personal contact is needed. Communications that do not require face-to-face meeting occur electronically.

The aged are cared for at home with devices like robots. Other communications devices enable families to know exactly what their older family member is doing, sensors feed back positions in the house, alert carers to falls or simply report that the person is resting. The interactive panel on the fridge door reminds them that it is time for a meal. When the prepacked meal is taken from the fridge it is scanned and an order placed with the online supermarket. The carer is also notified of this event. If the medications or carer robot is offline the electronic medications box reminds our person verbally to take the medication and how to take it: 'Take the blue pill now with a glass of milk'.

Well, maybe ... however, most of the technology introduced in this case study already exists or is a prototype in someone's laboratory; at this time it is not at the same place at the same time. Trends and future directions in healthcare and the use of technology are interdependent and are reliant on people as well as the technology.

Drivers accelerating automation

Although there will be increased spending on health and education and retaining health professionals, increasingly there will reliance on a more informal workforce, for example, more minimally trained or unqualified workers. Health systems are always in a constant state of evolution and this means that the environment in which the health worker works and develops is complex and ever changing (Australian Health Ministers' Conference, 2004). The number of health workers will decrease as the population ages and qualified health workers will be more specialised. The volatility of the health workforce will continue and professionals will no longer see healthcare as a career for life.

Individual preferences in lifestyle matters will demand greater flexibility in work practices and this in turn will affect retention. The workforce will be under greater pressure and scrutiny and burnout will become more commonplace. Increasingly, work will shift to computers and robots placing an emphasis on the need for interoperability and integration of systems and the use of quality, standardised information. Building a skilled workforce to meet this changing landscape is essential.

The changing workplace

The nature of healthcare will continue to change with specialisation and integration commonplace. There will be increasing audits of practice and safety. The trend to keep people out of institutions will grow, accentuating the need for community and home nursing care. Multi-disciplinary teams will work across traditional structures, creating new roles and new professions. The health professions may not look anything like they do now in ten years' time. Again, the key to this is the interoperability of electronic devices and an integrated communications network.

Information technology and 'labour-saving' technology will consolidate and expand key services. This may result in safer care and may help to attract and retain the best staff. However, governments will push the need to optimise return on information and communication technology investments. If optimising equates with a cost benefit analysis and purely fiscal judgements, then the healthcare system is in trouble. There are many other health outcomes that demonstrate the worth of a system and these cannot be measured in this way. Possibly in the future technology and the community will support research into ways that qualitative data can become as measurable as quantifiable data.

In the future, health service priorities will lean more towards improving access and increasing the knowledge base, while infrastructure such as buildings and other resources will continue to be downsized per head of population. Increasingly we will have to live within shrinking health budgets and a user pays model of healthcare. What then for the disadvantaged in our community?

In the near future we will see:
- integrated systems with electronic health record and point-of-care support
- mobile clinical support service delivery systems that include fully integrated medication management systems
- ubiquitous computing in healthcare
- decision support and communications with knowledge management capabilities as the rule rather than the exception
- integrated management of all resources with eBusiness and resource management
- comprehensive and searchable knowledge-bases at the point-of-care
- empowered consumers who can take charge of their healthcare (if they wish).

The next twenty years will see advances in health technology that will greatly impact on demand, productivity and practice. There will be some technologies that have not been invented yet and we can only wonder at what they may be. However, the further development and integration of those considered cutting edge now will continue, with the treatment of many diseases and injuries substantially influenced in the future by:

- nanotechnology (the ability to assemble materials molecule by molecule)
- gene technologies (genetic screening and gene therapy and individual knowledge of the genetic profile)
- robotics
- e-technologies (impacting on the way care is delivered, the storage of information and data, and communication) (Australian Health Ministers' Conference, 2004).

Emerging trends in clinical information systems
– Bob Ribbons

Given the economic and clinical imperatives to reduce expenditure and improve the quality of patient outcomes, most government agencies and healthcare providers are recognising the need for capital investment in health information technology infrastructure.

The health IT market in the United States is being driven by the need to invest in PACS and e-Orders followed by the purchase of other clinical systems such as patient documentation, medication management, pharmacy, documentation management and clinical repositories. It has been predicted that the United States health IT market will exceed US$30.5 billion by late 2006 (Dorenfest & Associates, 2003). In spite of this, the *Economist* (2005) reports that the United States health care industry is spending only around two per cent of its revenues on information technology, compared with 10 per cent of revenues in other information intensive industries.

A survey of the Australian e-Health market revealed figures that are certainly comparable to those of the United Sates (CHIK Services, 2004). This survey indicated a trend toward the implementation of clinical information systems in Australian acute health care settings. In addition, it identifies the adoption of wireless and handheld technologies as the primary emerging hardware technology trend in healthcare.

The emergence of these technologies is directly related to the developing requirements for point-of-care clinical systems. The increasing sophistication of the systems will require hospitals to invest in a variety of mobile technology platforms providing more accurate, timely communication of patient information. These platforms will certainly, in the short term, include such devices as trolley mounted laptops, personal digital assistants and tablet devices. In the longer term, point-of-care devices may well take the form of a hybrid system.

Hybrid technologies evident in today's consumer electronics market (for example Internet enabled digital video phones) will increasingly find they way into use in healthcare to incorporate a patient entertainment system, telephone, nurse call, Internet access together with clinical information system access, all housed within the one device.

In order to work effectively on such platforms, clinical information systems will need to make greater use of thin client applications employing three-tier architecture, utilising interface engines to integrate disparate data sources ranging from legacy to best of breed systems. A number of vendors currently employ these technologies, using a web portal approach that allows for a single user login, patient-centric view of health data.

Essentially, this means that the clinician only has to log into the clinical information system and, once authenticated, has access to specific patient information extracted from a variety of back-ended databases. A feature of these systems is their ability to extract data while retaining the same patient context across these multiple systems. The key benefit for the clinician is a single login to obtain patient information.

A number of clinical systems also provide access to programming and configuration objects that enable health facilities to customise various components of the application. This provides hospitals with greater flexibility, ensuring that the clinical system is able to adapt to local business practices and clinical workflows. Integration engines also allow hospitals to integrate additional data sources quickly and cost effectively, while the ability to adapt to 'local conditions' leads to increased 'ownership' and, subsequently, greater clinical acceptance.

The continued move to consumer-oriented health care will see the development of consumer-focused collaborative care delivery models (Harsanyi et al., 2000). These models make it possible to transform traditional healthcare roles and responsibilities, furthering collaboration and cooperation across multiple care settings. A move to a health consumer focus will allow individuals access to intuitive web-based interfaces to view personalised information on their health conditions via a secure network connection.

Individuals will be able to update their health record, upload physiological data such as blood sugar levels, and receive health care education as well as obtain direct access to health care providers. The move towards bridging the gap between data held in acute clinical information systems and those held in the primary care/ community care sector has already begun. The results of Health*Connect* trials in Tasmania and the Northern Territory provide an insight into the trend in this area of clinical informatics in Australia (Commonwealth of Australia, 2005).

Given Australia's ageing population, and the economic pressures this will place on the healthcare system, it is clear that the focus on preventative care will increase. This trend will see clinicians working in more of a collaborative partnership with health consumers in order to reduce health care costs and improve quality of care. This will ensure improved access to patient information for clinicians in acute care areas. In the future, should an individual present to an emergency department, staff will be able to access information such as current medications, immunisation record, allergies and chronic health conditions. Having this information to hand in an emergency situation will not only save time and money, but more importantly, it will save lives.

The development of multimedia health records, video-store and forward systems (Ball, 2000) and the move towards greater use of hospital-in-the-home facilities means that clinical information systems must have remote access to hospital systems. The traditional notions of organisational boundaries will also need to give way to the often mooted but not yet implemented concept of 'healthcare without walls'.

Future of telehealth – *Sisira Edirippuligé and Richard Wootton*

Chapter 19 demonstrated that telehealth could be used successfully to improve healthcare delivery. It permits health care to be delivered in circumstances where it was previously difficult or impossible, and can do so in a way that is cost-effective. Telehealth may actually be superior to traditional mechanisms in some circumstances, for example, in the exchange of health care information, especially for educational purposes. On the other hand, if used inappropriately, expensive resources can be squandered on telehealth – a not unfamiliar problem in health IT generally.

Much of the telehealth work to date has consisted of pilot trials. No health service anywhere in the world has yet managed to bring telehealth into the mainstream of routine operations. If and when this can be achieved, telehealth will not *replace* traditional healthcare. Rather, it will be integrated into healthcare as a complementary method of providing services to previously under-served communities. Before this can happen, there is a number of barriers to overcome. Among them is the important issue of the dearth of evidence-based research.

Factors in future development

Future development depends upon a number of factors, none of which are impossible although many will take tenacity and good will, and all of which are essential. These are:

- resources – people and fiscal
- adequate capital cost and funding initiatives, key systems and applications
- shared vision, leadership and governance
- standardisation of core clinical and business systems
- education for all health workers and consumers
- an engaged and contented workforce
- the success of distributed health records systems
- interoperability and integration of systems
- settling the public policy debate over confidentiality and security of information
- policy development that keeps pace with advances in technology
- training and development in public policy areas to keep policies, procedures, and technology up-to-date and effective.

The Australian healthcare system is labour and technology intensive, geographically dispersed, and focused on trying to meet diverse community health needs. Trials and systems implementations have demonstrated the benefits of information technology, but while the provision of healthcare 'must be safe and in line with community expectations, it must also be grounded in economic and financial reality'(Australian Health Ministers' Conference, 2004, p.8). Most of the innovations in healthcare today reach far beyond just being health applications. They could potentially touch just about every aspect of today's society.

Conclusion

Health informatics has developed so quickly that legalisation and policy development are lagging behind. In fact, in some areas, projects are being implemented before trials have finished. There are substantial challenges ahead. The health workforce is changing and the solutions we have historically used are unlikely to succeed for much longer. Health informatics brings challenges of its own, but will continue to transform the way in which health services are delivered, the way that health workers work, and the way that consumers access healthcare.

Review question

What challenges lie ahead for health with respect to the deployment of information technology?

Exercises

- Describe three future population trends in Australia and discuss the potential impact of these trends on the development of new healthcare information systems.

- Identify and briefly describe four major issues, trends or developments you see taking place in the next five years.

References

Australian Health Ministers' Conference (2004). *National health workforce strategic framework. Canberra*, Commonwealth of Australia, Canberra.

Ball, M.J. (2000). Emerging trends in Nursing Informatics, in M.J. Ball, K.J. Hannah, S.K. Newbold and J.V. Douglas (eds), *Nursing Informatics: Where caring and technology meet*, 3rd edn, Springer-Verlag, New York, pp.301–4.

CHIK Services (2004). *Australian eHealth market: acute care 2003–2005*, CHIK Services, Gosford, New South Wales.

Dorenfest Integrated Healthcare Delivery System (IHDS +) Database (2003). *Healthcare information technology spending is growing rapidly*, Dorenfest & Associates, Chicago.

Economist (2005). Economist looks as the barriers to Health IT, 5 May, p.45.

Commonwealth of Australia (2005). *HealthConnect*. Retrieved 3 June, 2005, from http://www.healthconnect.gov.au/.

Harsanyi, B.E., Allan, K.C., Anderson, J., Valo, C.R., Fitzpatrick, J.M., Schofield, et al. (2000). Healthcare Information Systems, in M.J. Ball, K.J. Hannah, S.K. Newbold and J.V. Douglas (eds), *Nursing informatics: where caring and technology meet*, 3rd edn, Springer-Verlag, New York, pp.264–83).

Glossary

AS5021–2005 – *The language of Health Concept Representation* released by Standards Australia is a very useful resource as it also provides definitions for the most commonly used concepts in health informatics. The direct link is http://www.standards.com.au/catalogue/.

Access control	The prevention of use of a resource by unidentified and/or unauthorised entities.
Acuity	A measure of the relative workload placed on carers as a result of the client's ability for self care, interventions required to manage the presenting condition of the patient, and standards of practice required of the profession.
Aggregate terminology	An aggregate terminology groups similar concepts, using relationships that may be hierarchical and/or uni- or multi-dimensional. AS5021–2005
Application server	In a three-tier client seven network, the computer that provides the client with access to a specific application. The application server then passes a query onto a database server.
Architecture	A term applied to both the process and the outcome of thinking out and specifying the overall structure, logical components, and the logical interrelationships of a computer, its operating system, a network, or other conception.
Archetype	Archetypes are models of clinical or other domain-specific concepts. They define the business rules (constraints) for valid values of a concept. AS5021–2005
Asynchronous communication	A mode of communication between two parties, when the exchange does not require both to be active participants in the conversation at the same time, e.g., sending a letter. See also: Synchronous communication
Audit trail	Record of resources that were accessed and/or used by whom. This may involve a formal monitoring technique for comparison between the actual use of a medical information system and pre-established criteria. (IT-EDUCTRA)
Bandwidth	Amount of data that can be transmitted across a communication channel over a given period of time..
Barcode	Pattern of thick and thin parallel lines printed on objects and containing coded information that can be read by a light pen or similar device and translated into an electronic form. (IT-EDUCTRA)
Bayes' theory	Theorem used to calculate the relative probability of an event given the probabilities of associated events. Used to calculate the probability of a disease given the frequencies of symptoms and signs within the disease and within the normal population.

Bridges	A bridge is a device that connects a local area network (LAN) to another local area network that uses the same protocol. Bridges are able to decide whether a message from one person is going to another person on the same local area network in the same building or to someone on the local area network in the building across the street. A bridge examines each message on a LAN, 'passing' those known to be within the same LAN, and forwarding those known to be on the other interconnected LAN (or LANs).
Broadband network	General term for a computer network capable of high-bandwidth transmission
CEN	Comite Europeen de Normalisation. European Standards Organisation
Change and stress	The critical issue is not this stress but managing it to obtain an optimum and productive level for the change required.
Client	A program that can request services from another computer called a server.
Client-server	Where the processing power is distributed and different but linked computers are used, invisible to the end-user, to deliver the technical functionality. Client-server agent model – this is a model of a distributed application process in which various activities are carried out by different entities. The client is that entity requesting a service. The server is that entity providing the service. An agent is that process acting on behalf of the client or server. (IT-EDUCTRA)
Clinical information system	A large computerised database system that manages clinical data including its storage and communication to support the planning, implementation and evaluation of patient care and clinical decision-making derived from various feeder systems
Clinical pathways	A suggested multidisciplinary plan or map for the care of a patient with a particular diagnoses. Designed to standardise and optimise the care provided, based on evidence of best practice for the cohort. Clinical pathways can be automated to include alerts that notify clinicians when specific requirements for a particular pathway have not been attended to.
Closed system	A self-contained system: outside events are separated from the system
Computerised physician order entry	See: order entry.
Concept	A unit of knowledge created by a unique combination of characteristics. In terminology work, the concept is identified as abstract from the language, and the term is a symbol that is part of the language. AS5021–2005
Consumer sovereignty	The assumption that consumers act rationally in trying to maximise their utility or satisfaction gained from the available resources. It assumes that all consumers have complete knowledge, information and understanding about all products availailable

Controlled terminology	A terminology that is constrained and is or has been maintained. AS504
Controlled vocabulary	A constrained set of words or phrases, generally in a list. In the context of HL7, controlled vocabulary includes development and maintenance of code sets. AS504
Data	Representation of real world facts, concepts or instructions in a formalised manner suitable for communication, interpretation or processing by human beings or by automatic means. AS5021–2005
Database server	A computer on a network that houses a database application and provides access to this database by clients.
Decision-support	Part of an information system that presents information in such a way so as to assist in the decision-making process.
Developmental change	This represents the simplest approach to change and consists of fine-tuning or improving existing processes. It is based on skills development and acquisition and is the least stressful and demanding on individuals, management and the organisation in general
Dissonance	The difference between espoused theory (what people say) and theory-in-use (what people actually do)
Double-loop learning	We learn to change the field of constancy itself by challenging the appropriateness of existing approaches. Double-loop learning addresses the values and norms of an organisation and provides the basis for moving from knowledge to the higher levels of attitudes, individual and group behaviours
DRG (Diagnosis Related Group)	In Australia, the system used is the AnDRG (Australian version) which is an adaptation of the international dataset to capture local healthcare variations. Version numbers change over time as new groups are added or superseded ones deleted
Dumb terminal	A device consisting of a screen, a keyboard and sometimes a light-pen and/or barcode scanner. It cannot do any processing or storage of data
Elasticity	A measure of demand and supply responsiveness to changes in price and any other factors that affect demand or supply
e-ordering	See: Order entry
e-prescribing	An electronic system that automates the process of prescribing medications
Espoused theory	The view of the world and values and beliefs a person believes she/he follows in their normal behaviour (what people say)
Expert system	A computer program that contains expert knowledge about a particular problem, often in the form of a set of if-then rules, which is able to solve problems at a level equivalent or greater than human experts
Granularity	Level of detail (complexity or crudeness).

Graphical user interfaces (GUI)	Graphical User Interface. That part of a computer application seen and interacted with by its user. Specifically, that part of the interface that is based upon visual structures like icons, which act as metaphors for the different functions supported by the application, e.g., deleting a file is enacted by dragging a visual symbol representing the file onto a trash can icon
HL7 (Health Level 7):	An international standard for electronic data exchange in healthcare that defines the format and content of messages that pass between medical applications
Hybrid technology	Any technology that consists of an amalgam of the other technologies. An example is an Internet enabled, digital video telephone
Iatrogenic complications	Mistakes made by doctors and nurses including such things as administering the wrong medication and amputating the wrong limb
Inference engine	A set of programs using knowledge for reasoning
Infoglut	An overload of information
Information silos	A term typically used to describe data contained in a database housed on one computer only and usually available only to a limited number of users. Data that is not available in a distributed fashion.
Infostructure	Information infrastructure for health that provide, shared resources and standards for healthcare agencies/parties that enable information to flow in appropriately structured identifiable (unambiguous) and secure ways. (CEN)
Internet	Technically, a network of computer networks. Today, associated with a specific global computer network that is publicly accessible, and upon which the World Wide Web is based
Intranet	A computer network, based upon World Wide Web and Internet technologies, but whose scope is limited to an organisation. An intranet may be connected to an Internet, so that there can be communication and flow of information between it and other intranets
ISO	International Standards Organisation
Knowledge-base	A structured repository for knowledge, consisting of a collection of knowledge elements such as rules and their associated data model, or ontology. A knowledge-base is a core component of an Expert System
Knowledge management	Managing knowledge created by clinicians in technology-based information systems that facilitate the communication and sharing of such knowledge among clinicians both within and across organisations
Knowledge representation	The process and the result of formalisation of knowledge in such a way that it can be used automatically for problem solving
LAN	Local Area Network. A computer network limited to servicing computers in a small locality. See also: Intranet

Legacy systems	Operational application systems that still have a useful life but do not meet the technological environment for development, for example, were not written in Windows.
Life cycle	From design to implementation, maturity and obsolescence, duration of the operability of the device.
Local Area Network	A localised network of computers located in the same building or within a limited geographical area.
Mainframe	A large computer that has access to significant quantities of data and is able to process these data very quickly. In many health care organisations, mainframes have been replaced by client server networks.
Marginal analysis	The evaluation of the costs and benefits of providing an additional unit of activity.
Marginal revenue	The additional income or revenue received for providing an additional unit of activity.
Medication management	The process by which medication prescribing, dispensing and administration is supported by an automated system providing clinical decision support to the clinician at each step of these three phases.
Mapping	A relationship between the code or term used to represent a health concept in one system, and the code or term that would be used to represent the same concept in another coding or terminology system. AS5021–2005
Metadata	Data describing data. AS5021–2005
Metathesaurus	The Metathesaurus is a database of information on concepts that appear in one or more of a number of different controlled vocabularies and classifications. In general, the scope of the Metathesaurus is determined by the combined scope of its source vocabularies. The Metathesaurus preserves the meanings, hierarchical connections, and other relationships between terms present in its source vocabularies, while adding certain basic information about each of its concepts and establishing new relationships between concepts and terms from different source vocabularies. AS5021–2005
Minimum data set	The least number of data elements required in a data set to do a particular job/s. AS5021–2005
Mobile computing	A situation in which a computer or information technology device is capable of being used without the need to be physically plugged into the network in order to receive data. This frees the user from the constraints of having to sit at a workstation, allowing them to access data on the move.
Model	1. Formal representation of an object, concept or process. 2. An abstraction of something for the purpose of understanding it before building it. (IT-EDUCTRA)

Model 1	These organisations and their management maximise eliciting negative feelings and are focused on being rational at the cost of emotionality.
Model 2	Is based on valid information, free and informed choice and internal commitment to the choice and constant monitoring of the implementations.
Network	Set of connected elements. For computers, any collection of computers connected together so that they are able to communicate, permitting the sharing of data or programs.
Network operating system	An operating system (software) designed to allow computers on a network to share resources such as hard drives and printers.
Nosocomial infections	Infections introduced in the hospital.
Occurrence of change	It occurs on a regular basis, is planned or unplanned, only the scale and level of planning differs in each case.
Ontology	The set of concepts understood in a knowledge base. A formal ontology specifies a way of constructing a knowledge base about some part of the world. An ontology thus contains a set of allowed concepts, and rules that define the allowable relationships between concepts. See also: Knowledge-base.
Open system	Open systems are those that conform to agreed standards defining computing environments that allow users to develop, run and interconnect applications and the hardware they run on, from whatever source, without significant conversion cost.
openEHR	A framework for building scalable, robust and future-proof health records that are open-source and standards-based.
Operating system (OS)	A set of program routines containing basic instructions that provide an environment in which applications software can access disk, keyboard, screen and printer. The operating system is the first loaded before you run other programs, controlling them and providing them with services.
Organisational change	Any response to internal or external pressure or force by the organisation, from the whole of the organisation or any of its parts.
Order entry	Order entry is a computer application that allows providers to order medications, diagnostic investigations or other clinical services electronically rather than handwriting these orders. Such systems are superior to traditional manual ordering by utilising decision support systems. When integrated with decision support, order entry systems can check for duplicate orders, drug interactions in addition to dose and allergy checking, thereby reducing the potential for errors and over servicing.

Organisational defensive routines	This is an environment in which the organisational dynamics include quasi-resolution of conflict, uncertainty, avoidance, mistrust, conformity, face saving, inter-group rivalry, invalid information for important problems and valid information for unimportant problems, misperceptions, miscommunication, and parochial interests.
Patient administration system	An information system designed specifically to manage non-clinical aspects of a patient's episode of care. For example, demographics, GP, Medicare number, health insurance details, billing details.
Perfect competition	A hypothetical market condition in which no producer or consumer has the power to influence prices in the market. It assumes that all producers and consumers have complete knowledge and information about all products available.
Personal Computer	An inexpensive type of computer frequently used by an individual in an office or home environment.
Physician order entry	See: Order entry.
Picture archiving and communication systems	A subsystem of the radiology information system designed to facilitate the production, management, transmission, storage and archiving of digital radiology images.
PKI (Public Key Infrastructure)	A combination of information technology and procedures enabling secure exchange of electronic data (enables authentication, confidentiality, non-repudiation and integrity. (http://www.hic.gov.au/providers/online_initiatives/pki_security.htm)
Point-of-care systems	Information systems located as close as possible to where care takes place; in most circumstances, at the bedside.
Point-to-point communications	Established physically between two units' speakers either human or electronic.
Protocols	The rules two computers must follow to exchange messages.
Radiology information systems	An information system that performs the management functions related to digital radiological investigations.
Reference Information Model (RIM)	An information model that relates to a specific domain and that shows the relationships between the key concepts within the knowledge domain. AS5021–2005.
Results reporting	Usually a module within a clinical information system that specifically deals with patients' results (for example, laboratory results or radiology reports). Results reporting functions allow clinicians to cumulate and graph patient results.

Risk analysis	A method for assessing risk. This may be used to subsequently compare the cost of achieving something (such as hospital system security) against the risk of losing something.
ROM (Read Only Memory)	Permanent memory that is built into a computer. Provides a means to boot-up when switched on.
Routers	A device that forwards data packets along networks. A router is connected to at least two networks, commonly two LANs or between a LAN and the Internet. Routers are located at gateways, the places where two or more networks connect.
Server	A program that provides a service to a client.
Semantic network	Semantic network is a formalism (often expressed graphically) for representing relational information, the arcs of the network representing the relationships and the nodes the objects in the network. (IT-EDUCTRA)
Semantics	Definition of meaning and the meaning of symbols and codes.
Single-loop learning	A consequence of focusing on superficial learning, where the underlying assumptions are treated as fixed and we learn to maintain the field of constancy by learning to design actions that satisfy existing governing values.
Smart card	Basically made of plastic, look like a credit card, but as their name suggests they have electronic integrated circuits in their sub-stratum. Patient smart card is a computer readable card held by or related to a patient used for some purpose connected to the receipt of health services.
SNOMED	The Systematised Nomenclature of Medicine. A commercially available general medical terminology, initially developed for the classification of pathological specimens
Social welfare or efficiency	Looks at the impact of a project from a total society point of view. Most public projects create winners as well as losers. An increase in social efficiency occurs when the project results in an overall gain to society
Software	Collecti ve term for all computer programs
Software design	The process of going from what a system is intended to do, specified in the requirements and functional specification (analysis), to how it is to do it. In this stage the designer transforms the functional specification into a form from which the programmer can more easily code the problem represented by the requirements and functional specification into a list of programming instructions. (IT-EDUCTRA)

Software engineering	The establishment and use of sound engineering principles in order to obtain economically viable software that is reliable and works efficiently. Software engineering is concerned with the development of software systems by teams as well as individuals, and encompasses a range of technical and non-technical aspects. (IT-EDUCTRA)
Spreadsheet	A program that mimics large tables of numerical information. The program will allow the user to perform mathematical functions on sections of the table and to manipulate the data in a variety of ways
Standard	A standard is an accepted or approved example or technique against which other things are judged or measured, or which sets out a set of criteria that serves as a guideline for how something should be done
Synchronous communication	A mode of communication when two parties exchange messages across a communication channel at the same time, e.g., telephones. See also: Asynchronous communication
Telehealth	The use of computer information and telecommunication technologies to provide health care in situations where the provider and the patient or client are not in the same physical location
Telematics	Telematics is the discipline combining telecommunication technologies and informatics
Telemedicine	Clinical activities undertaken with an element of distance/remoteness between health care providers and the patient. Investigation, monitoring and management of patients that facilitates ready access to expert advice and patient information, irrespective of the distance between the location of the patient and the expert, expertise or relevant information
Theory-in-use	The view of the world and values and beliefs implied by the individual's actual behaviour and actions (what people actually do)
Thesaurus	A thesaurus provides a way of linking similar items (near-synonyms) together, to help the user find the precise term required. The term also can apply to the repository of linked terms themselves, in fact a structured keyword catalogue
Thin client	In client/server applications, client software designed so that the bulk of the data processing occurs on the server. Although the term usually refers to software, it is increasingly used for computers supplied without a hard disk drive, whereas a fat client includes a disk drive
Three-tiered architecture	A client/server architecture in which there is an intermediate computer between the server and the client

Transitional change	This intermediate stage is larger in scale than developmental change and involves a change in thinking, or the introduction of new technologies. The approach starts with the evaluation of the existing system, development of the new system, introduction of the new system, piloting, re-evaluation of the system, implementation, training and then complete departure from the old and reliance on the new.
Transformational change	This is the most complex level of change and is often forced on an organisation due to extreme financial or external pressures. Because it requires higher order innovation it is often more difficult to manage.
User interface	Method of interaction between users and information systems. This includes Graphical User Interface (GUI), dialogue model, particular devices and general ergonomic features.
Virtual Reality	Computer simulated environment within which humans are able to interact in some manner that approximates interactions in the physical world.
WAN	Wide Area Network – A kind of computer network linked by telecommunication links. The network is over a wider area than with Local Area Networks (LAN) that are not connected by telecommunications links.
Wireless LANs	A local area network that uses radio waves to connect devices on the network rather then using cables.
Whiteboard systems	An information system that presents information in a similar format to that presented on traditional whiteboards, but which integrates information from a number of different sources.

Contributors

Peter Adkins	MBBS. General Practitioner. Birkdale Medical Center.
Diane Ayres	RN RM M.Info.Comm.Tech., B.Admin.(Nurs). Manager, Client Partnerships NSW Health.
Cath Cameron	RN RM PhD BN, MN, Grad Cert HE. Lecturer. Griffith University.
Stephen Chiu	PhD, FACS. Associate Professor of Health Informatics. University of Auckland, Auckland, New Zealand.
Moya Conrick	RN, RM, PhD, MclED, BN, DipAppSc. Griffith University. Convenor Nursing and Health Informatics. Chair Nursing Informatics Australia.
Helen Cooper	Assoc Dip MRA (Cumberland College of Health Sciences), B Bus (Marketing) QUT, MTM (Griffith).
Paul Donaldson	RN PNC BHlthSc(Nurs) MSchMgmt. Manager Clinical Information – Nursing. The Prince Charles Hospital.
Richard Dixon-Hughes	BSc BE(Hons) MEngSc DipLaw MLS(Hons) FIEAust CPEng FAICD MACS. Managing Director, DH4 Pty Ltd.
David Evans	MBBS, FRACMA, AFCHSE, CHE, MSIA, BBus Health Admin, Grad Dip IT, Grad Dip OHS. Medical Superintendent. Queen Elizabeth II Jubilee Hospital.
Sisira Edirippuligé	PhD, MSs. Lecturer Postgraduate Courses. e-Healthcare Center for Online Health, The University of Queensland.
Ian Edwards	B.Bus (HRM) QUT, MHA UNSW. Queensland Health is Senior Business Analyst. Health Service Executive. Lecturer, Griffith University
Joanne Foster	RN, Renal Cert, DipAppSc (NsgEdn), BN, GradDipClEdn. Queensland University of Technology. Secretary Nursing Informatics Australia.
Isobel Frean	RN, MS. Visiting Fellow. Health Informatics Research Centre. University of Wollongong.

Rod Gapp	PhD., BSc, BAppSc.
	Director Masters of Management (Innovation & Change) & (Research). Department of Management. Griffith University – Gold Coast.
Heather Grain	AssocDipMRA CaulfieldLincoln, GDipDataProc Caulfield.
	Coordinator Health informatics. School of Public Health. Consumer Representative.
Karen Guest	BA CQU, BInfTech GU.
	School of Information and Communication Technology. Griffith University, Nathan.
Sam Heard	MBBS, MRCGP, FRACGP, FACHI. General Practitioner.
	Adjunct Professor of Health Informatics at Central Queensland University. Senior Visiting Research Fellow at University College London. Vice-Chairperson of the openEHR Foundation and CEO and Clinical Director of Ocean Informatics.
Evelyn Hovenga	RN, PhD, FCHSE, FRCNA, FACHI, MACS.
	Professor, Faculty of Informatics and Communication.
	Central Queensland University. Rockhampton.
Sheree Lloyd	B Bus(Computing) QUT, Assoc Dip MRA (Cumberland College of Health Sciences). MTM (Griffith). Honorary fellow QUT.
Anyes Marsault	MMS, GradDipCommM, BBS.
	Project Manager PMP® – EDS Australia.
	[2005 PMI Project Manager of the Year]
David Mitchell	PhD, MEI.
	Research & Business Leader, Biotechnology & Health Informatics CSIRO.
Ron Natoli	PhC, FPS, FAIPM.
	Community pharmacist. Fellow/Councillor FPS of the Pharmaceutical Society of Australia NSW Branch.
Christopher Newell	AM, PhD, BA, BD, MA (Hons), MPET, FACE.
	Consultant ethicist and Associate Professor of Medical Ethics within the School of Medicine, University of Tasmania.
Malcolm Pradhan	MBBS, PhD.
	Director of Health Informatics, Faculty of Health Sciences, University of Adelaide.
David Rhodes	B Social Studies, Grad Cert Health Services Management.
	Director, Allied Health Services.
	Hunter New England Area Health Service.

Bob Ribbons	RN, ICCert, BAppSc (Nur), MEd (Computing), FACHI. Manager, Clinical Informatics, Peninsula Health. Frankston. Honorary Senior Lecturer, Faculty of Medicine, Nursing and Health Sciences, Monash University.
Bruce Roggiero	Aboriginal Community Health. Katherine District Health Services.
Peter Scott	MBBS, BA. National Centre for Classification in Health (Brisbane).
Jan Stanek	MD (Comenius Univ.), GradDipIT (UniSA). Health Informatics Research Group. Advanced Computing Research Centre, University of South Australia.
Stella Stevens	PhD. Senior Lecturer, Public Health. Griffith University Gold Coast Campus.
Michael Strachan	BBus HIM (QUT)/Grad Cert Health Informatics (Monash). Director, Health Information Services. Mater Health Services, Brisbane.
Jeff Soar	BA (Hons), GDipCommDP, GDipEd, MEd, PhD, MACS. Associate Professor, Information Systems. Director Collaboration for Ageing and Aged Care Informatics Research (CAAIR). University of Southern Queensland.
Sue Walker	MHlthSc, GradDipPH, BAppSc (MRA). Associate Director, National Centre for Classification in Health.
Jim Warren	PhD, BS. Chair of Health Informatics. University of Auckland.
Richard Wootton	PhD, DSc. Professor. Director of Research Center for Online Health.

Index